# CHANGING THE CULTURE OF COLLEGE DRINKING

## A SOCIALLY SITUATED HEALTH COMMUNICATION CAMPAIGN

**Health Communication**
Gary L. Kreps, series editor

Communication in Recovery: Perspectives on Twelve-Step Groups
  *Lynette S. Eastland, Sandra L. Herndon, and Jeanine R. Barr (eds.)*

Communicating in the Clinic: Negotiating Frontstage and Backstage
  Teamwork
  *Laura L. Ellingson*

Media-Mediated Aids
  *Linda K. Fuller (ed.)*

Cancer-Related Information Seeking
  *J. David Johnson*

Changing the Culture of College Drinking: A Socially Situated Health
  Communication Campaign
  *Linda C. Lederman and Lea P. Stewart*

*forthcoming*

Communication and Cancer Care
  *Dan O'Hair, Gary L. Kreps and Lisa Sparks (eds.)*

Cancer Communication and Aging
  *Lisa Sparks, Dan O'Hair and Gary L. Kreps (eds.)*

# CHANGING THE CULTURE OF COLLEGE DRINKING

## A SOCIALLY SITUATED HEALTH COMMUNICATION CAMPAIG

Linda C. Lederman, Ph.D.
*Rutgers University*

Lea P. Stewart, Ph.D.
*Rutgers University*

HAMPTON PRESS, INC.
CRESSKILL, NJ 07626

Libarary of Congress Cataloging-in-Publication Data

Lederman, Linda Costigan.
   Changing the culture of college drinking : a socially situated health
   communication campaign / Linda C. Lederman, Lea P. Stewart
        p.cm. -- (Health communication)
   Includes bibliographical references and indexes.
   ISBN 1-57273-592-9 (cl) -- ISBN 1-57273-593-7 (pb)
      1. College students--alcohol use--Prevention. 2. Binge drinking--
   Prevention. 3. Health risk communication. 4. Universities and colleges--
   Health promotion services. I. Stewart, Lea. II Title. III. Health
   communication (Cresskill, N.J.)

HV5135.L43 2005
378.1'978--dc22

                                                              2004060637

Hampton Press, Inc.
23 Broadway
Cresskill, NJ 07626

# CONTENTS

Foreword - *Gustav Friedrich*                                              *vii*

Preface                                                                     *ix*

Acknowledgments                                                             *xi*

### Part I
### Background of the RU SURE Campaign–Brief Overview  1

1. The Culture of College Drinking: A Health Communication      *3*
   Issue
2. Baseline Data Collection: Conducting a Needs Assessment      *11*
   Before Designing a Health Communication Campaign
3. The Conceptual Model: College Drinking as Socially          *27*
   Situated Experiential Learning

### Part II
### Design and Implementation of the RU SURE Campaign
### –Brief Overview   47

4. Campaign Language: Understanding How to Get Students         *49*
   to Personalize Campaign Messages
5. The Design of the RU SURE Campaign: The Top Ten             *59*
   Misperceptions Media Campaign
6. Implementation of the Campaign: A Curriculum Infusion       *73*
   Design

### Part III. Outcomes of the Campaign–Brief Overview   97

7. Interpersonal Strategies for Campaign Message               *99*
   Dissemination

8.  Continuous Evaluation of the Campaign                              *119*

9.  Unanticipated Results: The Impact of Campaign                      *133*
    Messages on the Messengers

10. The RU SURE Game of Choices and Consequences:                      *145*
    A 1-Hour Brief Intervention Alcohol Decision-Making
    Tool

11. Extending the Campaign and Its Socially Situated                   *165*
    Experiential Learning Approach to Other Campuses

**Part IV**
**The Larger Context for Prevention: Invited Contributions–**
**Brief Overview    177**

12. An Integrated Environmental Framework: Education,                  *179*
    Prevention, Intervention, Treatment, and Enforcement
    – *Fern Walter Goodhart and Lisa Laitman*

13. An Overview of the Social Norms Approach                           *193*
    – *Alan D. Berkowitz*

14. Managing Multicampus Campaigns Using a Social                      *215*
    Norms Approach – *Linda R. Jeffrey and Pamela Negro*

15. A Case Study in Using a Social Norms Approach Within               *233*
    a Brief Intervention for Identified High-Risk Students
    – *Patricia Fabiano*

16. Drinking Stories as Learning Tools: Socially Situated              *243*
    Experiential Learning and Popular Culture
    – *Thomas A. Workman*

References                                                            *255*
About the Authors                                                     *275*
Author Index                                                          *279*
Subject Index                                                         *287*

# FOREWORD

## Gustav W. Friedrich

**Dean, School of Communication,
Information and Library Studies
Rutgers University**

I am delighted to be writing this foreword for Linda Lederman and Lea Stewart's book because it provides an opportunity for me to share publicly my high regard for the two authors and for their contribution to communication scholarship.

Linda and Lea are the founding directors of The Center for Communication and Health Issues (CHI) at Rutgers. CHI is a wonderful collaboration of communication scholars, health professionals and researchers, and students, focused on understanding the interaction of communication and health issues in the college-learning environment. This collaboration is unique in multiple ways: (a) the partnership of communication scholars with campus health professionals, (b) the involvement of students, (c) the insistence that research be driven by both theory and practical concerns, and (d) the smooth integration of the three major domains of academic life (teaching, research, and service).

This book describes such collaboration as it plays out in studying the "culture of college drinking" on college campuses. It describes how Linda and Lea, and their CHI colleagues, build on the construct of socially situated experiential learning to conceptualize, design, implement, and evaluate a communication campaign (RU SURE) targeted to this issue. Their successes are documented in the research projects described in their book. Their accomplishments are also demonstrated by the significant funds that external sources have provided in support of their work and the recognition awarded by the U.S. Department of Education's designation of RU SURE as a Model Program.

This book is but another indication that Linda Lederman and Lea Stewart are talented communication scholars who know how to integrate and effectively utilize their balanced strengths in teaching, research, and service. I am confident in predicting that you will find the book stimulating to read and that you will learn a great deal from it.

# PREFACE

In 1982, Brent Ruben, then chair of the Department of Communication at Rutgers University, assigned us to co-teach a course called "Administrative Communication." Being relatively new assistant professors, we couldn't say no to his request but we both thought that working together would never work. Of course, we didn't share this thought with each other, but neither of us could figure out how a person who is a global thinker trained in qualitative research and experiential learning whose favorite phrase is "What did you learn from this?" could ever work with a methodical quantitative researcher with a traditional organizational communication background whose favorite phrase is "What's your evidence for that?". After spending countless hours challenging each other's ideas, we developed SIMCORP (a semester-long instructional simulation) and THE MARBLE COMPANY (a simulation/game used both in the United States and internationally as a management training tool) and haven't stopped working together since.

Our work on innovative instructional methods has received international recognition. In 1991, Linda delivered the keynote address at the International Simulation and Gaming Association meeting in Kyoto, Japan on communication, simulation, and intercultural differences. Among many other awards, she was named a Distinguished Research Fellow (2001) and recognized as an Outstanding Woman in Communication at the 75th Diamond Anniversary Conference of the Eastern Communication Association (ECA) (1984). She also served as a Center Associate with the

U.S. Department of Education, Higher Education Center (2001-2003). Lea received the Warren I. Susman Award for Excellence in Teaching (Rutgers highest award for teaching excellence) in 2003. She was named to the Eastern Communication Association Committee of Scholars (1989) and received the ECA Past Presidents' Award (1987) for mid-career achievement. Together, we were named Founding Fellows at the Rutgers University Teaching Excellence Center (1992-1993). In addition to numerous other awards, we have been principal or co-principal investigators on more than $7 million in competitive grants from the U.S. Department of Education Safe and Drug-Free Schools Program, New Jersey Consortium on Alcohol and Other Drug Education and Prevention, New Jersey Department of Health and Senior Services, U.S. Department of Justice, National Institute on Drug Abuse (NIDA), among others.

The RU SURE Campaign is the latest result of our very successful collaboration and was named a model program in 2001 by the U.S. Department of Education. RU SURE is a dangerous drinking prevention campaign developed after a decade of research on alcohol-related behavior on the Rutgers campus and based on our Socially Situated Experiential Learning (SSEL) Model. The innovative nature of this campaign combines social norms messages with interpersonally based experiential activities delivered by college students to their peers. In this way, students become the co-creators and carriers of carefully designed prevention messages and, thus, create a more credible campaign for a college audience. This book describes the development of this campaign including its theoretical framework and innovative design. Suggestions are also given for implementing a similar campaign on other campuses. In this way, we hope to add to the work on alcohol prevention on college campuses and create a safer learning environment for all students.

# ACKNOWLEDGMENTS

There are so many people to thank and acknowledge publicly for their encouragement, support, or collaboration over the years. Perhaps the first people we need to acknowledge are Ron Rice, who suggested that we write this book and who helped us shape and nurture it into its present shape, and Gary Kreps, our series editor, whose work over the years has inspired our own interest in health communication and the adaptation of our experiential learning approach to the advancement of that important area of the communication discipline.

We also would never have begun the RU SURE project, which is the focus of this book, if we had not formed a partnership with Fern Walter Goodhart, Lisa Laitman, and Richard Powell, outstanding health prevention and treatment specialists at Rutgers who helped us learn so much about alcohol abuse and alcohol prevention. The five of us began the Communication and Health Issues Partnership for Education and Research that grew into the Center for Communication and Health Issues (CHI). CHI is our "home away from home," the ongoing collaboration that motivates us to seek the external funding we need to support the research upon which all of our communication-based approaches to prevention are based. Working with Fern and Lisa (Richard has recently retired), and with Adrienne Coleman, a newer member of the health education team at Rutgers, has been a model of inspiration, mutual trust, and respect for which we are more grateful than these few words can express. All of us owe a debt

of thanks to David Burns, then assistant vice president for student life at
Rutgers, whose project on alcohol prevention began the association between
professionals at the Health Services and faculty in the Department of
Communication.

Perhaps no one in the Department of Communication over the past several years has been more supportive and influential in the growth and development of the CHI than our colleague Harty Mokros who, as chair at the
time, encouraged us to pursue our interests in alcohol use as a health communication issue and even provided some seed money for us to develop the
survey and coursework necessary for this venture. Together with a mini-
grant from the Rutgers Health Services that Fern Goodhart was able to
secure, our work began on a shoestring and has ended up receiving millions
of dollars in external funding. We owe these folks thanks for believing in us
and sharing our vision of a healthier campus, free from the illusion we call
the *culture of college drinking.*

So many other colleagues have supported us directly and indirectly. We
appreciate the input of our colleague Itzhak Yanovitzky whose campaign
evaluation expertise has helped shape the ways in which we are able to articulate the conceptual model driving our work. Our current chair, Jenny
Mandelbaum, has given us support and also access to a myriad of large lecture classes from whom we could collect data about their drinking-related
thoughts, attitudes, and behaviors. We thank the colleagues who made time
for us to gather data in their classes, especially David Gibson, Mark Frank,
Kathryn Greene, Itzhak Yanovitzky, Bill White, Lynn Cockett, and Jim
Katz.

It would undoubtedly have been impossible to test out our conceptual
model and the campaign that developed from it without the encouragement
and support of many administrators. We are particularly grateful to our
dean, Gus Friedrich, whose own understanding of communication and
learning encouraged us in our explorations of experiential learning with our
students, and to Joan Carbone, associate dean for student services at Rutgers
College for her support of our campaign and the access she made possible
for us to first-year students who were our target audience.

Our first external funding came from the New Jersey Higher Education
Consortium on Alcohol and Other Drug Prevention and Education supported by the New Jersey Department of Health and Senior Services and the
project leaders who guided our early campaign design were Linda Jeffrey
and Pamela Negro, both of whom we thank for all of the fine work they do
for the state of New Jersey in funding projects at various colleges. We, too,
thank the people at the U.S. Department of Education who encouraged our
work and recognized it in 2000 with a Model Program Award (including
Lavona Grow, our project director) and Bill DeJong and Beth DeRicco of
the Higher Education Center for the work in environmental management

that has been an underpinning of the ways in which we at CHI address all the work we do, including the campaign in this book, which was embedded in the array of other prevention, treatment, and enforcement activities on campus. Other researchers noted for their work in the alcohol prevention and treatment fields, such as Alan Berkowitz and Wes Perkins, Pat Fabiano, Robert Pandina, and Helene White have all contributed to our thinking and we appreciate them for their excellent work.

And finally, and so incredibly importantly, are the graduate and undergraduate students with whom we have had the honor to work over the past 6 years. There isn't a facet of the campaign, its conceptualization, implementation, or evaluation that has not benefited from the input and often the hard work of students who worked with us. They wanted to learn about the role of communication in health issues and how to create and implement campaigns. What they didn't know was that even as we taught them we learned so much from their insights and ability to help us really come to understand the culture of college drinking at Rutgers so that we could try to change it. Every class of Advanced Health Communication with whom we worked since 1998 has been filled with students whom we thank. And each year we relied on the efforts of talented and dedicated graduate students to help run the project including Lynn Kennedy who was involved in the baseline data collection effort. We most particularly want to thank Sherry Barr and Marlene Matarese, each of whom has gone on to her own successful career, and Shakira Johnson, who is currently finishing her masters degree and embarking upon her own career. Special thanks to Anna Timoshkina for help with the references, to Travis Russ for the graphic design of the SSEL model, and to Anastacia Kurylo for proofreading assistance.

The project described in this book has been and continues to be a labor of love. We have both invested significant amounts of our time and energy, often at the sacrifice of time we wanted to spend on other projects or with our loved ones. We thank and appreciate those people who are dear to us and who have shared the experience of the entire project, as well as the writing of this book, a project in itself. We are particularly grateful to Alan Stewart, Joshua Lederman, and Robert Kully for more than needs to be said here.

L.C.L.
L.P.S.

# Part I

## Background of the RU SURE Campaign

---

### Brief Overview

This book describes the development, design, implementation, and evaluation of the RU SURE Campaign at Rutgers University and the conceptual model used as the theoretical grounding for the campaign. The first part of the book focuses on the background for the campaign and the development of the conceptual model. This framework guided each stage of campaign development, design, and evaluation as described in subsequent chapters.

Chapter 1, The Culture of College Drinking, provides the background to the problem addressed by the RU SURE Campaign. The chapter describes health communication campaigns as omnipresent in the American culture and explains the case study presented in this book as an instance of enhancing health communication efforts by incorporating interpersonally based strategies with a media approach to health campaigns. The chapter goes on to describe the problem of college drinking and the ways in which various experiences, images, perceptions, and misperceptions form and shape what we refer to as the culture of college drinking (Lederman, 1993).

Chapter 2, Baseline Data Collection, reviews the background information and research into the drinking-related behaviors and perceptions at Rutgers. The chapter begins with the earliest research on college drinking conducted in the late 1980s at Rutgers and reviews all research up to the present. It is designed to provide a review of the data on which the RU SURE Campaign and all other interventions that we created were made.

Finally, Chapter 3, College Drinking as Socially Situated Experiential Learning, explicates the construct of socially situated experiential learning (Lederman & Stewart, 1998) and describes and explains the conceptual model which incorporates that construct and the construct of the culture of college drinking into the conceptualization, design, implementation, and evaluation of the RU SURE Campaign. The chapter presents a step-by-step discussion of the five steps in the model. The model is then used as the organizing framework for the chapters on the design, implementation, and evaluation that follow in Parts II and III of the book.

# 1

# THE CULTURE OF COLLEGE DRINKING

## A HEALTH COMMUNICATION ISSUE

Health communication, as an area of study, has focused on two primary areas—how it is provided (e.g., analyzing doctor-patient communication, studying how information provided on the Internet affects patients' decisions) and promoting public health (e.g., analyzing, designing, and evaluating media campaigns to persuade people to adopt specific behaviors and attitudes that are thought to lead to more healthy lifestyles). Public health campaigns are ubiquitous in contemporary society. Topics such as preventing the spread of HIV/AIDS, cigarette smoking, and drug abuse have received attention from health communication researchers (Rice & Atkin, 2001). Everyone has seen a message encouraging people to stop smoking, to eat healthy foods ("Got milk?"), to have a designated driver ("Friends don't let friends drive drunk"), or to avoid illegal drugs ("This is your brain on drugs"). Millions of dollars are spent each year on these campaigns, and some of them are extremely memorable. Whether or not these campaigns have been effective (or even necessary or appropriate) is a more complex question (Salmon & Murray-Johnson, 2001; Snyder, 2001). If we assume, however, that there are some issues of such societal significance that it is important to address them through health communication campaigns, there are effective ways to design, implement, and evaluate these campaigns.

In order to improve the chances of developing meaningful and effective health communication campaigns, it is important to implement "a wide range of different prevention messages and campaign strategies targeted at relevant and specific (well-segmented) audiences" (Kreps, Bonaguro, & Query, 1998, p. 14). Thus, when thinking about developing a campaign about a particular issue or health-related behavior, it is also important to determine the nature of the specific audience for the message. Once this analysis is completed, communication strategies that incorporate multiple levels and channels of human communication can be developed (Kreps et al., 1998).

College students have become the focus of several health communication campaigns in recent years both because college campuses may be sites for unhealthy behaviors and also because of the specific nature of this target audience. Thus, communication researchers and others are increasingly turning to the college campus as one venue in need of health communication messages and one where these campaigns have been effective.

A typical health communication strategy to address an issue of relevance to any audience, including college students, would be to design an educational campaign to present information to the target audience with the explicit goal of modifying their knowledge, attitudes, beliefs, or behavior concerning a particular issue (Salmon & Murray-Johnson, 2001). Before disseminating any messages among the college population, however, it is important to assess the perceptions of the target audience because the most effective health communication campaigns address the "specific vocabulary, perceptions, and values of the target population" (Simons-Morton, Donohew, & Crump, 1997, p. 544).

One value of this audience that is often taken for granted is its view on the use of alcohol. Everyone knows (or at least thinks they know) that college students perceive alcohol to be a natural and, even, necessary part of college life. This perception helps reinforce "the culture of college drinking," which consists of both the actual alcohol-related behavior of college students and the misperceptions that surround this behavior (Lederman, 1993; NIAAA, 2002). The next section of this chapter contains a description of relevant research in this area and a discussion of our understanding of the implications of this research in shaping people's misperceptions of the norms of drinking on college campuses today.

## IMAGES AND REALITY OF COLLEGE DRINKING

It is difficult to think of drinking on college campuses without imagining excessive drinking. Thus, the image of excessive drinking becomes intertwined with the popular conception of college life in America. This perception is reinforced through various mediated messages including television (such as the episode of *The Real World* on MTV that featured a college-age woman who passes out and has to be taken to a hospital after a night of bar hopping), films (such as the "classic" *Animal House*), and the news (including reports of alcohol-ignited rioting at major universities throughout the country). In many ways, college culture itself vigorously communicates and perpetuates the myth that this type of behavior is the norm and that excessive drinking is an integral part of every college student's life (Lederman, 1993).

The image of excessive drinking and perpetually inebriated college students is a cliché in the media and contemporary American culture. It often seems as if the popular view of the college student is somehow incomplete without a reference to the "typical" alcohol-doused, rowdy college party. (See Chapter 16 for a more detailed discussion of the effects of popular culture on perceptions of college drinking.) This perception creates a broad conception of college life as one in which alcohol is constantly and freely used—most often abused—by everyone. Of course, there are popular misconceptions and clichés about various segments of society, but when it comes to college life and alcohol, the college culture itself is most vigorous in communicating and perpetuating its own myths about how excessive drinking is an integral part of student life.

Although every student does not drink excessively, dangerous drinking does occur on college campuses and does pose a risk to the student population. *Dangerous drinking* is the term that is used throughout this book to describe the well-documented phenomenon in which college students consume unhealthy quantities of alcohol (particularly in social situations) that can lead to negative consequences for themselves or for others (Lederman et al., 1998). Although much of the research literature is based on the concept of *binge drinking* defined as five or more drinks on one occasion for males and four or more for females (Wechsler, Lee, Kuo, & Lee, 2000; Weitzman, Nelson, & Wechsler, 2003), college students do not believe this term applies to them. For example, in one study, researchers found that 92% of students did not think of themselves as binge drinkers, even though 35% of these students drank at levels that conformed to the operationalization of binge drinking in the literature (Lederman, Stewart, Laitman, Goodhart, & Powell, 2000). Thus, if researchers and prevention specialists are to use terminology that resonates with our target audience, the term *binge drinking* is insufficient. (Nevertheless, when reporting research literature, we use the term preferred by the author of the study if necessary to maintain clarity or consistency. Chapter 4 includes a more detailed discussion of this issue.)

The U.S. surgeon general indicates that the excessive use of alcohol continues to increase on college campuses nationally. In some cases, minority groups, such as African Americans and Asian Americans, whose rate was once markedly lower than White students, report an increasing use of alcohol (U.S. Department of Education's 12th Annual National Meeting on Alcohol, Other Drug, and Violence Prevention in Higher Education, 1998). In 1998, the National Advisory Council to the National Institute on Alcohol Abuse and Alcoholism (NIAAA) established the Task Force on

College Drinking. Reports commissioned by this task force confirm that alcohol-related problems continue to plague college campuses across the United States. Recent estimates (O'Malley & Johnston, 2002; Wechsler et al., 2000) indicate that well over 80% of all college students nationwide drink and that 50% engage in dangerous drinking. For example, Wechsler et al. (2000) found that 44% of college students reported a recent episode of binge drinking (using Wechsler's standard measure of five or more drinks in one sitting for males and four or more drinks for females).

The period of late adolescence and early adulthood is epitomized by a variety of developmental tasks that must be confronted and integrated as part of the maturation process, such as identity formation and the establishment of more mature interpersonal relationships (Danish, Petitpas, & Hale, 1993; Erikson, 1968). Failure to master these tasks successfully can result in frustration and stress, which can lead to a variety of unhealthy behaviors, including, potentially, alcohol abuse. Paradoxically, alcohol abuse often impedes the successful mastery of such tasks (O'Malley & Johnston, 2002).

Besides increased stress and freedom, other factors may lead to initiation or escalation of substance use among students. This is especially true of first-year students. First-year students may perceive that drinking and drug use are normative behaviors among college students. Researchers at a variety of U.S. institutions of higher education, for example, report that the percentage of students who drink dangerously is far lower than the perceived norms on the campus (Haines, 1993, 1996; Jeffrey, Negro, Demond, & Frisone, 2003; Perkins, 2003c).

Additionally, many students go to college with ideas about the positive effects of alcohol. They often believe that alcohol use can help them make friends or symbolizes a way to achieve a more mature status and a way to explore personal identities (Maggs, 1997; Paschall & Flewelling, 2002). Because of increased anxiety as a result of school and peer pressures, students may turn to alcohol or other drugs to cope with stress and associate with other students who use these substances as coping strategies (Paschall & Flewelling, 2002). Often, there is a rapid increase in dangerous drinking for first-year students over a relatively short period of time, which can contribute to difficulties with alcohol and with successful adaptation to the college environment. In fact, about one third of first-year students drop out which may be due, in part, to increases in alcohol and drug use at the beginning of their college experience (NIAAA, 2002; Perkins, 2002b).

In addition to school retention problems, college students are at high risk for a variety of other alcohol-related negative consequences. Dangerous drinking among college students is associated with negative consequences that can have long-term effects on physical and psychological well-being, including fatal and nonfatal injuries, academic failure, violence and other crime, unintended pregnancies, and sexually transmitted diseases (Goldman,

2002; Hingson, Heeren, Zakocs, Kopstein, & Wechsler, 2002; Perkins, 2002a; Wechsler et al., 2000). Excessive drinkers also create problems for other students and for residents of local neighborhoods including physical and sexual assaults, vandalism, needing to be taken care of by others, insults and humiliation, or preventing others from studying and sleeping (Hingson et al., 2002; Perkins, 2002a; Wechsler et al., 2000).

These negative effects of alcohol use contribute to the fact that students believe dangerous drinking occurs even more than it actually does and believe that the majority of their peers are supportive of excessive alcohol use (Burns, Ballou, & Lederman, 1991; Perkins, 1997; Perkins, Meilman, Leichliter, Cashin, & Presley, 1999; Perkins & Wechsler, 1996). Our research has demonstrated that Rutgers students, like their counterparts at other institutions, suffer from misperceptions about alcohol use as normative. Although less than 33% of Rutgers students drink dangerously, 84% of the student respondents in a 1998 survey reported that they believed the social atmosphere on campus promotes drinking (Lederman, Stewart et al., 1998). Also alarming is the finding that a majority of students reported that they felt faculty members reinforce the assumption that college students drink excessively. (This idea is discussed in more detail in the Chapter 2.) These misperceptions lead students, faculty, parents, and alumni to believe that college is a place where everyone drinks a great deal. Dangerous drinking as the perceived norm fosters the creation and maintenance of the cultural image of drinking as a rite of passage, as an inherent facet of college life.

One pervasive and powerful environmental factor in creating and maintaining this cultural image of drinking as fundamental to college life is students' own social interaction. The myth of dangerous drinking as pervasive is perpetuated by students sharing war stories about the "night before" (Burns & Goodstadt, 1989), faculty making jokes in class about students' partying (Lederman et al., 1998), and social events that encourage alcohol abuse (Burns & Goodstadt, 1989; Cohen & Lederman, 1998). If drinking and talking about getting drunk help students achieve their social and interpersonal goals, the data suggest that students can be expected to continue these behaviors.

## LEARNING THE NORMS ABOUT DRINKING

Perceptions in a culture or social organization, such as a college campus, are created by language and basic communication practices. Existing culturally determined labels for situations, for example, affect the way individuals perceive a situation (Whorf, 1956). In an even more complex view of cultural organizations, the view group members hold of reality can be shaped by the language patterns, the verbal cues and labels the culture has historically applied to any number of events (Brown, 1973). On a college campus, this perception results in notions such as interpersonal comfort being fostered by drinking or that recreation involves activities at the local bar. In this view, the absence of alcohol diminishes the entertainment value of any activity, and important occasions are celebrated with the consumption of massive quantities of alcohol. Such is often the case on many college campuses, especially in various college subcultures like clubs, cliques, fraternities, and sororities. Universities are, in reality, collections of such various subgroups, but the rising reports of campus dangerous drinking (Wechsler, Davenport, Dowdall, Moeykens, & Castillo, 1994) suggest most of these groups have long been structuring the meaning of the "college experience," with its myriad of social activities, as activities involving alcohol use. As noted earlier, studies indicate that the cliché of drinking dangerously permeates most college campuses. (See Chapter 14 for an additional discussion of the pervasiveness of this misperception.)

Students learn far more about drinking in the dorms and fraternity houses, in parties and in post-hoc discussions of those parties during the "morning after" than in classes or health education seminars. Through these interactions, students construct and reconstruct the "rules" for drinking that they learned in these social venues. For example, many students report believing that they are more socially attractive when they are drinking. This belief reinforces the notion of the desirability of dangerous drinking. (This concept is discussed in more detail in Chapters 2 and 3.)

Dangerous drinking is used by undergraduates as a means of fulfilling social interaction needs. One focus group study of high- and low-risk female respondents demonstrated that self-destructive alcohol consumption is negotiated as an acceptable risk for the sake of making friends and creating social circles among undergraduates who are new to vast, potentially overwhelming, and alienating environments like a large college campus (Lederman, 1993). The inhibition-lowering and perceived interpersonal competency-aid of alcohol may be used by incoming students to make contact with new friends and potential sexual partners.

If simply getting drunk helps students achieve their social and interpersonal goals, these data suggest that students will continue to get drunk. Even if severe intoxication causes illness, if alcohol generally is the key to some ultimate pleasure, the downside of drinking can be endured as long as it is not worse than the rewards gained. Furthermore, when communicating about alcohol use, overuse, or health problems related to alcohol, network analysis has shown that students more readily turn to their peers for information, rather than to professors, counselors, parents, or any other authority figure (Marshall, Scherer, & Real, 1998). Thus, in the instance of each of these findings, it becomes clear that the college culture itself has a powerful hand in shaping students' perceptions about correct and incorrect alcohol use and that a strong influence in the creation and maintenance of that culture is social interaction (Lederman & Stewart, 1998).

## OVERVIEW

This book describes the design, development, implementation, and evaluation of a health communication campaign addressing dangerous drinking on the college campus—the RU SURE Campaign. This campaign was selected in 2001 as a U.S. Department of Education model program and is based on Lederman and Stewart's (1998) Socially Situated Experiential (SSEL) model that brings together ideas from interpersonal communication with social norms theory and experiential learning theory to provide a comprehensive framework for a modern prevention campaign. Although this campaign was developed at Rutgers University, it is applicable to colleges throughout the country (as discussed in Chapter 11).

Part I of this book provides a discussion of the background of the development of the RU SURE Campaign including collection of baseline data (Chapter 2) and the conceptual model (Chapter 3) on which this campaign is situated.

Part II focuses on the design of the campaign describing both the *Top Ten Misperceptions at Rutgers* (the media component of the campaign) as well as the unique interpersonally based experiential strategies for message dissemination. Chapter 4 argues for developing campaign language that resonates with students in order to help insure the effectiveness of the campaign for them. In Chapter 5 the design of the *Top Ten Misperceptions at Rutgers* as the media component of the campaign is described in detail. Chapter 6 details the curriculum infusion component of the campaign in which students participate in all facets of message dissemination to their peers, and Chapter 7 presents the interpersonal strategies that are used in the RU SURE Campaign for that dissemination.

Part III focuses on the outcomes of the campaign. Chapter 8 details the evaluation process that was used as a basis for developing, implementing, and evaluating the success of the campaign. Because students are involved in dissemination of the campaign message, important outcomes include the effect of this participation on the campaign messengers. Thus, Chapter 9 describes the results observed with some of these messengers. Chapter 10 provides a description of a bi-product of the campaign, the *RU SURE Game of Choices and Consequences* that can be used as a 1-hour brief intervention to help students understand their alcohol-related decision making. Chapter 11 discusses how the media component of the RU SURE

Campaign, the *Top Ten Misperceptions at Rutgers*, can be adapted for use on other college campuses.

The final part of this book, Part IV, includes chapters by some of the leading scholars and practitioners in the field of alcohol studies today. Chapter 12 is written by Fern Walter Goodhart and Lisa Laitman, alcohol specialists at the Rutgers University Health Services who provide the context in which the RU SURE Campaign was embedded at the university and the environmental approach used at the university. In Chapter 13, Alan D. Berkowitz, one of the two founders of social norms theory, provides a comprehensive review of social norms theory and its success in reducing dangerous drinking on college campuses from coast-to-coast. In Chapter 14, Linda R. Jeffrey and Pamela Negro, Rowan University, describe a consortium of educators from institutions of higher education throughout New Jersey who have worked for several decades to reduce dangerous drinking on their campuses. Patricia Fabiano, a leading health practitioner at Western Washington University, describes her highly successful program based on social norms theory in Chapter 15. Chapter 16, written by Thomas A. Workman, University of Nebraska-Lincoln, presents his research on social networks, such as fraternities on campus, and the ways in which their drinking stories reinforce myths about college drinking.

Thus, this volume is designed for both scholars and practitioners. The construct of socially situated experiential learning and the conceptual model in which it is presented in the book, which are based on almost two decades of research at Rutgers University, provide the conceptual foundation for the RU SURE Campaign. Because all elements of the RU SURE Campaign were designed in collaboration with research faculty, University Health Services staff, and students, the design is both theoretically sound and capable of implementation with a relatively small investment of university resources. This book demonstrates that successful prevention efforts can be developed by bringing together the expertise of a variety of individuals who have a vision of making the campus a safer place for all students.

# 2

# BASELINE DATA COLLECTION

## CONDUCTING A NEEDS ASSESSMENT
## BEFORE DESIGNING A HEALTH
## COMMUNICATION CAMPAIGN

As noted in the previous chapter, successful health communication campaigns are based on a foundation of solid research that often includes both qualitative and quantitative data collection. Qualitative data (such as that collected through interviews, focus groups, and observation) are used both to collect initial impressionistic data that inform the development of specific quantitative data collection instruments and to provide meaningful insights into the results of the quantitative data collection efforts. Quantitative data collected through surveys can serve as both a baseline measure (or starting point) to chart the progress of the campaign and as evidence of the campaign's effect (discussed further in Chapter 8). This chapter focuses on the baseline data collected at Rutgers University that served as both the impetus for developing a comprehensive campaign to address dangerous drinking on the campus and as a foundation for evaluating the effectiveness of the campaign. Although our research included reviewing the existing literature on college drinking, and we include some of that in this chapter, our primary concern was researching our own campus and learning about our own environment and its needs. In this sense, the Rutgers' experience is presented in this book as an elaborated case study in the use of research-driven communication theory as the basis for the development health communication campaign.

# EARLIEST COMPREHENSIVE STUDY AT RUTGERS

Since the early 1980s, Rutgers University, the eighth oldest institution of higher education in the country, has committed itself to dealing vigorously with alcohol abuse treatment and prevention for members of the Rutgers community. (See Chapter 12 for a detailed description of the history and the context within which the research in this chapter took place.) In 1989, a team of health educators and research faculty received funding to create a comprehensive prevention campaign on the campus. The project, the first systematic, funded, alcohol prevention research on the campus, included a 3-year comprehensive study with two major goals: (a) to develop an understanding of students', parents', administrators', and faculty's perceptions of the nature, extent, and origins of students' alcohol-related problems; and (b) to develop effective interventions based on this research.[1] The study consisted of the following components: (a) a major campus-wide survey of students, parents, and staff; (b) a multiphased research component; and (c) the design of major prevention interventions.

## Rutgers Student Alcohol and Drug Survey (1987)

In 1987 the Student Drug and Alcohol Survey, a pilot study for a major component of the 3-year study funded in 1989, was created and pilot-tested with convenience samples of students in undergraduate classes. After analysis of the instrument and refinement of it, it was administered in 1989 in a random mail survey of Rutgers' undergraduate students, under the direction and supervision of the university's Eagleton Institute for Public Opinion Polling. The following year, a funded research team, led by David Burns and Michael Goodstadt, created a survey instrument with the help of Eagleton that was mailed to a random sample of students, parents, faculty, and staff. The questionnaire was a multi-item measure designed to gather quantitative data to provide a picture of how the attitudes, behaviors, and expectations of students, other students, parents, faculty, staff and administrators as well as the surrounding community affected student drinking behavior. Data were collected during a 2-year period to examine how these different university populations influenced student drinking and to determine how best to mod-

[1]This research was funded, in part, by a grant from the U.S. Department of Education Fund for the Improvement of Post-Secondary Education (FIPSE) with supplementary grants from the Rutgers University Health Services, the Rutgers University Teaching Excellence Center, and the School of Communication, Information and Library Studies Research Subgrant Program.

ify the alcohol and drug policies and programs that existed at the time with respect to the information obtained.

There were several key findings from this comprehensive survey (Burns & Goodstadt, 1989). Although less than one third of students reported high-risk or dangerous drinking, there was a perception among students that heavy drinking and, consequently, "hooking up" (one night sexual encounters) were the norm on campus. Conversely, parents perceived that the use of alcohol was much lower than the actual rates of alcohol use. The majority of faculty and staff surveyed at that time did not concern themselves with students' alcohol use, concluding that students' substance problems were not their responsibility.

This study also found that parents expected that students were going to "experiment" with alcohol because they were away from home and their parents for the first time, because of peer pressure, and because students needed to find and test their limits. Furthermore, parents felt that, since students were just experimenting and probably would not continue this behavior, they should "get away with it" the first time. It is not surprising then that parents made a distinction between first and second offenses when asked about punishment for alcohol violations, contending that second violations deserved more attention.

On an interpersonal level, the study found that alcohol functioned as a social facilitator for students by making it possible for students under the influence to initiate relationships or have interactions they might not normally have. Many students reported that alcohol made them feel less inhibited and helped them overcome shyness and, in doing so, allowed students who were too shy or feeling isolated, lonely, or alienated from their peers to make connections with others. They saw drinking alcohol as an adult thing to do and felt that they were now expected to act more like adults and were given more responsibility with less guidance. These images were reinforced for them by alcohol advertising, media messages, and sports events in which beer/alcohol sponsorship was evident and specific as well as alcohol-related promotions for particular times of the academic year, such as spring break.

It was during this study that researchers at Rutgers first found that students' perceptions of drinking behaviors were distorted (Burns et al., 1991; Burns & Goodstadt, 1989). Students often did not recognize their drinking as excessive because their perception was relative to those around them — and they believed that the people around them were drinking excessively as well. For every student who drank, there was another who seemed to drink more frequently and to have more drinks per occasion. The study found, for the first time at Rutgers, however, that the perception of all college students as high-risk drinkers was incorrect. This perception existed, in part, because the high-risk drinkers were drinking quite visibly. In fact, more than half the students were low-risk drinkers or abstained from drinking altogether

(Burns & Goodstadt, 1989; Lederman, 1993). So surprising were these find-ings initially, that a review of the literature found few researchers were reporting similar results and seeking ways to address them (Berkowitz & Perkins, 1986a). More recently, however, particularly in the last 10 years, national studies echo the findings at Rutgers, and we at Rutgers have been informed in our work by the research of others around the country (e.g., Baer, Stacy, & Larimer, 1991; Berkowitz & Perkins, 1986a; Haines & Spear, 1996; Lo & Globetti, 1993; Perkins, 2002b).

## Survey of Parents

During the same study, researchers at Rutgers added an important compo-nent to their understanding of college students' behavior and perceptions by including parents in this research effort. Often, researchers studying issues relevant to college students focus their data collection efforts solely on the college population. Although this is understandable because college students are presumably the target audience for whatever message is to be disseminat-ed, there are often other stakeholders who are important influences on the attitudes and behavior of college students. Viewing parents as one important group that influences college students, the study included a survey of this constituency.

Surveying parents resulted in a finding that, like their sons and daugh-ters, parents saw alcohol use as a rite of passage. Many parents reported allowing their children to drink at home, but when their children were at college parents did not want them to drink in their dorm rooms. Because many parents, as well members of society at large, drink alcohol, their own behavior contradicts their "do not drink at school" message.

Although almost 75% of parents in this survey reported that they felt 21 should be the legal drinking age, they found it difficult to understand harsh punishments for underage drinking and felt the punishment did not necessarily fit the crime. This finding seemed to be an additional factor in understanding students' attitudes toward alcohol consumption on campus in that many parents reported having a difficult time criminalizing drinking and enforcing the legal age for drinking.

## Focus Group Interviews

Because the surveys raised almost as many questions as their findings answered, the study included an extensive qualitative component designed to get at the reasons behind some of the responses found in the surveys. Sixteen focus groups were conducted to determine the "why" behind the behavior of college drinking and the role alcohol played in their lives (Burns et al., 1991; Burns & Goodstadt, 1989; Cohen & Lederman, 1998). Although students articulated negative consequences from the excessive consumption of alcohol (e.g., hangovers, vomiting, being taken advantage of physically and/or sexually), they reported ignoring these factors because they saw drinking as a rite of passage into adulthood (i.e., limits testing).

These qualitative analyses also highlighted that alcohol consumption was used by students as a way to fulfill their need to socialize. Results of focus groups of high- and low-risk female students indicated that self-destructive alcohol consumption was negotiated as an acceptable risk for the sake of making friends and creating social circles among undergraduates who were new to vast, overwhelming, and alienating environments like a very large college campus (Burns et al., 1991; Burns & Goodstadt, 1989). (In this study high-risk was defined as having five or more drinks on one occasion and low-risk as zero to one drink.) The inhibition-lowering, and perceived interpersonal competency-aid of alcohol, in turn, was used by incoming first-year students to make contact with new friends, colleagues, and lovers. In other words, students felt that the consumption of alcohol resulted in a lowering of their inhibitions, which resulted in feelings of being more inter-personally competent, which led to more success in their social encounters.

Thus, one factor that contributed to whether or not students engaged in dangerous drinking was their recognition of the symbolic role of alcohol in their lives. Both groups of students in these focus groups (high-risk and low-risk) were very much alike in many ways, with the same needs and desires, yet they used alcohol quite differently. Members of both of these groups, however, had similar social goals that they needed to fulfill. They were looking to establish social lives. They needed human contact, friend-ship, and companionship. They both went about pursuing these goals through the network of college parties, bars, and fraternities. The high-risk drinkers, however, proceeded to use alcohol as a means to fulfill these goals, whereas the low-risk drinkers did not. But many of the low-risk drinkers felt that they were unusual and that most of their peers drank a great deal more than they did.

Thus, if simply getting drunk helps students achieve their social and interpersonal goals, as these data suggest, they can be expected to keep get-ting drunk. Even if severe intoxication causes illness, if alcohol generally is the key to some ultimate pleasure, the downside of drinking is endured as long as it is not worse than the rewards gained. However, alcohol is no longer abused when the students gain the pleasure of social contact and friendship without having to drink (Cohen & Lederman, 1998; Lederman, 1993).

### The Role Alcohol Plays in Students' Lives. Primarily, alcohol functions as a social facilitator by making it possible for students under the influence

to initiate relationships or have interactions they might not normally have. In our research, students reported that they thought that alcohol disinhibited them and helped them overcome shyness and, in doing so, allowed those who were too shy or feeling isolated, lonely, or alienated from their peers to make connections with others. This was particularly true at a large university where it was easy for someone to get lost in a "sea of numbers."

According to students in these interviews, alcohol encouraged bonding by forcing students to depend on their friends. Often, a student got too drunk and needed, literally, to be taken care of (e.g., carried home, given a garbage can to throw up in, or extracted from a sexually threatening situation).

Alcohol functioned as "social glue," which students saw as creating bonds in situations that were normally more private or isolated. For example, many students consumed too much alcohol and vomited at the end of the night. When they were not doing this in full view of others in the common bathrooms, they reported that they made sure to tell their roommates and neighbors about it the next day. They often chose to display and/or share their stories of "hooking-up" experiences with others.

They also saw alcohol as excusing excessive sexual behavior. As one student put it:

> I think girls just use it as an excuse. I've seen like, in bed, one girl hook up and the next day she is like, "Oh, my God, I was drunk." And the next time I see her and she does it again, it is "Oh my God, I was drunk." And they just do it, and they think just because they were drunk it was ok.

Alcohol was also an excuse for "wild" behavior. Students said things like:

> You act weird and do whatever you want when you are drunk; you see it as an excuse to do anything.

> You have a couple of extra drinks and you can be an asshole, you can be obnoxious, you can try to blame it the next day on being drunk. That is another thing, a lot of people use it as an excuse to act wild, as long as they supposedly had a couple of drinks they can get away with it.

But mostly, students reported alcohol as a relaxant, as a social facilitator, and as social glue. It was not unusual for students to say things such as:

*The guys I live with I really, really connected with, I mean we've been through a lot together, just this semester alone. We partied together, got sick together, we've had problems, gone through everything.*

These findings are consistent with the results of more recent qualitative work (Cohen & Lederman, 1998; Workman, 2001a). Workman's (2001b) ethnography of college drinking discovered that drinking stories recounted by fraternity members were seen as performances that enacted a number of coming-of-age rituals for young men and, in effect, constructed the social reality of the masculine setting of the fraternity house. Where the fraternity house culture functioned as a transitional period for men from childhood into adulthood, the culture's rituals ultimately centered on a number of growth and self-discovery performances. As Workman noted, these performances were often alcohol related and the over consumption of alcohol was perceived to facilitate each act of self-discovery.

Among the functions of drinking that Workman (1999, 2001a) explored are risk-taking, entertainment, physical exploration that often involved being naked and exposing one's body to others, as well as the testing of one's limits of endurance and pain through fighting, the sickness of hangovers and vomiting, unplanned sexual encounters, and the participation in what was perceived as the quintessential college experience, a "once-in-a-lifetime experience." The war stories that the Rutgers' focus group participants recounted invariably dealt with how the over consumption of alcohol helped them enact one, or several, of these rituals. As Workman (1999) noted, "the social practice also represents the college experience; drunkenness is seen as a key confirmation of having been at the university" (p. 24).

*Rules for Alcohol Use.* Students also reported rules they developed regarding alcohol use. Students' rules were characterized by very specific instructions on how to prepare their bodies for a night of alcohol consumption. The thought of not drinking, rather than prepping the body to endure an evening of "safe" alcohol abuse, was not an issue. Rules included eating during the day to prevent getting sick, avoiding shots if drinking hard liquor, sipping rather than chugging, and, most significantly, learning through experience what each person could personally drink and how much each person could handle. As the students noted: "Beer before liquor, you'll get sicker. Liquor before beer, you'll stay clear."

Students also reported that their rules included watching out for others, not trusting people that they would not ordinarily trust, not drinking with strangers, and not letting somebody else get a drink for them ("because you don't know what they might put in it"). Self-admonishments were also a common part of the rules:

*Don't drink and drive.*
*Don't get the spins.*
*Don't do things you will regret.*

## PREVENTION EFFORTS BASED ON THESE FINDINGS

Based on these findings, Rutgers Health Services' personnel decided to revise and amplify some of their alcohol prevention activities. Since the early 1980s, Rutgers had been actively addressing college drinking with a variety of health education programs and access to treatment for students with addiction problems. One of the outcomes of the additional research was the design and implementation of prevention campaigns such as RU AWARE? (a social marketing campaign) and You're Not What You Think When You Drink (an awareness campaign.) (See Chapter 12 for a more in depth discussion of the history of alcohol prevention at Rutgers.)

## Identifying Young Adult Substance Abusers: The Rutgers Collegiate Substance Abuse Screening Test

It was obvious from both the qualitative and quantitative data collected in the late 1980s and from an examination of the prevention literature, that some college students' drinking is not only dangerous but can be classified as abusive. In the early 1990s, researchers at Rutgers focused added attention on the behaviors of alcohol abusers within the student population. Because survey instruments designed to identify substance abusers are typically normed on adult populations not in college environments it was important to develop an instrument that could be used successfully with this group of people. Thus, the Rutgers Collegiate Substance Abuse Screening Test (RSCAT) was developed for this purpose (Bennett et al., 1993).

This measure, based on the Michigan Alcohol Screening Test, consists of 25 true-false items tailored to the specific experiences of young adults. To determine its reliability and validity, three groups completed the RSCAT: a clinical sample of young adults who were problem substance users; a group of young adults who were referred to an assistance program but were judged not to have a substance problem; and a control sample of young adult, non-problem substance users. The RSCAT correctly identified the majority of participants as problem or nonproblem users and was effective in classifying participants when they were divided into distinct clinical and control groups. Finally, the RSCAT effectively distinguished between problem substance users and nonproblem substance users, all of whom had been referred for evaluation to the campus alcohol assistance program.

## The Personal Report of Student Perceptions

It is clear from the previous discussion that researchers and health services staff at Rutgers have been involved in a variety of efforts to more clearly understand the role of alcohol consumption in students' lives since the initial funded research back in 1989-1991. Early efforts had culminated in the development of a screening tool that would help identify students with substance abuse problems who could be offered treatment. But more was needed in order to understand what the climate of college drinking was by the late 1990s, and how, if at all, it had changed.

By Fall 1997, it became apparent that additional quantitative research would be helpful to more fully understand the scope of students' alcohol-related behaviors and the reasons for them. This information could be supplemented with items specifically focusing on the communication-related behaviors of students. Thus, the Personal Report of Student Perceptions (PRSP), developed by a team of researchers led by Lederman and Stewart (Lederman et al., 1998; Stewart & Lederman, 2002) was used to collect quantitative data to help get a clearer picture of current perceptions about alcohol use on campus, the extent to which these belief systems influence behavior, and the communication behaviors involved in this process. Additionally, the PRSP was conceived as a measure of perceptions of normative drinking behaviors among college students and how much these perceptions differ from actual drinking practices.

The PRSP was developed using questions from the 1987 Rutgers Student Alcohol and Drug Survey, relevant questions selected from the Campus Survey of Alcohol and Other Drug Norms (The Core Institute, 1996) adapted with permission, and specific questions designed for the Rutgers' student population. The questions included standard measures of students' alcohol and other drug use and attitudes toward these substances. Additionally, questions that addressed students' perceptions of their behavior and its consequences were developed.

The survey was pretested on a group of undergraduate student volunteers drawn from classes taught by the principal investigators. Student responses to the pretest were anonymous. After the pretest, selected items were deleted or modified to more accurately reflect students' reported behaviors and perceptions.

The final survey was sent to a randomly selected sample of 5,000 undergraduate students at both the Newark and New Brunswick campuses of Rutgers University. Responses to the survey were anonymous, and students were offered an incentive (a drawing for cash prizes) for completing the survey and returning a postcard to the researchers. Survey responses were received from 1,208 students for a return rate of 24%.

# Results

The results of the survey painted a mixed picture of student behavior and perceptions. On the one hand, the majority of students did not drink dangerously. On the other, students seemed to think that almost everybody else did. These findings are consistent with the findings of Berkowitz and Perkins (1986a), Haines and Spear (1996), Jeffrey and Negro (1996), and Perkins (2002a) and at odds with the findings of Weschler, Lee, Kuo, and Lee (2000) who suggested far higher rates of dangerous drinking than we found on the Rutgers campus. The Rutgers' data indicated that despite the fact that only 26% of the respondents in the study reported that their last drinking episode consisted of more than five drinks, more that 75% of the respondents believed the atmosphere on the campus did not discourage drinking. Half of the students believed that the campus atmosphere actually encouraged drinking. This was a surprising finding considering that alcohol is not sold on campus and the university has a policy that restricts alcohol use on campus.

When asked about their perceptions of the frequency of drinking, many students reported that they did not approve of habitual drinking, even one drink everyday, but they did condone what we would consider dangerous drinking (five or more drinks in one sitting) on the few occasions that they did drink. For example, students did not approve of continuous alcohol use in terms of drinking two to three or more times a week. However, drinking five or more drinks on one occasion was considered acceptable as long as it did not occur frequently (more than twice a month).

Additional findings from this survey are reported here.

*Demographics of Students As Drinkers.*   Based on the accepted definition from the literature, *heavy drinkers* were defined as males who reported that they consumed five or more drinks the last time they drank and females who reported consuming four or more drinks. This level of alcohol consumption marks the *binge* drinker, the individual who might not drink every night but did, in fact, overindulge in alcohol on the occasions when he or she drank. Demographically, heavy drinkers in this study were more likely to be White males. This finding is consistent with previous studies (e.g., Wechsler et al., 2002). The percentage of heavy drinkers declined slightly as the year in school increased, with 28.5% of the heavy drinkers being first-year students and only 17.3% of the seniors reporting heavy drinking. It is interesting to note that the drinking levels of first-year women were quite high but decreased more as they moved along in college years than the levels of their male counterparts.

*Drinking-Related Behaviors.*   Although less than 33% of students reported heavy drinking behaviors, and almost 17% reported that they abstained from alcohol use, a majority of students did report drinking between one and four drinks at their last time drinking. The mean number of drinks for respondents was 3.1. The reported range of quantity of drinks was from 0 to 24 drinks. More students (25%) reported a decrease in alcohol use within the past year than reported an increase (22%). The most frequent response, however, among those students who drank, was that their alcohol consumption remained the same (37%) in the past year. Slightly more than 16% reported that they had not consumed alcohol at all in the past year.

In addition, it is interesting to note that the majority of students in this study did not spend money on alcohol. As our previous qualitative studies have shown, much of the drinking among college students occurs in social surroundings, such as dorm parties and fraternity/sorority events, where alcohol is freely available. Although some parties may have an admission charge, students clearly do not equate this charge with "paying for alcohol." Students do spend more money, however, as they progress through school. This occurs, in part, because they become "legal" and are able to purchase alcohol in restaurants and bars. This finding, however, reflects only a change in the pattern of drinking, not in the quantity of drinking.

When asked to compare their drinking habits with those of their best friends, the problem of the blurring of reality, school culture image, and perception becomes apparent. Here, the responses indicated, as detailed in Table 2.1, that college students seemed to believe everyone else used alcohol the same way they did or, in some cases, everyone else drank more than they did. Nearly 17% of students felt they drank less than their best friends did, and only a very small percentage indicated they drank more than "other friends" and students in general. This finding supports Baer et al.'s (2001) contention that "current studies suggest that university students almost always perceive friends and members of social reference groups as drinking

Table 2.1.  Perceptions of Alcohol Use as Compared to Others.

|  | LESS THAN | SAME AS | MORE THAN | DON'T DRINK |
|---|---|---|---|---|
| In comparison to my best friend | 30% | 38% | 16% | 17% |
| In comparison to other friends | 48% | 28% | 7% | 16% |
| In comparison to other students | 62% | 17% | 5% | 16% |

more than themselves" (p. 584) and are consistent with the findings of Perkins (2002a), Haines and Spear (1996), and Jeffrey and Negro (1996), among others.

Relationships with others clearly influenced students' perceptions. The distance of the interpersonal relationship influenced the perception of others' drinking. The more distant the relationship, the more often students indicated that they drank less than others did. More students indicated that their drinking was the same as their best friends than said that they drank less than their best friends. When comparing their own drinking to their best friends' drinking, 45.9 % of the students indicated that they drink the same whereas 35.4% said they drink less than their best friends. Only 19% indicated that they drink more than their best friends. When comparing their drinking to other friends, 57.8% of the students indicated that they drink less than other friends, 33.9% said they drink the same, and only 8.4% said they drink more than other friends. When comparing their drinking to other students, 73.8% of the students indicated that they drink less than other students, 20.7% said they drank the same as others, and only 5.6 % said they drank more than other students. This relationship is illustrated in Fig. 2.1.

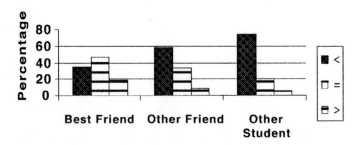

Figure 2.1.   Respondents' comparison of their drinking to others' drinking. (Data from New Brunswick students' PRSP, 1998.)

***Attitudes Toward Drinking.***   Although the respondents to this survey did not endorse heavy alcohol use as a means of solving personal problems, the majority were not concerned with the consequences of heavy drinking nor did they feel they had a drinking problem. Only 10% of the students did not agree that "drinking is fun," 14% felt they had a right to "blow off steam" by drinking a lot, and 65% did not feel they were "binge drinkers." Slightly more than half of the respondents (54%) said they were concerned over the consequences of heavy drinking, but 73% did not think they had a drinking problem. Although some of the actual percentages changed somewhat among respondents identified as heavy drinkers, the overall self-perceptions were much the same. For example, 43% of the heavy drinkers felt that drinking was fun. More than half of these students (60%) did not feel they were binge drinkers, and 30% believed they deserved to relieve stress or "blow off steam" by drinking. A small percentage (22.6%) curtailed their drinking owing to a fear of consequences, whereas 50.4% were concerned about the dangers of drinking but not ready to change their own behavior. A very large majority (87%) of this group also did not feel they had a drinking problem.

***Perceptions of Alcohol Use and Abuse.***   Perceptions of the role alcohol plays in the social life of these students shows that the respondents believed alcohol played a role in the social life of fraternity men, undergraduate men in general, sorority women, undergraduate women in general, and intercollegiate athletes. The role of alcohol among minority students was viewed as central by 48% of the respondents. Alumni and faculty/staff were perceived by a small percentage of the respondents as having alcohol as a central part in their social lives. However, about 50% of the respondents indicated a neutral opinion regarding the role of alcohol for these groups. Similar views of the role of alcohol were held regardless of the quantity of drinking reported by the respondent.

In general, students felt their friends disapproved of the heavy use of alcohol. Students overwhelmingly (71%) felt their close friends would approve of them having one or two drinks of alcohol occasionally. Only 9% of the respondents felt that their close friends disapproved of this behavior. Having four or five drinks was somewhat more objectionable, but only 43% of the respondents felt that their close friends would disapprove of this much drinking. Confirming previous findings about the college culture promoting substance abuse, the majority of students (53%) felt the social atmosphere on campus promoted the use of alcohol. What is even more startling is the fact that only 22% of the respondents disagreed with this statement.

On a positive note, this study demonstrated that most students had an adequate sense of the dangers of alcohol abuse, and, although they sometimes did not heed this sense, the respondents also gave a number of reasons for not drinking. The most frequent reasons for not drinking were that they planned on driving home (66%), that they just did not want to drink (65%), or that they did not feel well (60%). Slightly less than half of the respondents indicated that they did not drink because they had to get up the next morning (48%), did not feel safe (48%), or they were not with people they knew (42%). Only 35% of the students did not feel drinking interfered with campus life. The most frequently mentioned (23%) consequence of alcohol use by other students was that it "messed up" students' physical space.

Although the university has a clear alcohol policy for residence halls (discussed in Chapter 12), nearly 60% of the respondents did not know if resident assistants (RA)/Preceptors enforced the university's alcohol regulations. Only 17% felt the rules were uniformly enforced, and 42% felt there was either selective enforcement or mixed messages being sent by people responsible for enforcing the policies. In addition, although faculty members are not often seen as stakeholders in the alcohol-related behaviors of college students, they may be unwittingly participating in promulgating the image of excessive drinking to their students. The majority of the students in this study felt that faculty reinforced the assumption that college students drink excessively by joking about alcohol in class (58%) and by referring to Thursday night parties (43%). Few of the respondents (6%) indicated that direct actions of the faculty (e.g., drinking with students, holding class in a bar) reinforced the assumption about college students drinking excessively. Clearly, this perception is due to the relative lack of these activities not to the potential effect of these activities. Therefore, it appears that it is what the faculty say, not what they do, that reinforces this assumption.

## IMPLICATIONS FOR A NEW ERA OF PREVENTION ON CAMPUS

The data collected from the PRSP suggested that many of the attitudes, norms, and behaviors that had been identified back in the earliest campus survey in 1989 continued to exist on campus. The implication for the next step in reducing dangerous drinking on the campus was to formulate a conceptual, theory-based approach to the design, implementation, and evaluation of a prevention campaign designed to address both the dangerous drinking on campus and also the misperceptions that this excessive behavior was normative. What may be seen as the logical result of the perceived cultural norm of everyone drinking is the attitude held by many students that dangerous drinking is not a problem. At the root of college drinking lie perceptions, but perceptions are socially constructed. The challenge, thus, becomes how to design a health communication campaign to curb dangerous drinking that recognizes the social nature of college drinking, dispels the myths of excessive drinking as the norm, and is communicated in a manner that is most effective for a campus population. In the chapters that follow both the conceptual framework and the design, development, and dissemination of the campaign are discussed in detail.

# 3

# THE CONCEPTUAL MODEL

## COLLEGE DRINKING AS SOCALLY SITUATED EXPERIENTIAL LEARNING

Communication campaigns, as suggested in the beginning of this book, have long been accepted as a means for disseminating information, increasing knowledge, and changing social attitudes and behaviors (Rice & Atkin, 2001). Yet, according to Cappella (2003), the efficacy of even well-designed campaigns is often questioned and, for that reason, "understanding the mechanisms that activate campaign effects and, perhaps more importantly for the discipline of communication, the theoretical bases for the creation of effective messages to inform, persuade and motivate audiences is the sine qua non of the design and effective campaigns" (p. 160). In recognition of the profound importance of creating theory-driven campaigns, the design of the RU SURE Campaign began with the examination of theories of social interaction, experiential learning, and social norms as well as extensive theory-driven research into drinking on the Rutgers' campus.

Analysis of data collected over more than a decade at Rutgers (as discussed in Chapter 2) provided a grounded theory (Glaser & Strauss, 1967) understanding of students and their drinking behavior. Lederman (1993, 2002b) drew upon those data to formulate the construct of the culture of college drinking. According to Lederman, the *culture of college drinking* is the shared images, behaviors, attitudes, and perceptions that create a culturally specific sense that drinking heavily in college is an inherent and inevitable part of the college years. In the culture of college drinking, heavy drinking is viewed as a rite of passage rather than a health issue or social concern. In this view, drinking excessively is simply something that exists, has existed, and will always exist as part of growing up. In sum, the culture of college drinking is clearly a shared reality learned though drinking-related experiences, stories shared among students with one another, perceptions and many misperceptions of the behaviors and expectancies of one another, and a sense that belonging and bonding are so connected with drinking that the negative consequences are merely the admission price to belonging to the college culture.

To understand the role of communication in the culture of college drinking, Lederman and Stewart (1998) extended this conceptualization by creating a new construct that they refer to as socially situated experiential learning. According to Lederman and Stewart, *socially situated experiential learning* is the experience-based process of acquiring and interpreting social information (and misinformation) received from peers and other sources within the context of their direct learning experiences. The constructs of the culture of college drinking and socially situated experiential learning were incorporated into a conceptual model to describe the process of creating, implementing, and evaluating a prevention campaign (RU SURE) designed to address and change the culture of college drinking. The implication of this conceptual model is that prevention requires intervention into the types of interactional experiences that college students have on and off campus (including their interpretations of the meaning of those experiences) in order to influence and/or change their drinking behaviors over time. This chapter presents and describes this conceptual model and its role in driving the RU SURE Campaign.

## COLLEGE DRINKING AS SOCIALLY SITUATED EXPERIENTIAL LEARNING

The constructs of the culture of college drinking and socially situated experiential learning are central to the conceptual model of the components that coalesce to create the ways in which alcohol is used on the college campus and the development, implementation, and evaluation of the RU SURE Campaign as a prevention campaign designed to change college drinking. The model provided the basis for attempting to change that culture away from an image of college drinking as inevitable. Figure 3.1 presents the model.

The conceptual model of SSEL has five steps marked by numbers on the arrows in the model: The first step in the model is the use of theories of social interaction, experiential learning, and social norms theory/messages to begin to conceptualize and understand the culture of college drinking. The second step in the model is the use of these theories to conduct research into

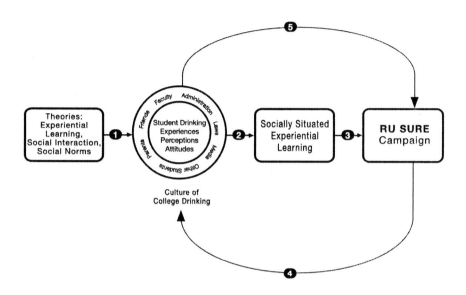

**Figure 3.1. Lederman and Stewart's Conceptual Model of Socially Situated Experiential Learning.**

and observation of the culture of college drinking in operation on the Rutgers campus that leads to the conceptualization of college drinking as socially situated learning. The third step is application of this analysis of the culture of college drinking and the construct of socially situated experiential learning to the formulation, design, implementation, and evaluation of the RU SURE Campaign. The fourth step is the implementation of the RU SURE Campaign as a brief intervention into student drinking-related attitudes, behaviors, and perceptions. The fifth step is the evaluation of the campaign's impact and the influence on the continued refinement of the construct of socially situated experiential learning. Each of these steps is discussed further in the next section.

## THE CONCEPTUAL MODEL: A FIVE-STEP MODEL

The conceptual model in which the RU SURE Campaign is embedded begins with the theories on which we drew to create the campaign and traces the conceptual pathways of all of the processes that were part of the thinking that went into the conceptualization, design, implementation, and evaluation of the campaign. Each step is discussed in detail here, and the part of the model representing that step is provided as a graphic to which to refer.

### Step 1: Application to the Culture of College Drinking

The first step in the model (Fig. 3.2) is the selection of relevant concepts from theories of social interaction/interpersonal communication, experiential learning theory, and social norms theory to draw upon in order to analyze the culture of college drinking (Lederman, 1993), most especially the shared ways in which students in college drink and think about drinking.

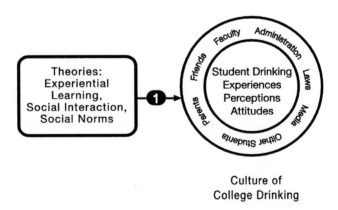

Culture of
College Drinking

**Figure 3.2.   Step 1 of the Conceptual Model.**

As reflected in Step 1 of the conceptual model, the development of the model began with an articulation of the theoretical basis on which all further research, analysis, and campaign design would take place. In some ways, from the beginning of the model, it is noteworthy that we departed from conventional wisdom in health communication. Much of the work done in health communication, and particularly health communication campaigns, draws on the Health Belief Model (HBM) which posits that preventive health behavior is influenced by five factors:

1. Perceived barriers to performing the recommended response.
2. Perceived benefits of performing the recommended response.
3. Perceived susceptibility to a health threat.
4. Perceived severity of a health threat.
5. Cues to action. (Witte, Meyer, & Martell, 2001, p. 34)

In other words, individuals weigh the costs of performing a particular action (e.g., wearing a seatbelt will wrinkle your clothes) against the benefits of the action (surviving a serious accident) and perform the behavior if there is a low barrier to its completion (seatbelts are available on every car and easy to use).

Although the HBM is useful in many circumstances, it is incomplete in helping to understand the culture of college drinking. As can be seen from the box in the conceptual model labeled "Culture of College Drinking," many factors (e.g., other students, friends, family, faculty, law enforcement) influence students' perceptions of their role in the culture of college drinking as well as their perceptions of the behavior of others. Given that these influences exist within social contexts, it is important to draw upon theories that shed light on the impact of social interaction and context on messages and meanings. Thus, the conceptual model posits from Step 1 that there are social interactional factors that need to be considered if effective health communication campaigns are to be designed to bring about changes in this culture.

The work of researchers in *social interaction* perspectives on interpersonal communication, for example, provides a lens through which to examine social behaviors. Although there are a variety of theories that address social interaction in the interpersonal communication literature, two streams of thought were particularly useful in creating the framework from which to view social behavior on the college campus. The first stream began with the work of Watzlawick, Beavin Bavelas, and Jackson (1967) and the transactional paradigm that grew out of their work. One of the axioms posited by the Palo Alto Group is that interpersonal communication involves two messages: the content and the relational. To the extent that students often use alcohol to deal with social relationships, this work is a vital part of the interpersonal communication theories incorporated into the conceptual model.

The second stream of interpersonal communication addressing social interaction that the conceptual model draws upon is the ethnography of communication or the application of ethnographic ways of viewing the communication patterns of individuals. The *ethnography of communication* articulates the assumption that a local cultural community creates a shared meaning and uses codes that have some degree of common understanding (Carbaugh, 1990; Philipsen, 1997). From this perspective, communication is the process through which social institutions and the norms and customs embedded in those institutions are created and maintained (Carbaugh & Hastings, 1992; Fisher, 1987; Workman, 2001b). Using these understandings of communication and its socially based nature to approach health communication behavior allows researchers to "enter socially situated scenes" (Carbaugh & Hastings, 1992). This creates the ability to take into account the ways in which individuals' attitudes, beliefs, and behaviors can be examined in relation to one another and as the product of the interpretive processes of the individual within the sociocultural community. Workman (2001a), for example, studied the narratives students used to describe their drinking-related behaviors as vehicles for insight into the role of drinking in students' lives.

In short, using these social interactional concepts allows for the examination of the college scene and its relationships in socially situated interactional patterns—to bring into view the locally distinctive symbols, symbolic forms, and meanings that the participants in that social scene consider significant and important. This view is a way to take the communicative activities, such as narratives (Fisher, 1987; Workman, 2001a), created by students in their social interactions and to use them to provide insight into the actual social construction and meanings attributed to a wide range of drinking-related attitudes, perceptions, and behaviors. Communication and the conceptualization of experience as grounded in social interactions (Manis & Meltzer, 1978), including the influence of group pressure to conform (Asch, 1951), are essential elements of the theories on which the conceptual model is based. These social interactional perspectives make it possible to examine the college culture itself as a powerful force in shaping students' perceptions about socially acceptable behavior (Stewart & Lederman, 2002; Workman, 2001a).

As suggested in Step 1, in addition to concepts of social interaction, the model draws upon concepts of experiential learning theory and the role of trial and error in college drinking, as well as social norms theory.

Experiential learning theory provides an additional set of theoretical concepts to understand college drinking. Experiential learning theory (Dewey, 1929; Kolb, 1984) argues that learning takes place in a cycle in which one has an experience; reflects on that experience; draws conclusions, and then acts during his or her next experience based on the initial experience-reflection-interpretation process (Lederman & Stewart, 1998). Learning from this perspective is cyclical. In fact, Dewey (1929) argued that all learning carries with it an experience and that experiences that lead one to withdraw from learning more are "miseducative."

*Experiential learning theory*, then, has implications for conceptualizing college drinking as part of the learning experience because experiences can provide both biased, as well as more accurate, occasions to learn what drinking norms actually are. First, students gain knowledge about drinking-related behaviors and attitudes on campus through their own experience, which includes observing and interacting with peers in social situations involving alcohol and substance use (e.g., in parties and social gatherings, in health education seminars, in the classroom, at work, etc.), and also seeing others' reactions. These experiences and others provide a framework for thinking about drinking. Next, students continue to reflect on their experience in relation to their own beliefs and behavior. Based on the outcome of comparing their own behaviors and belief systems to their perceptions (including misperceptions) of others, they may change (or maintain) their current expectations of using or abstaining from alcohol and other substances. This social comparison (Bandura, 1986), taken together with experiential learning theory, forms the basis of socially situated experiential learning, a process that begins with experience and then moves through reflection and interpretation to behavior the next time the experience presents itself.

Although classical experiential learning theory describes the learning cycle as if everyone learns similarly, data collected regarding the culture of college drinking at Rutgers painted a different picture. Regardless of their own level of drinking (low, moderate, or heavy), students believe that drinking dangerously is a "learning experience." When probed about what they learned from this experience, low and moderate drinkers noted that after an experience of getting sick they learned not to drink as much any more. When asked follow-up questions, these students reported that they rarely, if ever, drank that much again (Burns et al., 1991). In focus groups of heavy drinkers, however, the responses were different. Students reported that what they learned after getting sick was to "drink before you eat," "line your stomach with milk," or "don't mix beer and hard liquor." In other words, the lessons heavy drinkers took from their experiences did not influence the amount they continued to drink in the future (Cohen & Lederman, 1998).

In incorporating the experiential learning cycle into the conceptual model, therefore, we recognized the need to characterize learning as "socially situated" experiential learning, thereby drawing on Bandura's (1986) social cognitive theory to further explicate the experiential learning cycle. The implication is that learning takes place within a social context, and the interpretations and the behaviors to which it leads at the end of the cycle are a product of both the experience and the social context. Included in the social context is the individual's own sense of self. Part of the learning that takes place includes how the student thinks about him or herself, including his or her self-talk (Lederman, 1996; 2002a). When the environmental cues are con-sistent with the person's sense of self, the learning experience reinforces what the person initially thinks about his or her own behavior. When there is a discrepancy, the individual may be in a state of cognitive dissonance (Festinger, 1957). The conceptual model suggests that the way this disso-nance is resolved is socially situated. If, for example, a student who drinks passes out, is carried back to the dorm, and told the next day that he is a hero, this experience is only dissonant if he himself is ashamed of the behavior.

Furthermore, by drawing on social cognitive theory (Bandura, 1986) experiential learning theory can be expanded to include motives that can explain variability in alcohol use by college students. First, a student's attitude toward alcohol use both grows out of the student's own first-hand experi-ences and is a function of the perceived benefits and costs (i.e., expectancies) of performing this behavior weighted by the importance he or she places on each of these positive or negative outcomes (Fishbein & Ajzen, 1975). A strong positive attitude toward alcohol use (which is formed by a person's perception that alcohol use will lead to mostly positive and highly desirable outcomes) will predict a strong likelihood of performing this behavior, whereas a strong negative attitude will significantly reduce this likelihood. The second type of motivation for alcohol use, actual or perceived social pressure on students to use (or abstain from using) alcohol, is better explained by social norms theory (discussed later in this chapter). Central to many of these attitudes is the assumption that people actively seek social information that will allow them to form or modify normative or social judgments.

Individuals may be motivated to do so by the desire to express socially acceptable attitudes and behavior in public (impression motivation), the desire to hold attitudes that are consistent with reality (accuracy motivation), or the desire to find social information that reaffirms their pre-existing atti-tudes and behaviors (defensive motivation) (Eagly & Chaiken, 1993). In each case, the source and amount of motivation to seek and process social infor-mation determine a person's degree of susceptibility to social influence (Petty & Cacioppo, 1986). If a person is motivated to seek social information for objective reasons (e.g., for purposes of impression management), he or she is more likely to be susceptible to social influence than a person who seeks sim-ilar information to reaffirm his or her pre-existing attitudes and beliefs. Moreover, those who are highly motivated to seek and process social infor-mation are at the same time more susceptible to social influence if they process this information objectively (such as when the source of motivation is impression management) and less susceptible to social influence if they evaluate such information against their own preexisting biases and reject it if it contradicts their own attitudes, beliefs, and behavior (defensive motiva-tion). Thus, in Step 1 of the conceptual model experiential learning theory is incorporated as a way to take into account the various ways in which students are motivated to seek information and/or how they may filter in or filter out alcohol-related information that is not consistent with their previous beliefs.

In order to more thoroughly describe the processes in which students seek, acquire, and filter alcohol-related information, Step 1 also includes concepts from social norms theory about messages and shared misperceptions of college norms. The basis of social norms theory is the assertion that students measure themselves against others in assessing the appropriateness or acceptability of their own behaviors (Haines & Spear, 1996). Social norms theory describes situations in which individuals incorrectly perceive the attitudes and/or behaviors of their peers and others (Berkowitz & Perkins, 1986b; Haines & Spear, 1996; Perkins, 1997). It attempts to explain why individuals often perceive norms as different from their own behaviors when in actuality they are not. These mistakes are labeled "misperceptions." According to this theory, misperceptions increase as social distance increases. In the college environment this means that most individuals perceive that their friends drink more than they do and that students in general drink more than their friends (Berkowitz & Perkins, 1986b; Bourgeois & Bowen, 2001; Lederman et al., 1998; Perkins, 1997). (Alan Berkowitz provides a comprehensive discussion of social norms theory in Chapter 13.)

Social norms theory is employed in prevention campaigns by collecting data on the extent of misperceptions, successfully communicating this information to a targeted campus population, assisting them to understand the discrepancies between fact and myth, and making salient new behaviors and norms associated with the facts instead of the myths (Haines, 1996; Jeffrey & Negro, 1996; Perkins, 2003c).

Social norms strategies focus on social comparison and peer influence in relation to alcohol use, which has been found to be influential in shaping human behavior (Haines & Spear, 1996; Perkins & Berkowitz, 1986). Advocates of social norms-based approaches claim that students operate under the misperception that everyone on campus drinks excessively (Butler, 1993). Prevention programs based on social norms theory use a variety of mechanisms to convey to college students the actual norms on their campus. They are based on the assumption that learning the actual norms will reduce peer pressure by reinforcing the ability of those individuals who drink moderately or not at all to be more willing to express their real attitudes toward drinking. These interventions are based on the finding that many, perhaps most, students have healthy attitudes and that their mistaken notions, or misperceptions, of their peers' attitudes and behaviors influence their own sense of themselves and cause them to see themselves as the minority ("most people drink more than I do") rather than as the majority, which in fact they are (Berkowitz, 1997; Perkins & Berkowitz, 1986).

Thus, if college students routinely misperceive how much others are drinking, they are measuring their own drinking behavior against a misperceived norm. The most disturbing consequence of these misperceptions is the pressure that students then experience to increase their drinking in an effort to fit in with their social group by drinking more. A person's motivation to rely on normative judgments when making behavioral decisions is a key element in many social influence theories (for a review, see Petty & Cacioppo, 1986).

This tendency may be used to explain the consistent finding that rates of dangerous drinking are higher among first-year students than among older cohorts of students (Baer, 2002; Lederman et al., 1998; Wechsler, Lee, Meichun, & Lee, 2000). Many scholars identify the transition to the college environment as a detrimental factor contributing to this phenomenon but no single explanation of this effect has emerged. It can be argued that the transition to college is a stressful event for many young adults because it involves a significant change in social context and setting. However, a social influence approach would attribute the excessive use of alcohol by first-year students to the fact that the transition to college increases students' susceptibility to mechanisms of social influence and peer influence in particular.

From this perspective, the transition to a college environment is a defining structural event in the sense that students' social relationships and patterns of interaction with peers abruptly change and lead to heightened levels of social uncertainty. Some students (heavy drinkers in high school) are likely to project their own attitudes, expectancies, and behavior onto that of their peers. Others, who have little or no previous experience with heavy drinking, will be more motivated to seek accurate social information. In terms of alcohol use on the campus, these misperceptions occur when individuals overestimate how much others drink and underestimate the number of students who drink little if at all. D. Miller and McFarland (1987) referred to this phenomenon as *pluralistic ignorance*. Pluralistic ignorance has been found to cause individuals to change their own behavior to approximate their perceptions of the behavior of others (e.g., sharing war stories of the night before even though the individual actually did not drink excessively). From a communication perspective, pluralistic ignorance increases as individuals share their misperceptions with others, acting as "carriers of the misperception" (Perkins, 1997). Thus, social norms interventions attempt to correct the misperceptions in order to increase the actual norms, which tend to be safer (healthier) than the misperceptions about them. For social norms interventions to work effectively, however, the information they provide has to be credible to the intended audience.

One of the often raised questions with social norms interventions is which norms should be used. Groups (social networks) have their own or "local" as compared with the norms of the generalized other, the more distant "global" campus norms. Social norms theorists argue that it is important to select the most relevant and salient norms for a particular intervention and the appropriate strategy for changing those norms. Thus, the compatibility between social norms interventions and well-established communication theory is clear. Providing accurate information about norms creates cognitive dissonance (Festinger, 1957) by informing those who misperceive the actual campus norms. The stronger the dissonance, the more likely the students are to reduce their dissonance by dismissing the messages ("That's dumb, everyone drinks more than that!").

Using social norms theory together with social interactional views of interpersonal communication theory that posits that the socially situated nature of communication is a way to channel this cognitive dissonance into productive attitudinal change yields a more effective persuasive strategy. By understanding communication as socially situated, and the college community as created through experiential learning, then it is important to combine what is known about the process of learning from experience with what is known about the social construction of meaning (communication) and embed social norms messages within the social interaction of the campus.

Taken together, these theories and the concepts they include provide a communication-based way to look at the culture of college drinking and lead to Step 2 in the model, research and observation on the Rutgers' campus. To understand the culture of college drinking from a communication perspective, therefore, demanded taking into account the nature of social interaction, social influence, and student experimentation with drinking behavior. This required taking into account the following:

1. How social interaction and attribution theories help to explain how the dynamics of an organization, an insular culture, and one's peers form attitudes toward alcohol use and, in turn, create habits of drinking behavior.
2. How experiential learning theories provide insight into how these behaviors are adopted.
3. How social norms theory helps to explain the ways in which social construction of perceptions are distorted into misperceptions and shared in daily interaction.

These concepts are all part of Step 1 in the conceptual model and provide the theoretical basis for understanding how to change the culture of college drinking from one in which drinking excessively is perceived as inevitable.

## Step 2: Research, Observation, and Formulation of College Drinking As Socially Situated Experiential Learning

Step 2 of the conceptual model (shown in Fig. 3.3) takes the results of the theory-driven research into drinking at Rutgers and uses it to extend the conceptualization of college drinking by the additional formulation of the construct of socially situated experiential learning. As defined earlier, socially situated experiential learning is the experience-based process of acquiring and interpreting social information (and misinformation) received from peers and other sources within the context of their direct learning experiences.

It is Step 2 of the model that shows the grounded theory approach to the development of the construct of socially situated experiential learning. As discussed in the previous chapter, Rutgers researchers have been collecting both quantitative and qualitative data on students' alcohol use and consequences since the late 1980s. Based on these data, a more clearly defined sense of the culture of college drinking emerged. According to the concept of the culture of college drinking that was developed, in this shared cultural sense of the life of the students, students tend to feel that it is permissible to drink alcohol because "others" expect that they will drink. The "others" who contribute to the norms that create the perception that everyone is drinking are the media and advertisers, other students, parents, university faculty and staff, residents around campus, police and security personnel, and anyone else who believes that college students drink and will continue to drink regardless of the policy or law, as illustrated in Step 2 and suggested in the box labeled "Culture of College Drinking."

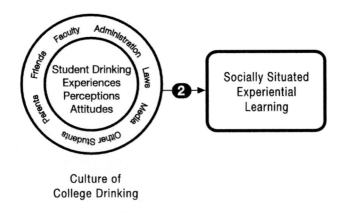

Figure 3.3.   Step 2 of the Conceptual Model.

Thus, students experience themselves as living in an environment that they perceive to support excessive drinking. For example, in one survey, they reported thinking that professors' comments in class about drinking ("I don't like to teach on Friday mornings—Thursday nights are party nights so everyone comes in hung over") encourage a drinking atmosphere (Lederman et al., 1998). Because students see themselves as engaging in an "expected" behavior, they perceive that the punishment if they get caught violating a campus alcohol-related policy will not be taken seriously by the enforcers (e.g., they will either be "slapped on the wrist" or, if they are punished at all, it will be with something that has a nonserious consequence such as doing 5 hours of community service).

The negative consequences students articulate as associated with drinking were hangovers, vomiting, or being taken advantage of physically and/or sexually (Burns et al., 1991). They ignore these factors because they see drinking as a rite of passage into adulthood (i.e., limits testing). "Doesn't everybody?" an interviewee asked during a focus group. Additionally, these consequences are much less than the social cachet they attach to drinking-related behaviors. The experience of alcohol as social glue, of bonding through the use of alcohol, is widely enough shared as to far outweigh waking up with a hangover. Furthermore, outcomes that are truly dangerous (e.g., fatal injuries, life-threatening situations) so rarely happen to students that their own sense of invincibility is reinforced.

Furthermore, students believe that others drink more than they do, no matter how much they themselves drink. Even many of the students who do not drink excessively behave as if they drink a great deal (e.g., nursing their drinks at fraternity parties, telling exaggerated "war stories" about the night before). All of these behaviors occur despite the fact that data consistently suggest that the percentage of students who actually drink excessively both at Rutgers and nationally is far below the shared misperception that "everybody does" (Burns et al., 1991; Burns & Goodstadt, 1989; Cohen & Lederman, 1998; Haines, 1996; Perkins, 1997).

Thus, part of the culture of college drinking is a shared, yet erroneous, conclusion about the value system of college environments. Research on social norms has repeatedly shown that students evaluate their peers as being much more permissive in their drinking habits and tolerant of illicit substances than themselves (Berkowitz & Perkins, 1986b; Bourgeois & Bowen, 2001; Far & Miller, 2003; Lederman et al., 1998; Perkins, 1997). In an attempt to live up to campus myths, students may, in fact, help those myths become a "self-fulfilling prophecy." (See Chapter 13 for a more extensive discussion of this phenomenon as addressed in social norms literature.) In other words, if students believe there is a (false) standard of behavior expected of them by their peers and then live up to those expectations, the very real atmosphere of alcohol abuse on a campus can rival the original mythic rates of "bingeing." For students whose own attitudes about drinking and substance abuse are permissive, a campus culture that exaggerates drinking norms can help push them into becoming habitual binge drinkers. Even for people whose drinking habits are moderate, an environment fostering an erroneous view of "everybody doing it" can become damaging by encouraging more drinking, abuse, and habitual bingeing (Perkins & Wechsler, 1996).

Along with the misperception of what is normative, those students who actually do drink excessively often do not recognize their drinking or other drug use as problematic. Many students believe themselves to be more inter-personally competent and communicative when drunk (Cohen & Lederman, 1998; Lederman & Stewart, 1998). Drinking is treated as a par-ticularly social experience, always done in public and with groups of friends, fostering the notion that it is "what you're supposed to be doing." The majority of students believe that drinking is a college-wide phenomenon, something the overwhelming majority of students are doing. Many students drink with groups of friends and drinking may be their chief recreational activity, whether they drink excessively or just nurse their drinks. For these students, in particular, their daily experiences reinforce their misconceived notion that they are simply doing what everyone does. As noted previously, this shared misperception is referred to as pluralistic ignorance (D. Miller & McFarland, 1987; Prentice & Miller, 1993).

Thus, many students think of drinking for fun as what the entire stu-dent population is supposed to be doing. And those college organizations, such as fraternities and sororities, for whom the overuse of alcohol has "historically" been an integral part of the organization's function can have a greater impact in prompting students to develop habits of alcohol abuse (Bourgeois & Bowen, 2001). Furthermore, when it comes to communicat-ing about alcohol use, overuse, or health problems relating to alcohol, stu-dents readily turn to their peers for information, rather than to professors, counselors, parents, or any other authority figures (Perkins, 1997). Thus, it becomes clear that the college culture itself may have the most powerful effect in shaping students' perceptions about appropriate alcohol use.

Whereas the need to belong to a peer group is very strong among young people, especially as they enter college, the need for acceptance by one's peers becomes so strong that it helps students accept a view of reali-ty prescribed by their targeted peer group. Students can learn to see and accept the world through the eyes of a group they desire to join. Thus, as counselors, parents, and school administrators repeatedly experience, stu-dents are more willing to heed the advice of friends and schoolmates than adults. This, unfortunately, is the case even if friends endorse dangerous drinking. Thus, it becomes clear that the best the approach to understanding drinking habits is to understand the college culture itself and the way it influences individual behavior.

Unfortunately, the reality of dangerous drinking is often far more costly and dangerous than the romanticized narratives enacted in the residence halls or fraternity/sorority culture. In contrast to the tales of harmless, youthful brawling, too often the result of dangerous drinking is very real and very destructive. In colleges across the country, dangerous drinking is repeatedly associated with serious physical injuries resulting from either fighting or motor vehicle accidents (Wechsler, Davenport et al., 1994). The reckless overconsumption of alcohol also claims many ancillary victims. The orbit of dangerous drinking college students includes their nondangerous drinking peers who experience "secondary dangerous effects," such as getting insulted, humiliated, hit, or pushed; having their property damaged; becoming sleep or privacy disturbed; being sexually assaulted or raped (Perkins & Wechsler, 1996).

The discussion so far has focused primarily on factors that increase the susceptibility of students to messages that encourage dangerous drinking. Nevertheless, an important element of the emergent culture of college drinking is the circumstances under which excessive drinking is not seen as necessary. In our research, the only time that students reported that alcohol was no longer abused was when they gained the pleasure of social contact and friendship without having to drink (Cohen & Lederman, 1998).

Taken together, these findings (discussed in more detail in the previous chapter) suggested to us that elucidating the mechanisms by which shared attitudes and normative perceptions are produced and maintained by individuals and groups of students through their social interactions with one another and their own experiences are pivotal to the explanation of the variability in drinking behavior observed among students.

The implication of this conceptualization is that college drinking is more than a health problem, more than a rite of passage. The culture of college drinking is an experience-based, socially situated set of attitudes, beliefs, and behaviors. It is the product of what students talk about, what they see around them, how they interpret the behaviors of themselves and others, and the socially and experientially constructed filters that shape those interpretations and beliefs about what is socially acceptable and attractive and what is simply required of them to fit into the college social scene.

Thus, Step 2 of the conceptual model uses the analysis of the culture of college drinking with the concepts articulated in Step 1 to articulate the construct of SSEL (Lederman & Stewart, 1998.) This construct provided the basis for decisions about the conceptualization, design, and implementation of the RU SURE Campaign that are part of Step 3.

## Step 3: Formulation of the RU SURE Campaign

The third step of the conceptual model (Fig. 3.4) is the use of the construct of socially situated experiential learning to formulate, design, and implement the RU SURE Campaign.

Because the campaign is theory-driven, it is not until Step 3 that the actual campaign was addressed. Only when the construct of college drinking as socially situated experiential learning had been formulated (Step 2), was it possible to begin to conceptualize what the campaign should be and how it should be formulated, designed, and implemented.

It was based on the conceptualization of college drinking as socially situated experiential learning that we formulated, designed and pilot-tested the campaign concepts. We approached the campaign design with the emphasis on social interaction. Mediated messages and campaign materials were seen as the means of creating conversation, and the heart of the campaign were those structured conversations that we planned to design. Having formulated, designed, and pilot-tested campaign concepts and materials based on the ways in which our thinking was shaped by conceptualization of college drinking, the model moves to Step 4, the implementation of the campaign. Step 4 is shown in Fig. 3.5.

## Step 4: Implementation of the RU SURE Campaign

As suggested in Step 4 of the conceptual model (Fig. 3.5), the campaign was implemented to intervene into the culture of college drinking, in order to change student drinking experiences and perceptions. The strategy of the

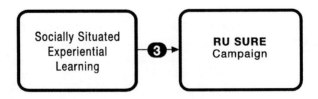

**Figure 3.4.   Step 3 of the Conceptual Model.**

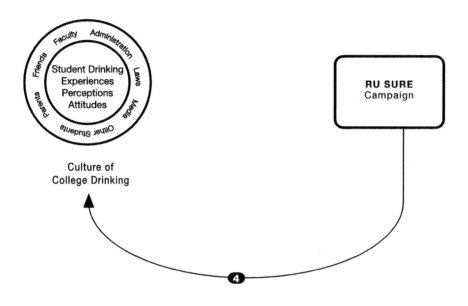

**Figure   3.5. Step 4 of the Conceptual Model.**

campaign was to create messages and messengers who will be able to participate in students' social interactions. This is perhaps one of the most graph-
ically important elements of the model. It suggests that that the campaign is
only one small component in the complex culture of college drinking, with
its multiple influences on student thinking and drinking.

## Step 5: Evaluation of the Campaign's Impact and Socially Situated Experiential Learning

As suggested by Step 5, the conceptual model is a process model that is non-
linear, noncausal, and continuously dynamic and changing, as people and
their behaviors, perceptions, and attitudes change. Step 5 of the model is presented in Fig. 3.6.

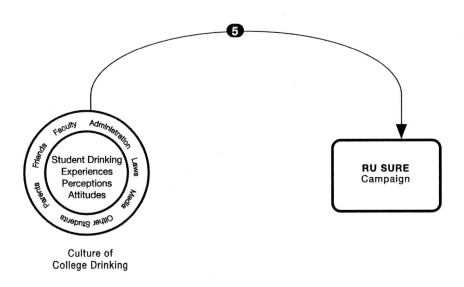

**Figure 3.6.    Step 5 of the Conceptual Model.**

As suggested in Step 5, knowledge of the culture of college drinking, as it expands with the evaluation of the impact of the campaign, was used to continuously re-examine and refine the RU SURE Campaign and its role in changing drinking-related behaviors, attitudes, and perceptions on the campus.

Continuous evaluation, both process and outcome, was used to track the progress of the campaign and its success. Evaluation tools included focus-group interviews, archival data analysis, questionnaires, and intercept interviews (developed specifically to meet one of the challenges of implementing the campaign). These methods are discussed in detail in Chapter 8. Additional chapters in Part III include a discussion of one of the unanticipated outcomes of the campaign—changes in the alcohol-related behaviors and attitudes of the campaign messengers (Chapter 9) and the development of the RU SURE Game of Choices and Consequences, a 1-hour brief intervention concerning students' alcohol-related decision making (Chapter 10).

Because part of the rationale for this book is to communicate our results to other institutions of higher education, Chapter 11 presents a description of how this campaign can be extended to other campuses.

## CONCLUSION

Lederman and Stewart's (1998) conceptual model of socially situated experiential learning provides an in-depth understanding of the socially situated nature of interpersonal and mediated communication, while taking into account both experiential learning and social norms theory. How and what students think about something, as well as what they learn from their experiences, all prepare them to accept, reject, or react to social norms messages. One of the reasons that heavy drinkers, for example, are more resistant to social norms messages is their own experience with friends who drink much like themselves and, thereby, reinforce their misconceptions. For this reason, the emphasis in the RU SURE Campaign is on changing the nature of this social interaction.

The conceptual model presented in this chapter is the basis of the work described in the chapters in Part II. In Chapter 4, we describe how the language of the campaign was designed to reflect the actual language usage and preferences of students. Chapter 5 details the design of the RU SURE Campaign, whereas Chapter 6 contains a description of the campaign implementation. Finally, Chapter 7 more specifically focuses on the innovative interpersonal strategies used for message dissemination.

## ACKNOWLEDGMENT

We would like to thank Itzhak Yanovitzky for his contributions to this chapter, most especially the reframing of the SSEL Model.

# Part II

# Design and Implementation of the RU SURE Campaign

## Brief Overview

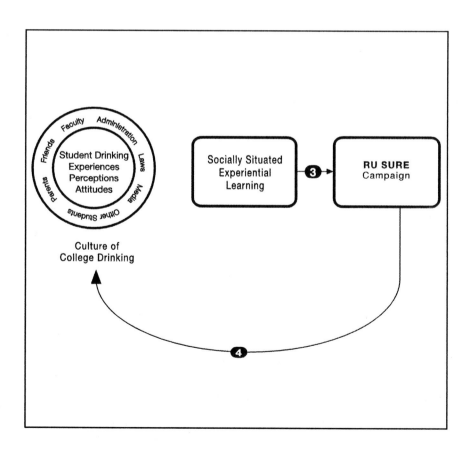

In Part II of this book, the design and implementation of the RU SURE Campaign are presented in detail. As described in Chapter 3, The Conceptual Model, Steps 3 and 4 of the model are design and implementation. In this part of the book, Steps 3 and 4 of the model are used to provide the context in which the chapters describe the design and/or implementation of the campaign.

Chapter 4, Campaign Language: Understanding How to Get Students to Personalize Campaign Messages, focuses primarily on Step 3 and the importance of the language used in the campaign to describe dangerous drinking. It presents a detailed discussion of language choice and the decision to replace the term *binge drinking* with a term more resonant with Rutgers' students, *dangerous drinking*. The chapter reviews the research with students that led to that decision.

Chapters 5, The Design of the RU SURE Campaign, discusses the design of the campaign components and the use of the construct of socially situated experiential learning to discuss how the campaign was conceptualized and designed. Although the chapter focuses on the media component of the campaign, the *Top Ten Misperceptions at Rutgers*, it also reviews in brief the other five components of the campaign: interpersonally based activities, a curriculum infusion plan, a public relations campaign, a Web site, and a campus coalition.

Chapters 6 and 7 concern themselves with the implementation of the campaign. Chapter 6, Implementation of the Campaign: A Curriculum Infusion Design, provides a detailed analysis of how the campaign was conceptualized and the role of students in its design. The chapter explains a semester-long simulation, Advanced Health Communication (AHC) Simulation, used in an advanced course in health communication, to engage communication majors studying health campaigns in the design, implementation, and evaluation of the campaign. The chapter includes specific descriptions of the course in which the simulation was run, its goals, objectives, and outcomes.

Chapter 7, Interpersonal Strategies for Campaign Message Dissemination, explains in detail the activities designed for students in the AHC simulation to use to engage members of the target audience for the campaign (first-year students) in conversations about the campaign messages. The chapter explains why these activities were used, how they embody the spirit of the socially situated experiential learning approach, and what exactly the activities are and how they were used.

# 4

## CAMPAIGN LANGUAGE

### UNDERSTANDING HOW TO GET STUDENTS TO PERSONALIZE CAMPAIGN MESSAGES[1]

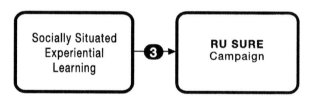

Figure 4.1. Step 3 of the Conceptual Model.

In order to design the RU SURE Campaign, it was necessary to understand the ways in which students thought about alcohol and talked about it in their social interactions with one another. To do this, we interviewed students to find out how they talked about alcohol use, including the terms they used to describe their alcohol-related experiences. An important part of Step 3 of the model, therefore, was to apply what we found in these inter-

[1]An earlier version of this chapter appeared in the *Journal of Health Communication* (Lederman, Stewart, Goodhart, & Laitman, 2003).

views to the language we used in the campaign design and implementation. Thus, the design of the RU SURE Campaign grew directly out of the formulation of the construct of socially situated experiential learning (Lederman & Stewart, 1998), as illustrated in Fig. 4.1. This chapter describes how students themselves think about drinking and how our insights into their thinking have been used to select the campaign language.

## BACKGROUND

One of the most important questions of language choice for the campaign was what to call the use of alcohol that we wanted to discourage. If the campaign was to be designed to communicate something to students about their drinking, we had to begin by making decisions about what kind of drinking we wanted to address in the campaign. We were sure from the start that we were not intending to create an anti-drinking campaign. What we wanted to do was to create a campaign that discouraged students from drinking in ways that were excessive and, therefore, potentially harmful to themselves and others—physically, mentally, and emotionally. We wanted the campaign we created to discourage problematic drinking on the campus.

Since the late 1990s, the term *binge drinking* had been used to describe college drinking that is problematic (Meilman, Cashin, McKillip, & Presley, 1998; Presley, Meilman, & Cashin, 1997; Thombs, Mahoney, & Olds, 1998; Wechsler, 1996; Wechsler, Fulop, Padilla, Lee, & Patrick, 1997). The drinking-related phenomenon that the term is used to describe is five or more drinks in a setting for a male and four or more for a female. Previously, the same drinking behavior was referred to in the scholarly literature as "at-risk drinking" (K. Carey, 1995a; Pasavac, 1993; Perkins, 1992).

Burns and Goodstadt (1989), however, found students reporting that they did not believe excessive drinking was a problem for them. "Problem drinking?" asked one student in an interview by Burns and Goodstadt (1989), "I drink. I get drunk. I fall down. No problem." In addition, their research indicated that students reacted to the term *high-risk drinking* as if it were positive. For these students, it seemed a badge of courage to refer to them as engaging in risky behavior.

Similarly, when surveying Rutgers' students more recently, Lederman et al. (1998) found that 92% of students did not think of themselves as binge drinkers, even though 35% of these students drank at levels that are what researchers operationalize as binge drinking. To them the term *binge* referred to far more drinking than that in which they themselves engaged, even when they themselves were drinking excessive amounts that researchers would operationalize as binge drinking. This reaction is consistent with the position taken by some scholars. Milgram and Anderson (2000), for example, argue that the term *binge* more accurately refers to a situation in which an individual consumes alcohol to the point of intoxication over a long period of time (e.g., 2 or 3 days). Furthermore, they point out that when *binge* is used to refer to a set number of drinks, it fails to take into account what the person is drinking, how large the drinks are, and how much the person weighs.

Because individual behaviors are based on constructs that are developed in a social context, it is important that health communication campaigns use language that accurately reflects the interpretive schemes that college students have developed (Delia, 1987; Littlejohn, 1996). If students do not relate to the phrase *high risk* as something to be avoided or the word *binge* as a descriptor of their behaviors, if these words have very different meanings and connotations for them than five or more drinks at a time, then to talk to them about high-risk drinking or binge drinking is not a very effective way to raise their awareness of their own behavior and to get them to personalize messages about their drinking. By using language that is outside the interpretive schemes of college students, researchers may be unwittingly contributing to a failure among students to identify their drinking as problematic, and even to report that behavior accurately on surveys.

## HOW COLLEGE STUDENTS THINK ABOUT DRINKING

Students know a great deal about drinking on campus, whether they drink or not. Drinking and/or observations of others' drinking-related behaviors are part of what students experience as college life. This is part of what has been referred to in the discussion of the SSEL Model in Chapter 3 as the culture of college drinking (Lederman, 1993). This is clear in several ways. Data collected from students at Rutgers (see Chapter 2 for a detailed discussion) and in surveys across the country support this contention (Workman, 1999). Through the analysis of the data gathered through survey research, students' knowledge of drinking on campus as well as their own self-reported drinking-related behaviors, attitudes, and perceptions is evident (Butler, 1993; Carey, 1995b; Harper et al., 1999; Klein, 1992; Marshall et al., 1998; Nezlek, Pilkington, & Bilbro, 1994; Rabow & Duncan-Schill, 1995; Thombs, Wolcott, & Farkash, 1997; Wechsler, 1996; Wechsler, Lee, Kuo, & Lee, 2000).

Students believe drinking plays a significant role in how they develop relationships and strengthen social bonds (Burns et al., 1991; Hanson, 1984; Lederman & Stewart, 1998; Rabow & Duncan-Schill, 1995). Even though excessive drinking can lead to a variety of health concerns such as motor vehicle accidents, accidental deaths, injuries (Engs, 1977; Milgram, 1993), or high-risk sexual activities (Butcher, Manning, & O'Neal, 1991; Cohen & Lederman, 1998), several studies have demonstrated that college students seem to associate drinking with sociability and positive outcomes. Nezlek et al. (1994) found that students who reported some level of binge drinking perceived they had more intimate interactions than those who reported that they did not engage in binge drinking. The social interactions that take place during drinking encounters appear to contribute to the ways students learn social norms and acceptable social behaviors while in college. Therefore, the behavior of peers plays a significant role in the choices students make when it comes to drinking.

One thing that has been learned from these studies is that college students who drink excessively do not usually characterize their drinking as problematic. This is consistent with the findings of Burns and Goodstadt (1989) at Rutgers. Many of the students in these studies do not think that five or more drinks is too much to drink, and most do not believe that they have a problem with drinking unless they drink every day (Butler, 1993; Haines, 1996; Lederman et al., 1998; Lederman et al., 2000; Perkins, 1994; Schall, Kemeny, & Maltzman, 1992; Senchak, Leonard, & Greene, 1998). Many of them think that, no matter how much they drink, there are others who drink more. Many also think that binges are things that happen to other people, not to them.

Furthermore, the studies that use the term *binge drinking* operationalize it as five or more drinks for a male in one sitting. The same operationalization of drinking exists for the term *high-risk drinking*. In operationalizing binge drinking as five or more drinks for a male and four or more drinks for a female, researchers create a way of looking at drinking that is simply foreign to most students. In reviewing all of the research at Rutgers, it was clear that this simply was not a term with which Rutgers students identified. Nor did they measure their drinking by how much they drank. Burns et al. (1991) interviewed students and found that they had a list of terms they used to describe how they felt and when they had had enough. "When I get the spins, I stop" was typical of the kinds of measures students reported. Nowhere was there any mention of quantity as a measure. Lederman, Stewart, Kennedy et al. (2001), in following up on the Burns et al. (1991) qualitative study, found in a random survey of Rutgers University students that 71% of respondents indicated that students measured their drinking by behavioral consequences, such as how they felt, rather than by the number of drinks they drank.

Although Wechsler and Kuo (2000) reported that the students they label as binge drinkers have a self-serving reason for their differences with the research definition of binge drinking, they do not take into account any of the real differences in the associative meanings or the connotations of the word *binge* to these drinkers.

If students do not think there is a problem with their drinking behavior, there is little hope that they will be motivated to change that behavior. It seems important, then, to look at the subject of college drinking through the eyes of college students (Burns et al., 1991; Klein, 1992; Lederman et al., 1998; Rapaport, Minelli, Angera, & Thayer, 1999). If what is wanted is to do more to change their behaviors, it is necessary to attempt to understand their drinking and their drinking-related behaviors through their own eyes. It is by understanding their attitudes and behaviors through their own ways of seeing that it is possible to become more effective in framing what is said to them about their drinking and in creating ways of communicating with them that will resonate with them.

## WHAT STUDENTS THINK IS PROBLEM DRINKING

Students have their own ways of thinking about problem drinking. In the most recent surveys at Rutgers University (Lederman et al., 1998), students reported that they thought that frequency rather than quantity was the measure of someone having a problem with alcohol. A drink a day is seen by these students as more problematic than eight drinks on one occasion once a semester. Many students do not think that drinking until they get "buzzed," "plastered," or "out of it" is a problem (Lederman, 1993). They do not use the word *binge*, nor do they relate to it when asked if they think of themselves as binge drinkers. Instead they use these other terms that are about the effects of drinking on them or the consequences of their drinking.

Students interviewed or surveyed at Rutgers classify problem drinking into four broad categories. Students label the first category of problem drinking as "Drinking Until You Are Out of Control." This is described as when there is an inability to stop or a loss of control—when there is too much emphasis placed on alcohol in your life, you are giving up everything to drink, if you can't say no, or if you can't go through a "dry" weekend (Burns et al., 1991).

The second category of problem drinking reported by students is based on "Frequency." This occurs when the number of times a person drinks during a given period of time is seen as "excessive," for example, when a person drinks every night. It is also described as when a person drinks all the time or is perceived as drinking continuously.

The third category of problem drinking focuses on people whose behavior is "Hurtful to Themselves or Others." This is described as the instance in which drinking causes behavior that is physically, emotionally, or academically hurtful to the individual or to others.

Finally, students describe another category of problem drinking called the "Motivation or Attitude Problem." A person's attitude toward alcohol can be a "tip-off" to a problem. In other words, if someone is drinking just to drink, that is a problem. If someone is drinking to relax or reduce stress, that is not a problem. Students say that even if they drink a whole case of beer to reduce stress, it is not a problem. The problem has to do with the motivation. This category is independent of quantity and reliant on motivation. Said one interviewee:

> It's why you drink. If it's cause you want to get messed up, that's a problem. Not like when you want to just let it all hang out after exams.

What is conspicuously absent from this list of drinking categories generated by students is any mention of quantity. This same finding occurred in later studies at Rutgers as well (Cohen & Lederman, 1998; Lederman, 1993; Lederman, Stewart, Kennedy et al., 2001). The quantity of alcohol consumed does not seem to affect what students define as a problem, hence students do not pay attention to limiting the amount they drink. Instead, they speak of limits in terms of impaired judgment and the resultant negative consequences or illness. They are also not fundamentally disturbed by the frequency of vomiting. This is understandable in light of students' perceptions of bonding around dealing with the consequences of drinking too much.

Thus, in order to get students to take into account the problems associated with the amount they drink, the amount has to be related to the effects and consequences of their drinking. Students can connect amount with consequences, and will, if the emphasis is placed on what happens when they drink too much. Students, even heavy drinkers, are aware of the consequences, or at least some of them, of excessive drinking. But the most important of these to them are expressed as relational consequences: getting taken advantage of (sexually or socially), getting into sexually intimate relationships too quickly, embarrassing oneself, or getting into situations that are violent.

Although, these may not be the consequences that appear on the police rosters or campus police data sheets, they are the things that students themselves report as consequential to them in individual and focus-group interviews (Burns et al., 1991; Cohen & Lederman, 1998; Harper et al., 1999). Although students report personal and physical consequences (e.g., vomiting, passing out, hangovers/headaches), these are not significant to them unless they have consequences for their relationships with others. Unfortunately, students reported that they thought that they simply had to learn about drinking from their own experiences (Burns et al., 1991; Cohen

& Lederman, 1998; Lederman et al., 1998). When asked who had taught them to drink in these ways, students repeatedly explained that they simply had to learn through/by experience what they personally could and could not do. They had to learn their own limits/capacity for themselves (Cohen & Lederman, 1998). For instance, in the original interviews conducted by the Burns team in 1991, one student reported:

> *The first time I got drunk I puked and I got really sick and ugly.*
> *I realized that drinking a lot is not a whole lot of fun.*

Drinking and learning to handle it was seen as a right of passage into adulthood. It was about testing limits and learning from those experiments. As a student working on a research report exclaimed when talking about first-year students:

> *I used to be just like those girls before I grew up. It embarrasses*
> *me to realize that 2 years ago I was one of them.*

In interviewing students, Cohen and Lederman (1998) found that students did not want to interfere in what they perceived to be other students' rights to learn from their own experiences. In more recent interviews with undergraduates, those who drink heavily find themselves skeptical that they are in the minority because they surround themselves with others who drink like them.

To drive home the danger of unwanted consequences, the literature indicates that it can be pointed out to students that it is not normative behavior (Berkowitz & Perkins, 1986a). As discussed in Chapter 2, students have misperceived notions of how much their peers drink. By pointing out to them that the majority drink moderately, the implied message is that by drinking too much the "danger" is in being different—in embarrassing oneself or in other ways getting into those situations that had the unwanted consequences of which they are aware. (See Chapter 5 for a detailed discussion of the construction of messages following these guidelines.)

## IMPLICATIONS OF WHAT WE LEARNED FROM STUDENTS

The problem of drinking on campus is complex—so, too, must be the answers and approaches. Some of the complexity is evidenced in the ways in which students think about their drinking and believe that they have to learn from experience. But the language being used to convey to students what is problematic about excessive college drinking is in itself a problem if it fails to get them to understand that their own behavior is what is being referred to. As we learned more about the primary audience, college students, and the ways in which they think, we were able to find a solid basis for making decisions about the appropriate word to choose to indicate problematic drinking. We concluded that although the most often used term to describe this situation currently is *binge drinking* (Weschler, 1996), there are two very different but important drawbacks to the word *binge* as the word of choice. These drawbacks are not theoretical. They arose from our research on students at Rutgers and the implications of their reactions to the term. First, it is inflammatory to them; it creates an image far worse than what is happening. Second, and related to the first, it is easy for them to deny that they binge by interpreting bingeing as what happens to others.

For our work at Rutgers, then, we were sure that we would not call the drinking that we were trying to discourage binge drinking. We also concluded that we could not use the term *high risk* for similar reasons and found that other terms, such as *excessive drinking* or *problematic drinking,* seemed also to fail to convey to students a kind of drinking about which they themselves would be concerned.

In interviewing students about their own ways of thinking and the words to express what they think captures the emphasis on consequences a term emerged from them. *Dangerous drinking* was suggested by our students as a more effective alternative to describe their behavior in a way that is more appropriate and difficult to deny. It was also a term that to them implied consequences.

## ADVANTAGES OF THE TERM *DANGEROUS DRINKING*

The term *dangerous drinking* has several advantages in the eyes of Rutgers students. First, it is a term that came from the students themselves. When a group of student leaders at Rutgers University was asked by a university-wide blue ribbon committee to identify what term, if any, they thought they could identify with more than *binge drinking*, they suggested *dangerous drinking*. They rejected *binge drinking* because they thought that students did not identify with it. They rejected *high-risk drinking* because they thought that some students thought that high-risk behavior was "cool." They rejected *irresponsible drinking* because they did not like the implied value judgment, pointing out to the committee that those members of the community with alcoholism were the drinkers who would be labeled irresponsible and that that seemed to them to be blaming the victim of a disease.

*Dangerous drinking* was a term they liked because they saw that it had differential application the way that *irresponsible drinking* does but without the value judgment. Instead they saw the term *dangerous drinking* as putting the focus where it should be—on outcomes. In studies designed to follow up on these recommendations it was found that a majority of students concurred.

The term *dangerous drinking* places the focus on the type of drinking that needs to be addressed, that which is dangerous, in an arena that perhaps most students and adults can agree. If a male student who weighs 190 pounds has five to six drinks during a party that starts at 11 p.m. and ends at 4 a.m., consumes food, and spaces his drinks out over this period, this is not necessarily problem drinking. If the same student has too much to drink in a short amount of time and needs to be taken to the hospital with alcohol poisoning, this should be defined as dangerous drinking. Yet, the definition of *binge drinking* does not include time or consequence as a factor—an issue that is often raised by students. *Dangerous drinking*, therefore, is a term that allows students to reflect on the consequences of their drinking and to be informed about the role of the quantity of their alcohol consumption in the effects of the alcohol on them, and the resultant consequences.

## CONCLUSION

The use of the term *dangerous drinking* grows out of what has been learned from employing our approach to research at Rutgers. It is our term of choice based on what has been learned about students from students. The term *dangerous drinking* grows out of a socially situated approach to college drinking (Lederman & Stewart, 1998). Fundamentally, the approach argues that students learn what they know about drinking in their social interactions with one another. It is an approach that focuses on understanding students' thinking in order to try to change their drinking. (See Chapter 3 for a more extensive discussion of this idea.)

Given that the people who need to be reached the most are those students who are the least likely to want to learn that their drinking is problematic, the words chosen to describe their drinking need to be carefully thought out. The word *binge* lets them off the hook; it is easy for them to think of binges as something that other people do, to associate them with alcoholics, and to think of alcoholism as something to avoid rather than as a disease. This means, of course, that when they go out to party and get "smashed" they may be ignorant of the real dangers associated with what they are doing—dangers that go beyond what they know about drinking and problems associated with drinking. The term *dangerous drinking* is a more effective way to get them to be more able to reflect on their own drinking-related choices than other terms used currently or previously, including *binge drinking*.

Based on the findings of the interviews with students, the RU SURE Campaign and all other prevention materials at Rutgers replaced the term *binge drinking* with *dangerous drinking*. Although we do not argue that the term is the ultimate way to describe unwanted drinking behaviors, its advantages outweigh those of the alternatives.

# 5

## THE DESIGN OF THE RU SURE CAMPAIGN

### THE *TOP TEN MISPERCEPTIONS AT RUTGERS* MEDIA CAMPAIGN

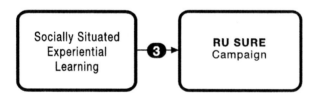

Figure 5.1.  Step 3 of the Conceptual Model.

The RU SURE Campaign was designed to be a multifaceted, dangerous-drinking prevention campaign. It was designed to build on, rather than compete with, other alcohol prevention work on campus (see Chapter 12 for a detailed discussion of the environmental approach to alcohol issues at Rutgers). As illustrated in Fig. 5.1, the design and implementation of the RU SURE Campaign grew directly out of the formulation of the construct of socially situated experiential learning (Lederman & Stewart, 1998). The purpose of the campaign was to reduce dangerous drinking on the Rutgers campus by raising student awareness that most students stopped before drink-

ing too much alcohol, and that they, therefore, did not have to drink dangerously either to fit in with the campus culture.

The RU SURE Campaign grew out of the preliminary research and
reconceptualization of the culture of college drinking described in Chapters
2 and 3 and the understanding of language use described in Chapter 4. This
chapter provides an overview of the actual campaign, its major components,
and how they were designed to be implemented.

## THE DESIGN OF THE RU SURE CAMPAIGN

There are six components to the RU SURE Campaign. Discussion of those
components begins with the articulation of the campaign goal.

### The Goal of the Campaign

We knew from our research that most students were concerned about the
unwanted consequences of drinking but also that they wanted to fit into the
culture that they perceived to require drinking dangerously. Our purpose
was to correct their mistaken image of college as a place where everyone
drinks excessively. By emphasizing that the actual drinking behavior of
their peers was moderate, the campaign was designed to get students to realize that drinking was a choice and that excessive drinking was not what
most of their peers were doing, and that they simply did not have to risk the
unwanted consequences of heavy drinking to fit in with their peers. And so
the goal of the RU SURE Campaign was to reduce dangerous drinking on
campus by getting students to know the actual norms of drinking on the
campus by encouraging lively discussion of the culture of college drinking.
We saw the discussion as the most critical part of the campaign; the dissemination of the information about actual norms was the necessary trigger for
those discussions.

To this end, the campaign used structured, interpersonally based strategies to create discussions about mediated messages created for the media
component of the campaign (the *Top Ten Misperceptions at Rutgers*) to
reduce dangerous drinking on campus. The mediated messages were
designed to be the agenda-setting aspect of the campaign, and the interpersonal interventions as the "conversations" that would infuse the social interactions and, thereby, compete with messages that misled students into
believing that drinking dangerously was the norm.

The notion of the media campaign as agenda setting and interpersonal
strategies as "conversations" to influence social interaction is a critical com-

ponent of the RU SURE Campaign approach as discussed in Chapter 3. Because the approach taken relies on the construct of socially situated experiential learning discussed at length in Chapter 3 it cannot be emphasized enough how central to the campaign were the interpersonal strategies. The media messages were the necessary but not sufficient condition to change the culture of college drinking; the interpersonal interactions were the interventions into the social scene on which change was envisioned.

In order to reach our target population with our messages, the RU SURE Campaign was designed as a multifaceted campaign with six related components: media campaign, interpersonally based strategies, curriculum infusion, a Web site, a public relations campaign, and coalition building. Figure 5.2 presents a graphic representation of the overall campaign

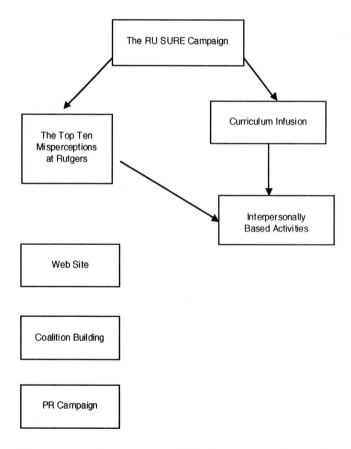

**Figure 5.2.   Components of the RU SURE Campaign.**

elements. This chapter emphasizes the media campaign, the *Top Ten Misperceptions at Rutgers*, and its development as the agenda-setting element of the campaign. The chapter also provides brief descriptions of the other campaign components as an overview of the RU SURE Campaign. Detailed discussions of the curriculum infusion (Chapter 6) and interpersonally based strategies (Chapter 7) are provided in chapters that follow.

## Review of Baseline Data

Before the RU SURE Campaign was designed or implemented, all of the baseline data collected in the previous decade were reviewed and analyzed to discover drinking-related attitudes, behaviors, and perceptions on the campus. So, too, was the work of other researchers such Berkowitz and Perkins (1986a), Haines and Spear (1996), Jeffrey and Negro (1996), and Weschler and Kuo (2000). In order to create a successful campaign that would get students' attention, it was necessary to know enough about those students and the ways in which they thought to create language and messages that would have meaning for them. In fact, as discussed in Chapter 4, starting with the words that were used to describe drinking (*dangerous drinking* rather than *binge drinking*), our focus was on students and their ways of thinking about drinking. It was through the analysis of data, especially the quantitative data from the campus surveys and the qualitative data from both individual and focus group interviews (described in Chapter 2 and Chapter 4), that it was possible to determine what was needed to reduce the dangerous drinking on campus that still existed despite other earlier attempts at prevention.

Because Rutgers is a large, public institution with more than 30,000 students on the New Brunswick campus where the campaign was to take place, we had to make some decisions about the actual target audience for the campaign. To try to reach all of the students with one campaign, and to make it effective given its emphasis on the interpersonal and mediated messages, it was important to segment the population and to identify a target population that was a manageable size.

## Identification of Target Population

There were several subpopulations that our research indicated were especially at risk for dangerous drinking. First-year students were a subpopulation of undergraduates who appeared to be most vulnerable in the baseline data collected. In data from the PRSP survey (Lederman et al., 1998), it was found that 31% of first-year students reported an increase in their alcohol consumption in the last year. Although 25% of the first-year students did not drink alcohol, the percentage of first-year students who drank dangerously was higher than the percentage of all Rutgers' students who engaged in dangerous drinking (34% of men, 17% of women). Nevertheless, only 7% of first-year students self-identified themselves as *binge drinkers*.

In interviews conducted with students in their last 2 years of college, it was reported that their drinking was at its highest in the first year. As one female interviewee put it:

*Guys at frat houses plied us with alcohol.*

Students reported when they got to their junior and senior years in college that they looked at the "cheesy freshman girls" and winced at their behavior. As one woman commented:

*Because I remember that I used to be like that before I matured.*

In terms of perceptions, both first-year men and women overestimated the degree to which alcohol consumption was a central part of the social life of other students. Although 75% of first-year women believed alcohol was central to the social life of students, this number dropped to 68% for junior women.

Thus, from these findings we concluded that first-year students were more likely to drink dangerously than other students (30% of first-year students vs. 25% of students overall) and that, although both men and women were reluctant to identify themselves as *binge drinkers*, first-year men are particularly misguided (36% of them drink dangerously, whereas only 5% of theme self-identify as *binge drinkers*).

All of the data at Rutgers were consistent with data collected nationally (Wechsler & Kuo, 2000), which indicates that first-year students are one of the most vulnerable populations on the college campus. Additionally, the Rutgers' data made it apparent that first-year students were particularly in need of information about the actual drinking on campus as well as some experiences to help them change their misperceptions about college drinking. In many cases this was true because students had little unsupervised experience with alcohol use before they came to college and often reported having to learn about drinking with their peers.

Based on these findings, first-year students were identified as an important population to reach. As a result, first-year students were selected as the target population for the campaign. Although we hoped that others, too, would get our message, the population on which we focused and the impact that we measured was on first-year students.

## Development of the Campaign Theme

As a result of analysis of the baseline data, it was learned that the majority of students, including the target population, did not drink excessively but that the perception of heavy drinking was pervasive. It was this finding that led to the articulation of the theme for the campaign that "Most students at Rutgers don't drink dangerously, and you don't have to either." Although this was the theme, it was not necessarily the phrasing that would be used in messages in the campaign. Instead, the theme guided all decisions about messages and message construction. No message, verbal or nonverbal (e.g., the visuals that accompanied words in ads), was used unless it advanced the campaign theme. For example, one of the members of the team working on campaign design found a very dramatic picture of a student bent over a toilet, throwing up, while another student held her hair back out of her face. It was pilot-tested and students responded to it as "social bonding," an instance of what happens on campus and how "you get to know who your friends are." Given that the theme of the campaign was that it was not necessary to drink dangerously, the photo had a message that reinforced drinking dangerously as an everyday occurrence and simply part of the campus culture. Thus, the photograph was rejected.

## Design of the Media Component:
### *The Top Ten Misperceptions at Rutgers*

Based on data collected from students about their preferences, it was decided to take a somewhat humorous approach to alerting students to alcohol-related misperceptions that might be influencing their drinking and drinking-related behaviors. It was found that students on our campus responded well to the tongue-in-cheek humor found in top 10 type lists. Therefore, the approach of the media campaign was to select familiar items to create a list that could be called the *Top Ten Misperceptions at Rutgers*. Thus, lists of commonly held misperceptions about college life were created in which alcohol-related misperceptions were included. This is discussed in greater detail later in the chapter.

## Phrasing and Pilot-Testing Key Campaign Messages

The next step in the process of designing the media component of the campaign was phrasing and pilot-testing the campaign messages. Because every step in the process was field-tested and piloted, it took almost a full year to develop the campaign and be ready to actually implement it. Although it was tempting at times to rush the process, the wisdom of taking that time has been proven in the years since the inception of the campaign by its ability to stand the test of time and to continue to be well received 5 years after its initial implementation. In part this is the case because the target audience is first-year students and each year the campus has a new first-year class. Continuous evaluative research (see Chapter 8) is conducted to make sure that the campaign continues to resonate with each new entering class. This was particularly true of the humor (discussed in more detail later in this chapter) embedded into the *Top Ten Misperceptions at Rutgers* list. Each year as the campaign has been implemented we have continuously tapped into our target population to make sure that they still find humor in the messages.

In developing the messages, persuasion theory and the axiom regarding repetition were relied on. This reflects itself in the decision to create two key messages that captured the actual norms of drinking on the campus and to repeat them in all media used in the campaign. The messages were: "Two out of three Rutgers students stop at three or fewer" and "Almost one in five don't drink at all." These messages grew directly out of the baseline data (discussed in Chapter 2). In fact, based on these data it would have been possible to say either three out of four students stopped at four or fewer or that two out of three stopped at three or fewer. Research with members of the target audience indicated that four (drinks) sounded to them like "a lot more drinks" than three (drinks) did. It also would have been possible to say 19% to 21% of students don't drink at all, but "Almost one in five" was selected for consistency in phrasing between the messages.

There was only one additional message added to the two key messages. It was: "We got the stats from you." Research indicated that students were impressed by the thought that the data had actually been collected from them on their own campus. The decision was made that wherever possible all materials disseminated for the campaign would include these two key messages and the phrase about the stats.

## Creation of a Formula for the
## *Top Ten Misperceptions at Rutgers*

Although we decided early in the design of the campaign to use humor, the creation the *Top Ten Misperceptions at Rutgers* itself took some time and effort. It was not difficult to come up with a list of misperceptions about college life that students would find funny, but it was a challenge to come up with a list that at the same time did not offend other members of the Rutgers' community. When, for example, research with students indicated that they wanted to include in the list that the buses on campus never ran on time (stated as a misperception: "You never have to wait for a bus at

Rutgers") the misperception was changed to "There's always an empty seat on the bus." The latter version gave the students who rode the overcrowded buses a laugh while at the same time it gave the administrators who ran the bus system evidence that they needed more funding for buses. Another example was the misperception that "No one steals silverware from the dining halls." Students reported that they often take plates and silverware to use in their rooms, but a consultation with staff members from Dining Services made it clear that they lose a considerable amount of money each year from this behavior and do not feel that theft is a humorous situation at all. Thus, this phrase was not used.

Because the list was going to be widely disseminated on the campus we wanted to be sure that it did not offend constituencies beyond our target audience. We saw all these other groups as secondary targets of our message and wanted them, too, to know that drinking dangerously was not the norm at Rutgers.

It was important to find commonly shared misperceptions about life on campus so that students could relate to them. After much experimentation for the formulation of the humorous messages and pilot testing versions of them with target-audience members and other audiences that were potentially affected by the messages, a formula was created. The formula consisted of (a) creating three alcohol misperceptions messages, (b) creating seven humorous statements to get students engaged in message processing, (c) embedding the three messages in a list of the *Top Ten Misperceptions at Rutgers* with the seven humorous messages, and (d) following the *Top Ten Misperceptions at Rutgers* with a norming message to give students accurate data.

Figure 5.3 presents the *Top Ten Misperceptions at Rutgers*, followed by the norming message. These messages combine statements that are generic to most campuses (e.g., "Used books are cheap") with some that are particularly unique to Rutgers (Fat Cat—a bacon cheeseburger with french fries in a bun, particularly popular as a late night snack). (See Chapter 11 for a more extensive discussion of the development of these messages.) Embedded within this list of statements are three misperceptions about drinking, each marked with an asterisk and printed in red (a school color) on our media materials. Below the list is an asterisk that links the misperceptions about drinking with the normative message.

## Creation of a Campaign Logo

Along with the key campaign messages and the *Top Ten Misperceptions at Rutgers*, a logo was needed to visually embody the message. After much experimentation, with many possibilities that students perceived as encouraging excessive drinking (such as an upside down shot glass) were rejected, a logo was created to which students responded positively. The RU SURE

1. Rutgers students don't write papers at the last minute.
2. It's easy to find a parking space on campus.
3. Everyone who parties gets wasted.*
4. FAT CAT = Fat Free and FDA approved.
5. There's always an empty seat on the bus.
6. Everybody at Rutgers drinks.*
7. Everybody goes to first period [8 o'clock] classes.
8. Most student at Rutgers drink to get drunk.*
9. You don't need shower shoes for the dorms.
10. Used books are cheap.

*"Two out of three Rutgers students stop at three or fewer drinks.
Almost one in five don't drink at all."

We got the stats from you!

**Figure 5.3.   The Top Ten Misperceptions at Rutgers.**

logo design (see Fig. 5.4) consists of four beer mugs with the last one containing the message "RU SURE?" with an additional line under the message that reads "Yes, 3 or fewer. We got the stats from you!" The visual message, as well as the words, was selected to convey the key campaign messages, followed by reference to the stats to reinforce the fact that these data were obtained from students themselves and that this message reiterates the reality of college drinking.

What seemed simple at first, an appealing visual, turned out to be complex to design. Students responded well to beer mugs as a visual but we did not want the message to seem as if we were encouraging beer as a drink of choice. Consequently, careful consideration was given to using beer mugs in the logo and to showing only one full mug and that mug leading to the question, RU SURE? It was with extensive pilot-testing of this image that we found that students felt the design was appealing but at the same time understood the anti-dangerous drinking message.

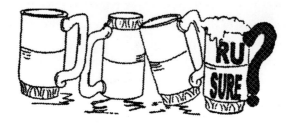

*Yes, three or fewer. We got the stats from you.*

**Figure 5.4.   RU SURE Logo.**

## Selection of Campaign Media

The goal of the media campaign was to deliver the campaign theme through the continuous dissemination of key campaign messages. A needs assessment of the target audience indicated that they were most likely to pay attention to ads in the campus newspaper (especially on certain days of the week), posters, flyers, and other artifacts. The two most popular artifacts that were created with the message were pens (students indicated that "pens are gold to college kids") and t-shirts. The t-shirts had the logo and key message on the front and the list of the *Top Ten Misperceptions at Rutgers* on the back. These messages were printed on t-shirts that were distributed in various campus locations including in front of the library, in dormitories, and at various student events. Over time it has been found that students respond favorably to receiving the t-shirts, think the logo is "cool," and have been observed wearing the t-shirts around campus. To reinforce this behavior, students who were seen wearing the t-shirt by a member of the project team were given a card with the RU SURE logo that enabled them to purchase $5 worth of merchandise at the college bookstore or food courts on campus.

## Dissemination of the Campaign Messages

The media selected were the channels through which there was distribution of the messages: posters, newspaper ads, flyers, pens, computer disks, magnets, stickers, t-shirts with key messages. In addition, the artifacts created for the media campaign were used in the other aspects of the RU SURE Campaign: interpersonally based strategies, experiential learning activities, coalition-building activities, a Web site, a public relations campaign, and curriculum infusion projects (as illustrated in Fig. 5.2).

## INTERPERSONAL COMPONENTS OF THE RU SURE CAMPAIGN

Although the *Top Ten Misperceptions at Rutgers* media campaign was the agenda-setting piece of the RU SURE Campaign, it was designed to be used in conjunction with structured interpersonal interactions. The media campaign was seen as the attention-gaining device, an attempt to set the agenda for the conversations that could be facilitated in a variety of interpersonally based strategies. Each of the other five components of the RU SURE Campaign are described briefly here.

## Interpersonally Based Strategies for Experiential Learning

Mediated messages have been shown to be highly effective in this type of misperception campaign, but given the focus on college drinking as socially situated experiential learning, a campaign of this type may not be truly effective in changing behavior without an interpersonal component to the message delivery. Thus, in order to facilitate the interpersonal process it was vital to the success of this effort to include an experiential component (see Chapter 7 for a description of the interpersonally based strategies used in the campaign) to get students to reflect on their drinking-related decisions. An example of this campaign component is RU SURE Bingo, in which students fill up a bingo-type card by finding other students who fit particular characteristics (e.g., were born in a large city, don't drink, have seen the misperceptions messages on campus, are majoring in a social science). Winners received prizes such as candy bars (with stickers containing the misperceptions on them) and t-shirts. This activity allowed students to have fun, interact interpersonally with other students, and reinforce the misperceptions messages. In this way, students modeled and learned the social skills that they might otherwise feel they needed alcohol to achieve. Using students trained in the campaign messages as facilitators, members of our target population were invited and came together in a group to meet each other, socialize, share food, and interact in an alcohol-free environment that reinforced that dangerous drinking was not a prerequisite for a fulfilling social life. Using activities like RU SURE Bingo, during a typical semester, students working with us on the campaign were able to interact with and provide information about the misperceptions campaign to approximately 600 students. (See Chapter 6 for a description of the use of students as carriers of the campaign message, and Chapter 7 for a more extensive discussion of these activities.)

## Curriculum Infusion

The purpose of most curriculum infusion plans is to find appropriate matches between theoretical course content and compelling contemporary social and health issues. Rather than taking what students learn in the classroom and using it in so-called "real-world" applications, curriculum infusion incorporates the study of issues from the real world into the classroom. Beyond adding richness and context to conceptual classroom learning, a curriculum infusion approach fosters opportunities for students to examine and reflect on their own attitudes and behaviors vis-à-vis compelling and relevant social and health issues. It is designed to use the classroom as a context in which to guide students through an examination of their own attitudes and behaviors in relation to that issue.

The curriculum infusion component of the campaign, described in detail in Chapter 6, incorporated alcohol-related issues into the college curriculum using varied strategies. Instead of limiting the dissemination of key campaign messages to outside the classroom, courses in health education, communication, and psychology were identified as suitable subjects in which to incorporate messages about the campaign. For example, in the Rutgers Department of Communication, two advanced courses, Advanced Health Communication and Communication and Learning, use the campaign as a major course component. These courses, offered each semester, focus on the design, implementation, and evaluation of a dangerous drinking prevention campaign as related to the courses' other primary objectives. The design of both courses is based on the assumption that dangerous drinking is not only a social and health issue, but is also a serious learning issue. Primary activities include: relationship building with residence life staff; disseminating campaign messages in first-year residence halls; designing interactive, interpersonal games and activities to be used in each of the residence halls; promoting the games and activities; monitoring campaign activities; and gathering data for assessment. The Rutgers Department of Health Education also offers course that utilizes the SSEL Model (Lederman & Stewart, 1998) to train social marketing peer educators. Peer educators incorporate the campaign messages into their alcohol presentations and are integrally involved in disseminating campaign messages. Additional curriculum infusion strategies have included incorporating campaign poster design into a senior level graphic design course and guest lectures addressing alcohol-related issues in undergraduate and graduate courses.

## Coalition Building

In order to embed the campaign within the Rutgers University environment, we worked extensively with the health educators and counselors at the University Health Services. It was through them that networking was possible with the New Brunswick Responsible Hospitality Resource Panel, which is comprised of university staff and faculty, local restaurant and bar owners, representatives from the New Brunswick and Rutgers police departments, the New Jersey Division of Alcohol Beverage Control, the National Committee on Alcohol and Drug Dependence, the town clerk, and high school and college students. As a result of this coalition, an initiative, "We Check for 21," was launched. Owners of local bars and restaurants signed pledges to support the "We Check for 21" program. By signing the pledge, restaurants and bar owners made a commitment to ensure that alcohol is not served to individuals who are under 21 years of age.

## Web Site

Because students increasingly use electronic means of information gathering, a Web site was used to disseminate the campaign message to students and to gather additional data from them. The Web site was an opportunity to both distribute accurate information about drinking on the college campus (and offer assistance to students who were having difficulties with their drinking through links to other Web sites providing information and/or counseling) and to assess students' awareness and recall of the misperceptions messages. In addition, announcements about campaign events and data collection opportunities were advertised on the Web site. Eventually, too, the Web site became the place that we reported on our campaign progress and findings.

## Public Relations Campaign

In addition to the activities on campus, a public relations campaign was designed to obtain more local coverage of the actual norms for college drinking in various media. The RU SURE Campaign received national and local television coverage including CNN, NBC Weekend Today, and News 12 New Jersey. The RU SURE Campaign also received coverage in *The New York Times, Alcoholism and Drug Abuse Weekly, The Focus* (distributed to all university faculty and staff), and several articles in the daily student newspaper.

## CONCLUSION

The RU SURE Campaign received the U.S. Department of Education's model program award in 2001 for both its innovative design and effectiveness in reaching college students with the message that dangerous drinking is not the norm on campus. The chapters that follow provide a description of the unique curriculum infusion design that was used to involve upper level students as campaign message disseminators, and the interpersonal strategies that were used as vehicles for involving first-year students (the target audience).

# 6

## IMPLEMENTATION OF THE CAMPAIGN

### A CURRICULUM INFUSION DESIGN[1]

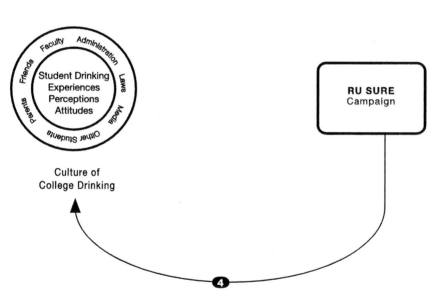

**Figure 6.1.  Step 4 of the Conceptual Model.**

[1]An earlier version of this chapter appeared in *Simulation & Gaming* (Lederman, Stewart, Barr, & Perry, 2001). Funding for this campaign was provided, in part, by the U.S. Department of Education Safe and Drug-Free Schools Program, New Jersey Consortium on Alcohol and Other Drug Prevention and Education supported by the New Jersey Department of Health and Senior Services, and the Rutgers University Health Services.

As illustrated in Fig. 6.1., the implementation of the RU SURE Campaign required competing with messages and influences from a vast array of other sources influencing college students. Thus, although we were aware that the primary way in which the culture of college drinking is being addressed on most college campuses is through health campaigns outside the classroom (Haines, 1993; Johannessen, Collins, Mills-Novoa, & Glider, 1999; Perkins, 1997), we wanted another approach. One alternative approach that has increasing popularity is the incorporation of alcohol prevention materials into curricular offerings, referred to as *curriculum infusion*. In the case of the RU SURE Campaign, curriculum infusion was used to create a collaboration in which students learned about a social issue (decisions around drinking and drinking-related behavior) while creating materials for other students to learn about these issues. This experience provided students with the cognitive and behavioral skills they needed to take the information from the campaign and incorporate it into their own living situations.

The purpose of this chapter is to present the curriculum infusion plan we developed that currently is in operation in the communication curriculum at Rutgers. It was through this curriculum infusion plan that we were able to work with groups of juniors and seniors (majoring in communication) to design and implement the RU SURE Campaign for their first-year classmates.

## CURRICULUM INFUSION IN COLLEGE CLASSROOMS

The purpose of most curriculum infusion plans is to find appropriate matches between theoretical course content and compelling contemporary social and health issues. Rather than taking what students learn in the classroom and using it in so-called real-world applications, curriculum infusion incorporates the study of issues from the real world into the classroom. Beyond adding richness and context to conceptual classroom learning, a curriculum infusion approach fosters opportunities for students to examine and reflect on their own attitudes and behaviors vis-à-vis compelling and relevant social and health issues. It is designed to use the classroom as a context in which to guide students through an examination of their own attitudes and behaviors in relation to those issues.

The problem of college drinking is a contemporary health and social issue that lends itself well to curriculum infusion because of its relevance to students. Rather than creating a course about alcohol use and offering it to students, a curriculum infusion approach incorporates the subject of college drinking into other course content to provide context and connections for students to examine their own drinking-related attitudes and behaviors. The literature indicates that courses totally dedicated to teaching about alcohol use are often not effective means of teaching students about their own drinking-related behaviors. In fact, the literature indicates that much of what students learn about drinking they know from their own first-hand experiences and/or their perceptions of the behaviors around them (Cohen & Lederman, 1998; Lederman & Stewart, 1998). Many students report that they need to learn about drinking by trial and error (Burns & Goodstadt, 1989; Cohen & Lederman, 1998). Unfortunately, excessive ingestion of alcohol is potentially deadly.

Although there are ethical and pedagogical concerns that any curriculum infusion effort must address, this approach is a means to help students personalize compelling and relevant social and health issues vis-à-vis their own attitudes and behaviors. In the case of college drinking, the subject is one about which even students who have a wealth of information may not have developed the intellectual tools to examine the validity and reliability of that information.

## THE INSTITUTIONAL SETTING FOR CURRICULUM INFUSION

Social sciences courses, such as psychology and sociology, are often the sites of curriculum infusion strategies. Usually the curriculum infusion takes the form of a particular lecture or class activity that can be tied to the social issue, such as alcohol use. Given that effective alcohol prevention campaigns rely on sound communication principles and interpersonal skills and interactions, courses in communication (e.g., health communication, interpersonal communication, mediated communication) provide a natural context in which to create an infusion program. These courses are particularly good sites for curriculum infusion concerning dangerous drinking because students are encouraged to examine the role of basic interpersonal communication processes in college drinking that can have a lasting impact on their social development. Additionally, faculty, who may not have seen themselves as responsible for dealing with student drinking and who have inadvertently added to the misperceptions of drinking as normative by references to drinking in class (Lederman et al., 1998) can become part of the solution.

At Rutgers in Fall 1998, we designed a new course for the Department of Communication in which the curriculum would be infused with college-drinking issues. The new course was in health communication and called Advanced Health Communication (AHC). Students eligible to take AHC were juniors and seniors majoring in Communication who had taken pre-requisite courses in health communication, interpersonal communication, and communication theory.

## THE CURRICULUM INFUSION DESIGN

### Course Description and Objectives

We designed AHC to provide students with hands-on experience in working on the RU SURE Campaign to change misperceptions of college drinking. The goal of the course was to provide students with a set of experiences in which they could apply their knowledge of communication, health communication, and public relations theory and practices to a specific health campaign, thereby emphasizing the real-world applications of these areas of knowledge. Because the goals of the course were to teach about communication and health campaigns and to use a specific health campaign to foster that learning, the course provided a perfect context in which to encourage students to address dangerous drinking on campus by working on a health prevention campaign.

The objectives of the course were as follows:

1. Familiarize students with the theoretical and pragmatic bases out of which college-drinking prevention campaigns grow.
2. Increase students' understanding of themselves as products and producers of culture, and the implications of both for them as instruments of changing the culture of college drinking.
3. Familiarize students with literature relevant to understanding college drinking and the misperceptions approach.
4. Conduct audience analysis research to test materials for the RU SURE Campaign with first-year Rutgers College students.
5. Implement the RU SURE Campaign slogans, posters, and messages for the print and electronic campaign.
6. Monitor and evaluate the RU SURE Campaign.
7. Apply what is learned to other health campaigns.

### Course Description and Requirements

The course was conducted as a workshop in which communication theory and practices were applied to the implementation and evaluation of the RU SURE Campaign. Students in the course were trained to participate in the design and implementation of the campaign. To prepare for implementing, monitoring, and evaluating the campaign, students were first assigned to read relevant literature on college drinking, social norms theory, experiential learning theories, and materials written to describe the work of The Center for Communication and Health Issues (CHI) at Rutgers University.

Students and the instructor worked together to simulate a real-world work situation in which an organization functioned to support a health campaign. Students were required to work in teams and to produce individual assignments, team projects, and total class presentations. In order to provide a context that simulated a work environment, AHC included a semester-long simulation of a work organization, the AHC simulation, designed by Lederman and Stewart as the campaign curriculum infusion component (Lederman, Stewart, Barr, & Perry, 2001). The semester-long simulation consisted of three phases of participation: Phase 1, Training Phase (4 weeks); Phase 2, Planning and Implementation (6 weeks); and Phase 3, Evaluation (4 weeks). Both the design of the course and all of the activities in which the students participated were guided by Lederman and Stewart's (1998) SSEL model discussed in Chapter 3.

On the first day in class, the course goals, the AHC simulation, and a syllabus were distributed to students. The simulation-based real-world work environment was described, and students were told that they had to be prepared to work with the team to which they were assigned for at least 2 hours a week outside of class. See the appendix at the end of this chapter for a summary of the major course assignments. The next section of the chapter describes the AHC simulation.

## The AHC Simulation

A simulation is best defined as a working model of reality or some aspect of reality (Lederman & Ruben, 1982). As reported in the literature on simulations and games since the late 1970s (Bredemeier & Greenblatt, 1981; Pierfy, 1977), simulations are particularly rich learning experiences for teaching about affect and behavior as well as conceptual materials. (See Chapter 10 for a more detailed discussion of the history of simulations.) Thus, the AHC Simulation was designed for two purposes: to involve students in the design of messages for other students who were the target of the campaign and to provide students with a learning experience about health campaigns, their design, implementation, and impact, as well as to influence their own behavior.

In order to make the simulation a good learning experience, it was designed to have both validity and reliability (Lederman & Ruben, 1982). In a simulation, validity is either face validity or construct validity. Face validity refers to a simulation that has the outward appearance of that which it models. Construct validity refers to a one-to-one correspondence with the concepts being modeled. AHC has construct validity. The parts students and instructor played, the ways in which they interacted, and the dynamics were all consistent with an organization like the one being modeled.

Reliability in a simulation refers to process (what participants do) or product (what they produce). AHC has both process and product reliability. Any time the simulation runs, students in the roles of employees/workers and instructor in the role of manager work together to produce materials, activities, or other campaign products. It also has a predictable outcome—implementation and evaluation of the RU SURE Campaign. Thus, it has product reliability. Despite the participants or instructor, the simulation is designed so that its processes and products are reliable.

The AHC simulation has the five characteristics of any valid and reliable simulation: roles, rules, interactions, goals, and outcome criteria (Lederman & Ruben, 1982). Table 6.1. summarizes those characteristics.

Each of the five characteristics are used to describe the ways in which students in the class worked with the instructor to learn enough to work on the campaign, implement and evaluate it.

**Table 6.1   Simulation Characteristics of AHC.**

| CHARACTERISTIC | FUNCTION OF THE CHARACTERISTIC | AHC FUNCTION |
| --- | --- | --- |
| Roles | Parts played in the simulation | Manager, assistant managers, and workers |
| Rules | Structures for operating | Who talks to whom, rights and responsibilitties within AHC |
| Interactions | Participation between roles | Work activities of managers and workers |
| Goals | Objectives of the participation in the simulation | To create, disseminate, and evaluate the RU SURE Campaign |
| Outcome criteria | The ending, how it finishes | Final presentation of campaign report to CHI |

## Roles

All participants in the simulation are cast in roles in the AHC organization. The organization, modeled after SIMCORP (Lederman & Stewart, 1983), was designed as a subdivision of an actual university organization, the CHI. AHC was designed to advance CHI's mission to conduct research on communication and health issues affecting college students and to design, implement, and evaluate campus and community-based prevention campaigns. The AHC simulation modeled a flattened hierarchical division that reported to its parent, CHI. Because CHI was an actual campus organization, and the RU SURE Campaign was an actual and ongoing campaign that CHI is funded to produce on campus, the students in the simulation had a reality-based experience in participating in experiential learning.

The roles included a manager (the course instructor), assistant managers (graduate students), and team members (undergraduate students). Figure 6.2 presents an organizational model of AHC. Class sessions were run as if the students were workers on the RU SURE Campaign and the course instructor was their manager. The hierarchy was set in motion by the instructor,

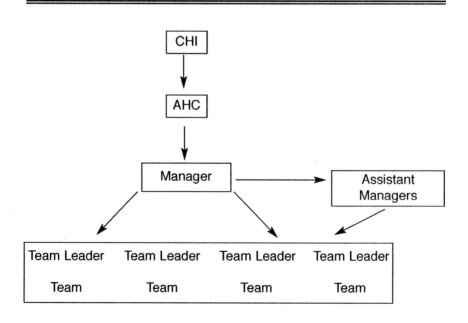

Figure 6.2.   AHC as a Subdivision of CHI.

acting as manager. The students worked in teams with imput from the manager and the assistant managers. All during the work day (class time), the instructor worked in the role of manager. At the end of each workday, the instructor called for a time out, and students and instructor dropped their organizational roles and were led by the instructor through a self-reflexive discussion of participation and what was learned from it.

To keep participants, including the instructor, aware of role demands, all participants "dressed for work." The simulated dress code involved wearing name badges created for AHC. It was also customary for the participants to arrange the chairs in the classroom into groupings that simulated team workspaces. Each day when they "reported to work," participants arranged the space so that they could meet and work in the same designated area. When time outs were called at the end of the "work day" the space was rearranged as a classroom and, in the roles of students and teacher, the discussion about the day's happenings was held.

## Rules

The rules for participation were kept to a minimum. Most rules were in regard to who communicated with whom and through what channels. Rules were also set in place for work expectations (i.e., keeping billable hours; working within a budget; signing in for work and signing out when working "outside" the office—the copy or computer room, for example; having work finished on time; reporting to work on time). These rules were provided by the instructor in the role of manager of the employees. Most of the other rules emerged from the interactions among employees of AHC. This simple rule-base, with the majority of rules emerging as participants enacted their roles, is referred to by Lederman and Ruben (1978) as an internally parametered simulation. In an internally parametered simulation the structure and basic rules are provided, and the rest is created through the participants as they work through the interactions in the simulation.

## Interactions

The interactions in the simulation are the work in which the participants engage in the simulation. The work schedule and all due dates were presented in the course syllabus.

The AHC simulation and work in the simulated organization was designed to maximize cooperative, shared effort, and responsibility. There was an open and free flow of information with the teams working cooperatively among themselves on interdependent projects. One team, for example, was responsible for the design of the logo for the campaign and another team for marketing strategies for all campaign artifacts. Because of the interdependency of the teams, and because of the open managerial style that a flattened hierarchy evokes, all participants were encouraged to have a free flow of roles and work interactions with one another.

In addition to team-specific tasks, all students in the simulation worked on both the mediated and interpersonally based strategies that the campaign used to address the problem of dangerous drinking on the college campus (Lederman et al., 2001). Because they were trained in the conceptual bases of the campaign and briefed on all campaign aspects before participating in any activities, Advanced Health Communication students were able to design and pilot test interactive experiences to disseminate campaign messages and bring them to first-year residence halls. Advanced Health Communication students also regularly collected pre- and postactivity quantitative data to determine any measurable changes in drinking-related attitudes and behaviors among first-year students, and worked on the analysis of those data.

Students had central roles in designing, running, and evaluating the campaign. On the one hand, therefore, they were learning about health prevention campaigns and how to design, implement, and evaluate a health communication campaign. This was the content level of the course. On the other hand, they were learning about drinking and drinking-related behaviors in socially situated experiences that were restructured to carry the message of the campaign that not everyone on the campus drinks dangerously and that students do not have to drink dangerously to fit in the college culture. This was the curriculum infusion level of their learning.

A typical workday involved arriving for work, arranging the chairs in the room to simulate a workplace space, and beginning teamwork. Work began on time whether the manager was there or not just as it would in the workplace. Most workdays, unless otherwise directed by the manager, students, in their roles as employees, had team work to do and knew what to do without having to wait for managerial approval. At the manager's initiation, team work would stop and teams would "brief" (update) the manager and other teams on their progress. After the briefing, teams would go back to work on their tasks. The manager would walk around "the office" stopping to work with individuals or teams who needed guidance. At the end of the work day (an 80-minute class) and usually 15 minutes before class ended, the students dropped their roles as employees and the instructor guided the class through a reflective discussion of what they had been doing during class and what they were learning from it.

All teams had designated times outside of class that they could complete work. It was a requirement of the course that each team had at least one time they could meet each week outside of class. Teams were created based, in part, on the times they were available to meet outside of class. As the semes-

ter went on, these times outside of class were used to implement the RU
SURE Campaign activities that the teams had been designing under the
supervision of the manager (instructor).

## Goals

The goals of the AHC simulation are to teach undergraduates about
drinking-related behaviors and the design of prevention campaigns to
address these behaviors. This was accomplished by having participants assist
CHI in changing first-year college students' misperceptions of excessive college drinking as the norm. The work that participants in the simulation did
was designed to change first-year students' misperceptions by increasing
awareness of the real norms of all students' college-drinking behavior. This
was done through a media campaign, through engagement in interactive
experiences designed to increase communication skills and reflective skills
training, and through interpersonally based experiential learning activities.
All of these activities are part of the RU SURE Campaign (see Chapter 5).

The simulation's goals were accomplished through a three-phase plan:
training, planning and implementation, and evaluation.

*Phase 1: Training.*    Each semester began with a training phase in which
all participants were placed in work teams and then briefed on CHI and its
RU SURE Campaign. At the end of the training phase, participants were
required to demonstrate their mastery of all materials relevant to CHI, the
RU SURE Campaign, and the theories on which the campaign is built, by
making a formal presentation to the manager. Only those teams that were
successful in mastering the materials were permitted to work on the campaign. Teams that were not successful were given additional training. This
was taken very seriously because alcohol abuse is a life-threatening problem,
and students who were not well enough trained to understand the RU
SURE Campaign and its basis were considered ill prepared to meet the challenges that the instructor knew would present themselves. In some ways the
tone of seriousness of purpose of this phase was curriculum infusion in
itself: it was a clear presentation of information about how serious alcohol
abuse is and why the RU SURE Campaign was designed as it was.

*Phase 2: Planning and Implementation.*    The teams worked in this
phase to plan and implement campaign activities. Along with periodic ads
placed in the campus newspaper, AHC teams took the pulse of the campus
by conducting an environmental scan of the campus. An environmental scan
is a systematic observational investigation of the potential places on campus
where the campaign activities would be conducted. Through an environmental scan, the appropriate place, channels (e.g., Table Talk or Walk About), and

schedules were determined for the campaign activities to achieve the best results. The places selected were those determined to be where first-year students were easy to reach to expose them to campaign messages. Based on the findings of an environmental scan, it was also possible to develop effective promotion strategies (e.g., using lollipops or music to attract attention) to get the message out and to gain the audience's reception.

After completion of environmental scans and selection of sites, times, and personnel, teams created a work plan to design activities and a timeline for their implementation. Activities included interactive games (RU SURE Bingo, RU SURE Word Scramble), Walk Abouts (physically walking around campus handing out information to first-year students and engaging them in dialogue about drinking), and Table Talks (attracting students to a table set up with various campaign promotional items).

*Phase 3: Evaluation.*    The final phase of the simulation was the evaluation of the campaign and its effectiveness for the given semester it had been run. Teams worked with the instructor and professional evaluators from CHI to learn how to collect qualitative, quantitative, and anecdotal data regarding the campaign's impact. (Data from some of these activities are reported in Chapter 8.)

## Outcome Criteria

The outcome criteria for each semester's run of the simulation was the presentation of completed work to CHI, the campus organization of which AHC simulates a division. Each semester, the simulation ended with a presentation to the CHI Board of a formal report/presentation on AHC's products for CHI and its effectiveness in running the campaign. The report to CHI each semester included a summary of activities from the initial training period and environmental scan and work plan as well as the actual campaign implementation and evaluation.

## CURRICULUM INFUSION AND PARTICIPATION IN THE SIMULATION AND THE RU SURE CAMPAIGN

The Advanced Health Communication course was dominated by the simulation and work in it. Because all students were seniors majoring in communication, their communication background provided them with a wealth of learning on which they could draw. After the simulation ended, a week of class was left to assess what had been accomplished, what had been learned, and the implications of all of it for students' own life choices and careers in communication.

Beyond involving the students in the simulation to enlist them in the design and implementation of the RU SURE Campaign, the goal of the AHC simulation was designed to provide students with a learning experience about working in an organization that creates prevention campaigns designed to address college drinking. The design and implementation of a complex, semester-long simulation provided a rich and multifaceted learning experience for participants about health communication campaigns, about dangerous drinking in college, and about their own drinking. There were three ways in which their learning was demonstrated: (a) the production of campaign materials, reports, and activities; (b) the reflective papers they wrote and their guided analytic discussions at the end of each class session; and (c) their pre- and postexperience self-reports of drinking attitudes, perceptions, and behaviors. Each of these is discussed subsequently in detail.

## Course Products: Campaign Materials, Activities, Reports

One of the outcomes, or evidence of learning, was the materials, activities, and campaign reports/presentations that students in the simulated organization prepared and delivered. Each semester that the simulation has run, students participating in it have produced all of the items discussed here.

*Training Document (Briefing Document).* Each team had to write a briefing document that answered a series of in-depth questions about the campaign, its theory, purpose, target audience, competing messages, and goals before it was permitted to work on the campaign. In addition, each team had to make a 10-minute presentation of the highlights of that document and lead a 10-minute question and answer session. Teams had to use these materials to demonstrate their mastery of the campaign, and only those teams who did so were permitted to work on the campaign. In the rare instances when a team had not met the standard, it was given an opportunity to improve. (See the appendices at the end of this chapter for a sample briefing document.)

*Campaign Materials.* Teams created posters, flyers, t-shirt designs, and designs for other artifacts such as pens, computer disks, and stickers. If materials were already available from past semesters, they created additional flyers, posters, and give-aways to use with the existent materials.

*Campaign Activities.* Teams created plans for and implemented various activities to disseminate campaign messages and for them to have interpersonal interactions with members of their target audience. Documents describing activities and providing instructions for their use were regularly created by teams working on the project.

*Instruments for Data Collection.*   Teams worked with the instructor to create short surveys for intercept interviews and used them to collect data throughout the campaign. They also had forms on which they recorded anecdotal data.

*Presentational Materials.*   The final project for the teams was to work together to prepare and present a formal report to CHI on the entire semester's accomplishments. The report (and overheads/power point presentation) was made in a 45-minute oral presentation followed by 15-minute question and answer session and accompanied by a formal written report.

## Process Outcomes: Reflection Papers and Guided Discussions (Debriefing Sessions)

Although some of what the students were learning was evidenced by the products they produced, as discussed previously, much of the learning for them was *process learning.* Process learning is used here to mean the students' interpretations of the experiences they have in working together to create the materials and activities for the campaign or what they think they have learned from their experiences. They learned, for example, about the dynamics of participation in organizational life, their own drinking behaviors, working in teams, and the meanings they attach to the experiences they have, which need to be expressed so that the instructor can help them to reflect analytically on their learning and to assess the conclusions they draw from their experiences. In Advanced Health Communication this learning was explored in two ways: (a) required reflection papers and (b) guided periodic discussions (debriefings).

*Reflection Papers.*   All students wrote reflection papers three times during the semester. The papers asked participants to describe and discuss what they had been doing in the simulation, what they learned from what they had been doing, and the applications of that learning. It was from the debriefing sessions and the papers that it was possible to draw some conclusions about students' learning about organizational communication, public relations, and working on an actual campaign.

Participants reported that some of what they learned was immediate. Because the simulation was tied to a real-world campus organization (CHI) participants saw, for example, how their ideas were used or ignored. They saw how products that they had created were in use almost immediately on the campus. Students reported that much of what they learned was about themselves as workers on a campaign and the talents and skills they needed to bring to those jobs. As in most uses of simulations, the learning experience only began in the classroom. By wedding the simulation with an actual organization, the simulation was enhanced by the pressure to meet deadlines and produce quality products.

*Guided Discussions (Debriefing Sessions).*   The "work day" was divided into work time and reflective time. At the end of each work day (the last 15 minutes of class), students and instructor left their roles as organizational members, and the instructor guided the class through a reflective discussion of what they had been doing during class and what they were learning from it. This was referred to as the *debriefing*. (For an in-depth discussion of debriefing, see Chapter 10.)

## Pre- and Postexperience Self-Report of Drinking Attitudes, Perceptions, and Behaviors

All participants completed anonymous quantitative pre- and postexperiential surveys reporting their drinking-related perceptions and behaviors. They also participated in focus group interviews. All of these sources of data indicated a decrease in participants' misperceptions of dangerous drinking and a decrease in their own drinking-related behaviors. For example, in a focus group interview, one participant explained:

> *When I first started on this campaign, I found it hard to believe the statistics because most of my "night life" revolves around the bar scene or drinking. But when I actually started to pay attention to my surroundings, I realized that a lot of people did go to a party or bar to socialize, not drink. A lot of people did stop at three or fewer [drinks], as the statistics showed.*

When participants were asked to anonymously write how this campaign had influenced them, one student wrote:

> *I take note of people who drink and quantities. I feel more and more that drinking in excess is very unattractive and immature.*

(See Chapter 9 for an in-depth discussion of the results of both quantitative and qualitative data collected from AHC students.)

# ETHICAL ISSUES

Learning by participation in an activity is a powerful and long-term learning experience. Most students who have gone through the AHC simulation, as well as other simulations created by Lederman and Stewart (1985, 1987, 1991; Stewart, 1987; Stewart & Lederman, 1988), report the experience to be invaluable. In the use of a simulation, like any other pedagogical method, the instructor always has to be mindful of the ethical ramifications. This is particularly true of participation in a simulation in which the subject matter (dangerous drinking) can have such personal meaning to participants, many of whom may in fact be heavy drinkers. One of the advantages of this approach to curriculum infusion is that AHC and its parent CHI are part of the coalition that we built on campus that includes health educators and alcohol counselors. These individuals are always available if any student is identified as a high-risk student or in need of additional, individualized counseling.

Just as service learning allows students to take classroom concepts and give new meaning to them through their engagement in community experiences (Sullivan, Myers, Bradfield, & Street, 1999), participation in the AHC simulation allowed students to gain a greater understanding of the concepts of health communication theories in an applied setting that was extremely familiar to them—the college campus. In addition to learning about health communication campaigns, however, this curriculum infusion approach presented students with the opportunity to examine their own drinking behaviors. As can be seen from the previous discussion, the drinking behaviors of some of these students clearly should be labeled dangerous drinking.

Given the possibility in any college classroom for there to be students who drink dangerously, instructors who implement pedagogical strategies such as the one described in this chapter have a particular ethical responsibility to provide support for students who may be facing in depth self-examination on this topic. Clearly, it is not the role of the instructor to be on call to provide counseling to individual students. Nevertheless, the instructor must be aware of the potential need for such guidance. One successful way to offer this support for students is to disseminate information on services provided by the university health services. This information can be given to students at the beginning of the semester in an unobtrusive manner in their course reading packets. An alternative strategy is to maintain a course Web site with links to various information resources on student alcohol use and alcoholism. A guest lecture from a staff member who deals with student life issues may also be a way to present additional information to help students in their explorations of appropriate social behavior.

Although this type of teaching strategy provides numerous advantages for both the instructor and student, the instructor is compelled to engage in continuous reflection about the holistic effects that participation in this type of course may have on students' developing self-concepts and views of the world around them.

## CONCLUSIONS

The subject of college drinking is an important one in health communication. It is estimated that thousands of students die each year from alcohol-related causes on college campuses nationally. Health educators try to prevent these deaths and other alcohol-related injuries. Faculty, too, can contribute—especially those who are teaching subjects like health communication or interpersonal communication where curriculum infusion projects can introduce subject matter about drinking in relation to important course concepts. A powerful way to approach this task is by the inclusion in a course of a simulation designed to model the aspects of college drinking that the course can address. Simulations are powerful instructional tools. In the AHC simulation, students are provided with a mechanism for learning about work life in a complex organization, the design, implementation, and evaluation of a health prevention campaign for a client, and their own drinking-related perceptions and behaviors. The interface with a real client and a real campaign provided participants with added dimensions of the consequences and outcomes of each of their behavioral choices during the run of the simulation. On a macrolevel of analysis, participants learned to understand the conceptual basis of the campaign and its health implications. On a microlevel, they got to reflect on their own choices, including their own drinking behavior. AHC allowed for both the creation and implementation of a student-driven health campaign and was a vehicle for those students to learn about themselves in relation to those health issues.

# APPENDIX A:
# AHC COURSE ASSIGNMENTS

| Assignment | Activity | Materials | Point Value | Individual or Team Grade |
|---|---|---|---|---|
| 1 | Briefing Document and Presentation | Intercept Interview Instructions and Forms; Coding Sheet, Briefing Document Form | P/F | Team |
| 2 | Work Plan | Action Plan Form | P/F | Team |
| 3 | Individual Paper | Guidelines | 200 | Individual |
| 4 | Environmental Scan Report and Presentation | Environmental Scan Form and Presentation Instructions | P/F | Team |
| 5 | Campaign Evaluation | Intercept Interview Instructions and Forms | 250 | Team |
| 6 | Presentation to CHI | Guidelines | 250 | AHC |
| 7 | Final Paper | Guidelines | 200 | Individual |
| 8 | Work Ethic | | 100 | Individual |
| Total Value | | | 1000 | |

# APPENDIX B:
## BRIEF DESCRIPTION OF COURSE ASSIGNMENTS

**Assignment 1: Briefing Document and Formal Presentation** (15 minutes plus Question and Answer Session)

The RU SURE Campaign consists of a multimedia approach to getting the message out that dangerous drinking is not the norm at Rutgers. Media include newspapers, posters, flyers, t-shirts, pens, stickers, and other artifacts, a Web site, and interactive materials created for use with first-year students.

You will work in a team of four or five students. Read all assigned materials. Attend all class briefing sessions. Conduct research with first-year Rutgers College students (individual interviews, intercept interviews—see below). Then complete the Briefing Document Form. Each team will make a 15-minute formal presentation summarizing the highlights of the document and should be prepared to answer questions about the document. Presentations should include the use of visual aids (posters, overheads, etc.). *Only those teams that make a successful presentation indicating a real understanding of the RU SURE Campaign, the target audience, and the objectives will be permitted to work on the campaign.* Effective presentations (both content and delivery) will be the basis of job placement.

### Intercept Interview Questionnaire

The purpose of the questionnaire is to gather data from individual Rutgers College first-year students regarding their alcohol-related perceptions and behaviors as well as their media usage. Each team member is to copy the questionnaire and individually interview at least 15 first-year Rutgers College students. Collate and summarize the data with your team members.

**Assignment 2: Environmental Scan Work Plan** (1 page)

Each team will prepare a work plan for how they intend to scan the environment to determine where first-year students gather and, therefore, where are the best places to communicate our messages. The work plan will be an outline that includes all activities, when they will take place, how they will be done, and who will do them. These will be presented in class. Environmental Scan Forms need to be completed.

**Assignment 3: Individual Papers** (5–7 pages)

Write a brief paper discussing what you have learned about health communication, college drinking, and/or prevention campaigns so far this semester. Make a connection between what you have done so far and its application to your everyday life and in your major in communication. The paper will be graded on content, style, organization of ideas, clarity, insight, and analysis. Be sure to proofread! No paper will receive an A unless it is perfect in all aspects.

### Assignment 4: Formal Presentations/Report on Environmental Scan and Data Collection (15 minutes plus Question and Answer Session)

Teams will discuss their progress on the environmental scan and data collection. Each team should use the Environmental Scan Form to collect data. A report is to be a written, and the team will make an oral presentation on the findings of the environmental scan and data collection. Teams are expected to use this process as the foundation for campaign activities and materials development.

### Assignment 5: Preliminary Presentation/Report on Implementation/ Materials Development Strategies

Each team will present for 15 minutes on their activities and feedback/outcome results. Formal presentations are to be accompanied by reports that are not to exceed 10 pages. Reports should include a detailed description of all activities. In addition, the reports will include summative assessments of the campaign effectiveness. These results will include all data that were collected to monitor the campaign, individual interviews, and any other data that were gathered.

### Assignment 6: Formal Presentations to CHI (45 minutes)

AHC will make a formal presentation to CHI highlighting their activities for the semester. This is the major product of the semester. Guidelines will be a product of team efforts.

### Assignment 7: Final Paper (6–8 pages)

The final paper is to be the summary, description, and analysis of your participation in all class and group/team activities, your contribution, and what you learned from your experiences. Use it to demonstrate what you have learned this semester about health communication, health communication campaigns, the monitoring and assessment of campaigns, college drinking, social norms theory, misperceptions theory, experiential learning theory, group process, presentational skills, interviewing, group interviews, data collection, data analysis, report writing, yourself as a college student, your drinking-related attitudes and behaviors, and anything else that you think has been a significant part of your learning experience. The paper will be graded on content, style, organization of ideas, clarity, insight, and analysis.

### Work Ethic

AHC simulates a work place situation. Students are put into the role of employees and the instructor takes the role of manager. Class time is divided between working on AHC tasks in these roles and debriefing sessions. During the debriefing sessions the instructor assumes the role of teacher and facilitates a discussion with students about what they are doing and what they are learning in their participation in the simulated organization.

While in the role of employees, students get to learn about the expectations the manager has of them as workers and how to be valuable and productive workers. *Work ethic* is the term we will use to describe this. Coming to work (class) on time, being prepared, working hard, making oneself valuable to the team and to AHC, and engagement in the work at hand are all part of job performance and all signs of a good work ethic. Lateness, absence, or lack of effective participation are viewed as evidence of inadequate job performance and a poor work ethic. The purpose of adhering to these standards is to learn through this experience about oneself as a worker and about the demands of being a productive employee.

# APPENDIX C:
## SAMPLE BRIEFING DOCUMENT

### RU SURE CAMPAIGN BRIEFING DOCUMENT

| Group Name: | Date: |
|---|---|

What is CHI?

What is AHC? And how is it related to CHI?

What is the RU SURE Campaign? What is the objective of the campaign? (What problem is it designed to solve?)

What is the Socially Situated Experiential Learning (SSEL) Model, and how is it related to the RU SURE Campaign?

How will results be measured? By whom? By when? How will they be communicated?

What are the principal competing messages? (What are their strengths/ weaknesses? How are they positioned? How are they advertised?)

Who is our target audience? (Demographics, lifestyle, and other profiles or mindsets of target audience or their influencers)

How should the campaign be positioned against the competition? (How is this different from other current campaigns? Why is this a new, desirable position for the campus campaign?)

How will the campaign be perceived by first-year Rutgers College students?

What does our audience currently think and feel about college drinking?

What strategies are available to help us communicate this message? (What claims can we make? What research can be leveraged? What convincing proof can we offer? What competitive comparisons will make us look better?)

Why should our audience believe us? (What support or evidence do we have?)

What barriers do we have to overcome? (Current perceptions, category interest, competitive noise, client operational concerns?)

What do we want our audience to think, feel, and do as a result of the campaign?

What are social norms and how are they derived?

Where, how, and by whom will our message be communicated?

How can the message dissemination and impact be monitored?

What are the indicators of campaign success?

What are misperceptions? How, if at all, can they be changed?

# Part III

## Outcomes of the Campaign

### Brief Overview

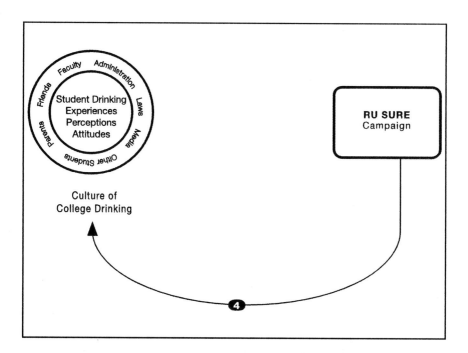

Part III of this book focuses on the evaluation the RU SURE Campaign and application of what was learned from the campaign to other activities and other campuses. In terms of the conceptual model discussed in Chapter 3, the focus of this part of the book is on Step 5, Evaluation. As evident in Step

5, the campaign and its results were continuously evaluated and that evaluation led to further refinement and implementation of the campaign. The chapters in this part of the book focus on evaluation or additional campaign applications that grew out of that continuous evaluation.

In Chapter 8, Continuous Evaluation of the Campaign, the process and outcome evaluation methods and results are presented and discussed in detail. The chapter reviews the various ways in which we collected data and the outcomes that we found. It provides the quantitative outcomes and the measurements that allowed us to determine the success of the campaign.

Chapter 9, Unanticipated Results: The Impact of Campaign Messages on the Messengers, presents outcomes of the campaign found in its evaluation in terms of the students working on the campaign and its impact on them. Although we did not design the campaign to have an impact on the students who worked on it, we discovered that indeed that happened. In debriefing interviews after the AHC simulation in which they participated for the semester, and through which they designed and disseminated campaign messages, students reported the ways in which they themselves were affected by the RU SURE Campaign messages.

In Chapter 10, The *RU SURE Game of Choices and Consequences*: A 1-Hour Brief Intervention Alcohol Decision-Making Tool, an application of the campaign is discussed. Based on what was found in the impact of socially situated experiential activities on the target audience, the brief intervention tool was developed and disseminated. It is a 1-hour simulation game in which students make typical alcohol-related decisions and are provided with feedback on the dangers associated with those decisions.

Finally, Chapter 11, Extending the Campaign and Its Socially Situated Experiential Learning Approach to Other Campuses, presents a step-by-step discussion of how the campaign can be implemented at other institutions. The chapter provides guidelines for consideration in adapting the campaign so that it fits into other environments.

# 7

## INTERPERSONAL STRATEGIES FOR CAMPAIGN MESSAGE DISSEMINATION

The RU SURE Campaign, which won a U.S. Department of Education Model Program Award in 2001, has been implemented for 5 years each semester at Rutgers University. As illustrated in Fig. 7.1, the implementation of the RU SURE Campaign required competing with messages and influences from a vast array of other sources that affect college students. One of the ways in which these competing messages were addressed was to work with senior-year students in Advanced Health Communication (AHC; see Chapters 5 and 6) who could use interpersonal interventions to talk to the target audience, first-year students.

In the early semesters of the campaign, students worked on message design and dissemination. In later semesters, students worked on message refinement and evaluation. When messages were designed, tested, and ready to roll out, AHC students in worked on creating interpersonally based strategies. These were mechanisms through which the communication students could take the campaign message out on the campus and talk to other students about dangerous drinking. The goal was to design activities that could create opportunities for AHC students who were seniors and juniors to talk with members of the target audience (first-year students) about the campaign.

In each semester, students working on the campaign do a needs assessment (referred to as an environmental scan), conduct a variety of interpersonally based strategies that include games, videos, or talks, and disseminate the campaign messages both in terms of the conversations they have with first-year students and in terms of campaign artifacts (pens, t-shirts, posters, key chains, etc.) that they distribute. At the end of the semester, when the dissemination data are tallied, the AHC students typically have run 16 to 24 of these events with 600 to 950 students attending and disseminated 2,000 to 3,000 campaign artifacts. All of these add to the message recognition and provide a way to intervene in the socially situated interactions of their first-year peers (our target population).

This chapter describes the mechanisms created by students to interact with first-year students in residence halls and on campus to disseminate the campaign message interpersonally. It is intended to be a guide to understanding and using interpersonal strategies to reduce dangerous drinking on campus. All of the interpersonally based strategies are described and instructions for creating and implementing them are detailed. These include the Walk About, Table Talks, RU SURE Bingo, RU Word Scramble, the RU SURE video, and RU SURE Coffee Breaks, which are all preceded by an environmental scan.

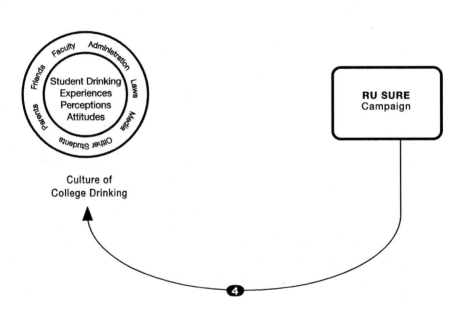

Figure 7.1. Step 4 of the Conceptual Model.

# ENVIRONMENTAL SCAN

Before engaging in any interpersonally based message dissemination, it was necessary for the students who would disseminate the campaign message to understand enough about the campus environment to know when and where it was best to attempt to engage members of the target audience (first-year students) in interactions. Although AHC members were themselves students and, therefore, familiar with the campus, the purpose of the environmental scan activity was to get them to look at the campus more critically—to view it as a context in which target audience members could be found and to analyze that context in terms of its potential for message dissemination. The analysis of the context in order to make that decision is referred to as an *environmental scan* (Lederman, Stewart, Barr, & Perry, 2001).

## Description of an Environmental Scan

An environmental scan refers to investigating the potential places where the interpersonally based campaign activities will be conducted based on an assessment of student usage and accessibility. Through an environmental scan, the appropriate place, channels (Table Talk or Walk About), and schedules for these activities were determined so that the activities could achieve the best results. The ultimate places selected were where first-year students were easily reached so that they could be exposed to the campaign message. Based on the findings of an environmental scan, it was also possible to develop effective promotion strategies (e.g., using lollipops or music to attract attention) to get the message out and to gain the audience's attention.

## Implementation of an Environmental Scan

An environmental scan had to be conducted each time the RU SURE Campaign was implemented. The steps for conducting an environmental scan were standardized so that replicability could be achieved each semester. Students were instructed to carry out the following tasks:

- Survey a series of places that groups of first-year Rutgers College students are known to frequent.
- Investigate the campus on foot to further determine a location useful for disseminating messages.
- Determine which areas present the best opportunity to interact with willing students.

- Conduct a process of elimination that will help finalize which area is used.
- Decide on the date and time for the activity, taking into account weather, holidays, and special events that could pose as competing messages.
- Propose the findings to the AHC organizational members and discuss a plan that will be most effective.

## Preparation Needed for an Environmental Scan

Before conducting an environmental scan, students were instructed to collect information about first-year Rutgers College students' lifestyles and interests. They were also asked to reflect back on their own experiences as first-year students to help sort out the potential locations for activities. Additionally, students were given an Environment Scan Plan Sheet that required them to fill in the times, places, and names of those who went to observe the environment, as well as the number of students present each time a place was observed and any comments to help explain the observation.

## Potential Problems and Their Solutions

Students were instructed to be aware of the impact of the weather on the decisions they would make about message dissemination activities as well as competing messages in the environment. The greatest obstacle they found that they had to overcome was finding a place that offered the best opportunity for dissemination of the message without the students feeling either overwhelmed or put off by thinking that the campaign is part of a sales solicitation.

They were also instructed to choose a location that would specifically target first-year students rather than the entire student body. They were asked to take all of this into account before deciding on the most effective area for an RU SURE Campaign activity and to be prepared to justify and explain it as part of their action plan for their interpersonal strategies.

## THE WALK ABOUT

## Description of a Walk About

A Walk About is an activity focused on disseminating information about the RU SURE Campaign by physically walking around campus handing out information to first-year students and engaging them in dialogue about drinking.

## Implementation of a Walk About

Walk Abouts were conducted throughout the semester during which the RU SURE Campaign was run. Given that AHC students worked in teams and that each team was responsible for two Walk Abouts each semester, depending on the number of teams, there were 8 to 12 Walk Abouts each semester.

These are the steps that were developed to be followed each time a Walk About was conducted. The following instructions were given to students:

- Arrive at the location 15 minutes prior to beginning the Walk About.
- Divide materials equally among team members.
- Spread team members out in the area to cover more ground.
- Approach members of the target audience (specifically first-year students) by asking if they would like free items, such as candy, magnets, key chains, etc.
- After catching a student's attention, ask if the student is familiar with the RU SURE Campaign, in an attempt to start a conversation about the main message of the campaign.
- Following this conversation, thank the student for his or her time and move on to the next student and repeat the procedure.
- In the event that a student does not have the time to stop, simply hand him or her an article with the message on it. This ensures that the student will receive the message even though you did not get a chance to share it verbally.
- Bring a notebook. Keep track of anecdotal data. This is important information that will aid in the next team's Walk About. One team member can be delegated to observe interactions and take notes. Other members should relay any anecdotal information to the notetaker.
- After running out of materials or when the allotted time is up, whichever comes first, make sure to clean up.

## Preparation Needed for a Walk About

One of the most important parts of having a successful interpersonal interaction was to make sure that the students engaging in an interaction on behalf of AHC were well prepared. For doing a Walk About they were given the following set of instructions, which were developed by students who had conducted Walk Abouts in the pilot-testing phase of the activities:

- Pick a date that works with all the team members' schedules.
- After picking a date, use the information from the environmental scan in order to pick a time and location for the event.
- Most teams will find the Walk About to be more successful if held outdoors. In this case, permission is not necessary. However, if a team chooses to hold a Walk About indoors, or is forced to go inside due to inclement weather, prior permission is required. Teams must decide what the back-up plan in this situation will be approximately one and a half weeks before the scheduled Walk About date in order to obtain permission from the proper authorities. Contacts can be found through the use of the Rutgers' Web site or from a representative of CHI.
- Decide how many items you will need during the Walk About. Here is a sample budget for a 2-hour Walk About: 50 magnets ($75), 74 pens ($75), 200 flyers (provided free by CHI), 50 keychains ($75), for a total of $225. Plan according to this sample. Contact a representative at the CHI office to arrange a time to pick up the materials (CHI supplied AHC with all materials for the dissemination activities).
- Also, still following the sample of a 2-hour Walk About, add to your budget the cost of about four bags of candy and other relevant materials (e.g., balloons, tape, etc.).
- On the day of the Walk About, the team should meet 15 minutes prior to the scheduled Walk About time in order to set up.

## Potential Problems and Their Solutions

Based on the experiences of AHC teams that pilot-tested the activity, a chart was created to illustrate problems that might occur and provide solutions for them (see Table 7.1). A "problem/solution" list was given to students preparing to do each of the activities in this chapter as a way of encouraging them to think through and be prepared for problems. These lists were created by students who pilot tested the activities and were students' advice to the next group of students on how to do the activities without any difficulties.

### Table 7.1.  Walk About Problems and Solutions

| PROBLEM | SOLUTION |
|---|---|
| Three team members in one space intimidate students. The students try to avoid walking past the team. | Spread out! Have team members stand alone or in pairs. You will cover more ground, and students will not feel as intimidated. |
| Students do not seem to be interested in stopping to talk about the campaign. | Try attracting students by announcing that you have "free stuff" for them. |
| Your team thought the location was a good one, but not many students are walking by. | Move on to your back-up plan. It's there for just such emergencies. |
| No one wants to take a flyer. | Roll up the flyers like a diploma and stick them through the loop of the key chains. |

## TABLE TALKS

## What is a Table Talk?

A Table Talk is a method of disseminating information to a target audience. This is achieved by attracting students to a table set up with various campaign promotional items (e.g., t-shirts, pens, magnets, posters, flyers, etc.) to be given out and talking to those students. Having a Table Talk promoted interaction between campaign representatives and the target audience, as well as aided in the dissemination of the RU SURE Campaign message through that interaction and the distribution of the campaign promotional items.

## Implementation of a Table Talk

Table Talks were conducted throughout the semester during which the RU SURE Campaign was run. Given that AHC students worked in teams and that each team was responsible for two Table Talks each semester, depending on the number of teams, there were 8 to 12 Table Talks each semester.

These are the steps that were developed to follow each time a Table Talk was conducted. The following instructions were given to students:

- Arrive at least 30 minutes prior to the intended start time to setup, including acquiring the table and chairs. Make sure to bring proper documentation if necessary.
- Begin decorating the table with banners, posters, and RU SURE Campaign promotional items.
- Position no more than two team members *behind* the table to avoid intimidating members of the target audience. Remaining team members should roam around trying to attract passersby to the table.
- Improvise and modify Table Talk if necessary—for instance, change the location of the table to a nearby, higher trafficked area.
- Continue to interact with students while continuing to disseminate the campaign message. Any way the group is able to get at least some form of the message out is a good way. Try implementing new ideas while observing the target audience's actions. For example, as another attractant try putting campaign flyers in *Daily Targums* [the student newspaper] that you put on your table.

## Preparation Needed for a Table Talk

One of the most important parts of having a successful interpersonal interaction was to make sure that the students engaging in an interaction on behalf of AHC were well prepared. For doing a Table Talk, they were given a set of instructions developed by students who had conducted Table Talks in the pilot-testing phase of the activities. The instructions were as follows:

- Using the Environmental Scan data, locate an area where a Table Talk would be most successful by identifying a site with a high traffic of first-year students.
- If permission is needed, contact the appropriate authority for permission—allowing at least 1 week for a response. If you are unsure whether or not permission is necessary, check with the division of the university that maintains that particular area.
- Plan a budget, anticipating the number of materials per student that will be given out, as well as the total number of students you plan on talking to. In addition, it is helpful to try to pre-

dict, based on your own group's preferences for campaign artifacts, what will be the most popular artifact given out and
accommodate that demand in your budget.

- Double check that all members of the group know the correct
date and time of the event, what to wear (RU SURE t-shirts),
and where the group is going to meet.

## Potential Problems and Their Solutions

Based on the experiences of the AHC teams that pilot tested the Table Talk
activity, a chart was created to illustrate problems that might occur and provide solutions for them (see Table 7.2).

### Table 7.2   Table Talk Problems and Solutions

| PROBLEM | SOLUTION |
| --- | --- |
| Location of the table was not ideal for attracting students and the location cannot be changed. | Have campaign representatives interact with students by passing out RU SURE Campaign promotional items and inviting them to the table. |
| Inclement weather will alter desired site location. | Be prepared with a back-up plan that includes the possibility of having to move the table talk indoors. |
| Reservation for the location and materials needed were not provided for. | Reconfirm all reservations with proper authority at least 2–3 days before the event is to take place. |
| Competing messages will hinder/hurt receptive nature of the target audience. | Survey the intended activity location to better predict what competing messages might affect the reception of the campaign. Choose a day that will have the fewest or no competing messages. |

# RU SURE BINGO

## Description of RU SURE Bingo

RU SURE Bingo is an interactive game activity focused on getting students to talk with one another and to find out about the key campaign message (Lederman & Stewart, 2001). The game can be played with any number of players and does not take more than 30 to 45 minutes to play. It is a fun way to give students an opportunity to break the ice with one another and also to find out some important things about drinking at Rutgers.

*The Game Board for RU SURE Bingo.*   The game uses a game board illustrated in Fig. 7.2.

## Implementation of RU SURE Bingo

RU SURE Bingo was designed to be used in residence halls or at the Table Talks that were conducted throughout the semester during which the RU SURE Campaign was run. Depending on the number of teams, there were 8 to 12 Table Talks each semester, many of which used the RU SURE Bingo game. The directions for playing RU SURE Bingo are included in Fig. 7.2.

## Preparation Needed to Use RU SURE Bingo

One of the most important parts of having a successful interpersonal inter-action was to make sure that the students engaging in an interaction on behalf of AHC were well prepared. For conducting RU SURE Bingo, they were given the following instructions, which were developed by students who had conducted the game in the pilot-testing phase of the activities:

- Pick a date that fits all team members' schedules.
- Pick an event, such as a Table Talk or Coffee Break, and use it to run the game.
- Most teams will find that the game will be more successful if held indoors. Prior to the event make sure to get whatever permission is required to run the game. Contacts can be found through the use of the Rutgers' Web site or from a representative of CHI.

| | | | | |
|---|---|---|---|---|
| Have you ever ventured into the dorm showers without flip-flops? | Have you heard of the RU SURE Campaign? | Do you currently possess dining hall utensils? | Have you ever made it to a Friday first period class? | Has your preceptor written you up? |
| Have you ever found yourself enjoying the food at a Rutgers dining hall? | Have you been to a football game? | Have you ordered pizza in the past week after 1 AM? | Did you know that 1 out of 5 students at Rutgers do not drink when they go out? | Can you name a freshman dean? |
| Do you have an RU SURE Top Ten Misperceptions t-shirt? | Have you been to every class this semester? | | Have you dropped a class? | Have you seen an RU SURE Top Ten Misperceptions ad in the *Targum* or a misperceptions flyer? |
| Have you consumed more than 2 meals from the grease trucks in one day? | Did you know that 2/3 of Rutgers' students drink 3 or fewer drinks when they go out? | Have you ever been inside the library? | Does your phone bill exceed $100? | Have you ever fallen asleep in class? |
| Have you signed up for a credit card after being offered free stuff? | Do you have back-to-back classes on different campuses? | Have you sold back a textbook? | Have you rearranged your dorm furniture more than 2 times? | Have you received an F grade on an exam or assignment yet? |

Figure 7.2.   RU SURE Bingo and Directions.

*DIRECTIONS for RU SURE Bingo*

**OBJECTIVE: TO GET A SIGNATURE IN *EVERY* BOX.**

<u>*Directions*</u>:   Find people who can answer "yes" to the questions in the boxes and ask them to sign that box. The same person can only sign one (or two) box(es). In other words, the same signature can only appear one (or two) time(s) on this paper. You may not sign your own game sheet!

When you get a signature in every box on your game sheet, shout:

> *"RU SURE? Yes, 3 or fewer."*

\*The first three people to complete the game win a Knight Express card worth $5.00.

\*Everyone who completes the game gets entered into our "WIN A DVD PLAYER RAFFLE."

**Figure 7.2.   RU SURE Bingo and Directions.** *(Continued)*

- Decide how many game boards and give-aways will be needed during the game.
- Create a budget for game boards and give-aways.
- Contact a representative at the CHI office to decide a time to pick up the merchandise. (CHI supplied AHC with all materials for the dissemination activities.)
- On the day of the game, the team should meet 15 minutes prior to the scheduled time in order to set up.

## Potential Problems and Their Solutions

Based on the experiences of the AHC teams that pilot tested RU SURE Bingo, a chart was created to illustrate problems that might occur with the RU SURE Bingo Game and provide solutions for them (see Table 7.3).

Table 7.3   RU SURE Bingo Game Potential Problems and Solutions

| PROBLEM | SOLUTIONS |
| --- | --- |
| Students do not seem to be interested. | Try attracting students by announcing that you have "free stuff" for them. |
| Your team thought the location was a good one, but not many students are joining in for the game. | See if you can get some of the students who are playing to round up some other friends. |
| No one wants to play. | Offer prizes to the first three people who volunteer to play. |
| People want to have snacks, but not play. | Let everyone know that *after* the game there will be soda, snacks, and prizes. |

# RU SURE WORD SCRAMBLE

## Description of the RU SURE Word Scramble

The RU SURE Word Scramble is a word puzzle that incorporates into the puzzle key words and messages from the RU SURE Campaign. It can be printed on separate flyers or handouts or in the student newspaper. It is a fun way for students to pass the time and start to think about some important things about college drinking. Figure 7.3 presents an example of one version of the RU SURE Word Scramble. Readily available computer programs can be used to generate alternative versions.

## Implementation of the RU SURE Word Scramble

The RU SURE Word Scramble was designed to be used in residence halls or at the Table Talks or Walk Abouts that were conducted throughout the semester during which the RU SURE Campaign was run. Many of these

```
M  Y  T  I  N  R  E  T  A  R  F  J  S  L
I  T  Z  L  Y  G  N  I  K  N  I  R  D  H
S  B  C  O  L  L  E  G  E  R  E  X  L  G
P  S  Y  T  H  L  L  Q  G  E  S  L  R  H
E  L  O  H  O  C  L  A  P  R  R  R  T  K
R  T  Z  C  K  D  R  D  Q  C  E  Q  K  R
C  W  S  R  I  P  E  C  X  S  G  B  H  X
E  P  D  Q  T  A  B  C  E  K  T  W  O  C
P  A  N  M  T  T  L  C  I  T  U  J  W  S
T  R  E  M  H  C  I  N  L  S  R  L  L  T
I  T  I  P  H  O  X  Q  O  V  I  K  D  L
O  Y  R  I  H  R  Y  X  B  R  R  O  L  V
N  K  F  C  J  L  D  N  V  Z  M  T  N  G
S  F  R  E  S  H  M  A  N  R  C  S  R  S
```

<u>WORDS</u>

ALCOHOL, CHI, CHOICE, COLLEGE, DECISIONS,
DRINKING, FRATERNITY, FRESHMAN, FRIENDS,
MISPERCEPTIONS, PARTY, PEERS, RUTGERS, SOBER

**Figure 7.3. The RU SURE Word Scramble.**

included the RU SURE Word Scramble. In addition, ads in newspapers and flyers were distributed with the RU SURE Word Scramble. In order to use the Word Scramble, AHC students were instructed to learn the word puzzle, to understand how it worked, and then to follow the steps for the particular activity (Walk About, Table Talk, or Coffee Break) where it would be used.

## Preparation Needed to Use the RU SURE Word Scramble

One of the most important parts of having a successful interpersonal inter-action was to make sure that the students engaging in that interaction on behalf of AHC were well prepared. For using the Word Scramble, they were given the following instructions developed by students who had used the Word Scramble in the pilot-testing phase of the activities:

- Do the Word Scramble.
- Learn how to explain the relevance of the references in the Word Scramble to the RU SURE Campaign message.
- Follow all of the instructions of the activity in which the Word Scramble is included.
- If it is going to be printed in the newspaper, find out the cost and make sure that CHI will provide the budget before making the commitment to the newspaper.
- Create a budget for what it will cost to make copies of the Word Scramble. Also, add to the budget RU SURE pens as give-aways with the Word Scramble.

## Potential Problems and Their Solutions

Based on the experiences of the AHC teams that pilot-tested the RU SURE Word Scramble, a chart was created to illustrate problems that might occur and provide solutions for them (see Table 7.4).

**Table 7.4   RU SURE Word Scramble Potential Problems and Solutions**

| PROBLEM | SOLUTION |
|---|---|
| Students do not seem to be interested. | Try attracting students by announcing that you have "free stuff" for them. |
| No one wants to take the time to do the Word Scramble. | Let them take it with them. Give them an RU SURE pen. |
| Your location doesn't seem inviting. | Try to see if you can move to another place that works better. |

# THE RU SURE VIDEO

## Description of the RU SURE Video

The RU SURE video is a 2-minute videotaped skit that uses humor and true-to-life college situations to convey the RU SURE Campaign's message of the realities of college drinking at Rutgers. The video was created by student members of CHI to be used as an educational tool targeting first-year college students at Table Talks and in classrooms.

## Implementation of the RU SURE Video

The RU SURE Video was designed to be used in residence halls or at the Table Talks or Walk Abouts that were conducted throughout the semester during which the RU SURE Campaign was run. Many of these included the RU SURE Video. The following instructions were given to students:

- Use effective methods to attract students. The video alone is not enough to draw students to a table, which is why the attitude of those staffing the table is extremely important. An upbeat, friendly, outgoing attitude is essential to attract students. Another method that can be used is going to each floor of the dorm with a box full of candy and handing it out to students who were in the lounges or in their rooms. (Each piece of candy had the RU SURE Campaign message attached.)

- Students can be shown the video and then given a short questionnaire about the video's content. Each student is "rewarded" for his or her participation with some type of merchandise—candy, RU SURE pens, magnets, or t-shirts.

## Preparation Needed to Use the Video

One of the most important parts of having a successful interpersonal interaction was to make sure that the students engaging in that interaction on behalf of AHC were well prepared. For using the video, they were given the following instructions developed by students who had created the video for the campaign:

- Obtain permission.

  **Table Talks:** Contact the Housing Department to reserve a table for your specified date.

  **Classrooms:** Contact the instructor of the course 2 weeks in advance to obtain permission to show the video during the class meeting. Ideally, the video should be shown to large, 100-level courses in order to target as many first-year students as possible.

- Obtain proper equipment.

  **Table Talks:** Contact the Housing Department 2 weeks before the Table Talk is to take place to insure that a television, VCR, and extension cord will be available.

  **Classrooms:** If the video cannot be projected (many lecture halls are "smart classrooms" that are equipped with the necessary apparatus), inform the instructor that a television, VCR, and extension cord will be needed on the day that the video is to be shown.

- Merchandise.

  **Table Talks:** The amount of merchandise you will need depends on the length of the Table Talk. Determine how much merchandise will be needed (i.e., pens, t-shirts, refrigerator magnets, keychains, etc.), obtain it from CHI, and bring it on the day of the activity.

  **Classrooms:** Because you will have a captive audience, merchandise is not necessary when using the video as part of a classroom discussion. However, if you choose to give away RU SURE Campaign merchandise in a classroom, ask the instructor how many students are in the class and plan accordingly.

- Double-check all reservations. Several days before the activity is to occur, contact the department or instructor to secure the date and time of your reservation.

## Potential Problems and Their Solutions

Based on the experiences of the AHC teams that pilot tested the RU SURE Video, a chart was created to illustrate problems that might occur and provide solutions for them (see Table 7.5).

Table 7.5   RU SURE Video and Potential Problems and Solutions

| PROBLEM | SOLUTION |
|---|---|
| Your location doesn't seem to attract attention. | Have a back-up plan of where to go. |
| Students do not seem to be interested. | Try attracting students by playing music. Also announce that you have "free stuff" for them. |
| Your team thought there would be the electric outlets you need but there are none. | See if you can get another space to play the video and use team members to attract students to that place. Or, just tell them about the video. |
| Poor equipment (e.g., bad sound quality/tracking/screen clarity). | Have a back-up plan of where to go. Test the equipment before use if possible—ask the instructor or the Housing Department when and where you can use the equipment before the Table Talk or classroom presentation. |

## RU SURE COFFEE BREAKS

### Description of the RU SURE Coffee Break

The RU SURE Coffee Break is an informal gathering in residence hall lounges hosted by AHC members where students are given coffee, cookies, and other snacks as well as materials on the RU SURE Campaign and the drinking norms at Rutgers.

### Implementation of the RU SURE Coffee Break

The RU SURE Coffee Break was designed to be used in residence halls throughout the semester during which a campaign was run. The Coffee Break was an alternative to the Walk About or Table Talk. It was an activity that could use the RU SURE Video, Bingo game, or Word Scramble, but could also just be used to generate informal discussion.

The following steps were developed to be implemented each time the RU SURE Coffee Break was used:

- Obtain permission from the resident advisors to come into a dorm on a certain evening and host a coffee break.
- Determine how many students are likely to be there and buy coffee and food accordingly.
- Prepare a budget and have CHI approve it prior to buying supplies.
- Determine what materials to give away and what activities (RU SURE Bingo or Word Scramble) to do. Remember: conversation with students is enough; no other activity is required.
- Be positive and upbeat, and go out to the first-year students to make them welcome.
- Clean up after the event and thank the resident advisor for access to the students.

## Preparation Needed to Use the RU SURE Coffee Break

One of the most important parts of having a successful interpersonal interaction was to make sure that the students engaging in that interaction on behalf of AHC were well prepared. For holding a Coffee Break, they were given the following set of instructions developed by students who had created the idea of the coffee break in the pilot-testing phase of the activities:

- Pick a date that works with all the team members' schedules.
- Get clearance on the date from the resident advisor and permission to be there.
- Create flyers and posters to advertise when you will be there and to invite students to participate.
- Make a budget for food and supplies and have it approved by CHI before buying anything.
- Buy food and coffee supplies and assign chores (e.g., making coffee, set up of refreshments and activities, clean up).
- On the day of the Coffee Break, arrive 15 minutes prior to the scheduled time in order to set up.

## Potential Problems and Their Solutions

Based on the experiences of the AHC teams that pilot-tested the Coffee Break, a chart was created to illustrate problems that might occur and provide solutions for them (see Table 7.6).

Table 7.6    RU SURE Coffee Break and Potential Problems
and Solutions

| PROBLEM | SOLUTION |
|---|---|
| People want coffee and want to take it and go. | Ask them to take flyers and talk to them for a few minutes. That's enough. |
| Students do not seem to be interested. | Try attracting students by announcing that you have "free stuff" for them. |
| Your team thought the location was a good one, but not many students are joining in for the game. | See if you can get some of the students who are playing to round up some other friends. |
| People ask questions you don't know how to answer. | See if another team member can. If not, get the person's e-mail and tell them you'll find out for them. And do! |

## CONCLUSION

These are the major interpersonally based strategies used to disseminate the message of the RU SURE Campaign. These strategies provide ways to carry the campaign messages to students and are mechanisms in which upper-class communication students get to talk to first-year students. As carriers of the campaign message, upper-class students have credibility that helps them get the message across to younger students.

It is recommended that all activities include data-collection mechanisms. Data-collection mechanisms include keeping track of how many people are encountered, how many items with the message are given out, and anecdotal data. In addition, surveys can be used to find out how effectively the message has been understood by the target audience (see Chapter 8 for a more detailed discussion of campaign evaluation strategies).

# 8

# CONTINUOUS EVALUATION
# OF THE CAMPAIGN

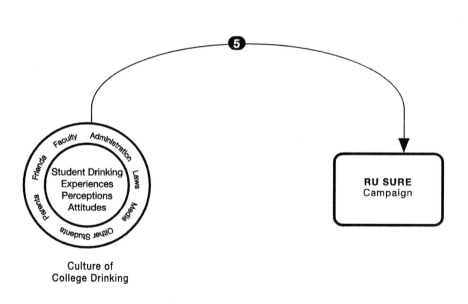

Figure 8.1. Step 5 of the Conceptual Model.

Health communication campaigns can be used to accomplish numerous beneficial goals. It is difficult to know, however, if these goals have been successfully met unless the campaign is evaluated in an appropriate manner. Successful evaluation efforts consist of three types of evaluations: formative, process, and outcome or summative evaluation (Witte et al., 2001). As illustrated in Fig. 8.1, the RU SURE Campaign was continuously evaluated and those evaluations led to further refinement of the campaign.

## FORMATIVE EVALUATION

*Formative evaluation* consists of testing campaign messages as they are being developed in order to make sure that they are applicable to the target audience. As discussed in Chapter 5, the RU SURE Campaign was developed with continuous input from undergraduate communication majors who were able to verify that the messages were "in the voice" of the students. In fact, all of the items in the *Top Ten Misperceptions at Rutgers* were suggested specifically by students, refined by the CHI team, and re-evaluated by students. In addition, input was obtained from university administrators concerned with specific areas (such as the dining halls and the bus system) to make sure that the messages did not offend them. Thus, all potential stakeholders in the campaign were consulted during the course of message development.

## PROCESS EVALUATION

*Process evaluation* involves collecting information during the campaign implementation that tracks the progress of the campaign and assures that the campaign is being conducted as designed. Table 8.1 lists the types of methods that were used to conduct a process evaluation of this campaign.

All facets of the campaign implementation were tracked. Table 8.2 summarizes campaign activities that were conducted for the first 4 years of the campaign. As an example of the scope of campaign activities, in the 2002–2003 academic year, for example, students in Advanced Health Communication who were responsible for implementing the campaign distributed 5,870 posters and flyers in first-year students' residence halls and high-traffic areas throughout the campus. Approximately 365 t-shirts and 3,500 additional giveaways all imprinted with the *Top Ten Misperceptions at Rutgers* messages were distributed to targeted first-year students and other

Table 8.1  Process Evaluation Components of the
RU SURE Campaign

| CAMPAIGN COMPONENT | FOCUS GROUP INTERVIEWS | DISTRIBUTION ANALYSIS | FREQUENCY TRACKING ANALYSIS | ARCHIVAL DATA |
|---|---|---|---|---|
| Media Campaign | | X | X | |
| Curriculum Infusion | X | | X | X |
| Peer-to-Peer Activities | X | X | X | |
| Web site | X | | | |
| Advisory Board | X | X | X | X |
| PR Campaign | X | X | X | X |

Table 8.2  Process Evaluation: Number of Events Held
and Artifacts Distributed

| EVENTS AND ARTIFACTS | YEAR 1 1999–2000 | YEAR 2 2000–2001 | YEAR 3 2001–2002 | YEAR 4 2002–2003 |
|---|---|---|---|---|
| Residence hall activities | 45 | 22 | 40 | 42 |
| Number of times first-year students participated | 3,800 | 3,250 | 3,050 | 6,500 |
| Posters and flyers | 6,872 | 9,484 | 1,300 | 5,870 |
| T-shirts | 600 | 1,000 | 200 | 365 |
| Give-aways | 3,000 | 3,000 | 2,300 | 3,500 |

members of the Rutgers community. In addition, approximately 6,500 students participated in 42 interpersonally based experiential learning activities that were held for first-year students during the 2002–2003 school year. Activities included coffee breaks in residence halls, facilitating experiential learning activities like RU SURE Bingo and the *RU SURE Game of Choices and Consequences* or doing Table Talks and Walk Abouts (see Chapter 7 for a discussion of these interpersonal interventions).

## OUTCOME OR SUMMATIVE EVALUATION

*Outcome evaluation* focuses on the effect a campaign has had on a target audience (Witte et al., 2001). All aspects of the RU SURE Campaign have been subjected to ongoing assessment including quantitative measures, such as the PRSP (Lederman et al., 1998) and the Core Survey (The Core Institute, 1996), and Intercept Interview Surveys (Stewart & Lederman, 2003) and qualitative assessments such as focus groups and debriefing interviews. Data have been gathered throughout the length of the campaign to determine its effectiveness in both raising awareness of this issue on campus, influencing students' misperceptions, and affecting students' behavior. Data include students' self-reports as well as environmental data such as number of alcohol-related arrests and amount of alcohol-related vandalism in the first-year residence halls. Table 8.3 summarizes the data-collection efforts that are discussed here.

### Table 8.3    Outcome Evaluation:
### Summary of Quantitative Data Collection

| DESCRIPTION OF INSTRUMENT | DATE | SAMPLE SIZE |
|---|---|---|
| The Core Survey | Spring 1999 | 529 |
| AHC Class Survey | Fall 1999 (September & December) | 15 (September); 11 (December) |
| RU SURE Bingo feedback form* | Fall 1999 | 327 |
| The Core Survey | Spring 2000 | 672 |

| DESCRIPTION OF INSTRUMENT | DATE | SAMPLE SIZE |
|---|---|---|
| AHC Class Survey | Spring 2000 (February & April) | 8 (February); 16 (April) |
| Intercept Interview Survey | Spring 2000 (February & April) | 206 (February); 72 (April) |
| AHC Class Survey | Fall 2000 (December) | 21 |
| Intercept Interview Survey | Fall 2000 (October & December) | 161 (October); 149 (December) |
| PRSP | Spring 2001 | 1,151 |
| The Core Survey | Spring 2001 | 571 |
| AHC Class Survey | Fall 2001 (September & December) | 15 (September); 16 (December) |
| Intercept Interview Survey | Fall 2001 (October & December) | 427 (October); 254 (December) |
| The Core Survey | Spring 2002 | 599 |
| AHC Class Survey | Spring 2002 (February) | 13 |
| Intercept Interview Survey | Spring 2002 (February) | 65 |
| AHC Class Survey | Fall 2002 (September & December) | 14 (September); 15 (December) |
| Intercept Interview Survey | Fall 2002 (October & December) | 508 (October); 450 (December) |
| The Core Survey | Spring 2003 | 536 |
| AHC Class Survey | Spring 2003 (February & April) | 24 (February); 19 (April) |
| Intercept Interview Survey | Spring 2003 (February & April) | 430 (February); 397 (April) |
| AHC Class Survey | Fall 2003 (September & December) | 23 (September); 22 (December) |
| Intercept Interview Survey | Fall 2003 (October & December) | 480 (October); 480 (December) |

*Discussed in Chapter 7

## Intercept Interviews

One of the most robust ways to assess the success of any health communication campaign is through the use of randomized, anonymous surveys. These surveys are often conducted through mailed questionnaires or telephone surveys. Care is taken to assure the randomness of the sample and that a large enough number of people respond to the survey to ensure reliable data analysis. Although they may be the "gold standard" of campaign evaluation, in the real world of research, they may not be practical or possible. In previous research, we determined that the mailed survey was not a practical way to reach our target audience. Because of their inconvenient location away from the residence halls, many Rutgers students infrequently check their campus mailboxes. Shared mailboxes also lead to potential problems with not receiving mail. Thus, we could not be sure that students would receive a mailed survey. Additionally, response rates to mailed surveys on our campus are often low.

Because our target audience members live in residence halls, other methods were sought to reach them in our data-collection efforts. Initially, we determined that a telephone survey could reach a random sample of our target population. To protect students' privacy, however, the university would not supply a list of student phone numbers, and it was deemed too time-consuming to comb through the student directory to isolate only the names of first-year students living in residence halls. In addition, many students now use their cell phones as their primary phones and are infrequently available via the telephone in their rooms.

To overcome these difficulties and still maintain the integrity of the evaluation process, we conducted a mailed survey (see the section on Personal Report of Student Perceptions discussed later in this chapter) but did not limit ourselves to this form of quantitative data collection. Additionally, we designed and implemented the Intercept Interview Survey methodology. Given the difficulty of gaining a substantial response rate from college students in a traditional mail survey, in the interests of obtaining a systematic sample of the target population, intercept interviews were conducted in first-year residence halls. Intercept surveys are most often used in market research to solicit information from members of a target population. Their key element is the ability to find and tap into systematically selected members of a target population with some immediacy. The Intercept Interview Survey (Stewart & Lederman, 2003) was created and pilot-tested as a means of reaching our target population. The intercept interview contained a short series of questions designed to assess the impact of the campaign on the drinking attitudes, perceptions, and behaviors of first-year students. Interviews were conducted by communication majors involved in the curriculum infusion component of the RU SURE Campaign to maximize the likelihood of responses to the interview because undergraduate students are often more willing to speak with other students than with either strangers or authority figures such as preceptors or faculty. It was decided that these students would be a good choice for administering the surveys owing to both their familiarity with the residence halls and the fact that they were not threatening to other students, perhaps reducing response bias. A survey consisting of questions to assess exposure to the campaign messages, comprehension of the messages, retention of the messages, and potential behavioral changes due to message exposure was developed.

*Training of Interviewers.* Students who were permitted to conduct the intercept interviews had to participate in a training program as part of the first phase of their preparation to work on the RU SURE Campaign (see Chapter 6 for more detail about the course in which they worked on the campaign). Along with the materials they were given to conduct the surveys, they were also trained in how to approach students, how to document any anecdotal data that might occur during the data-collection, and also in the ethics and seriousness of purpose of collecting these data. As part of the training, the instructor in the course worked with the students during the data–collection process, reviewing their data collection with them as it occurred, checking to make sure that the process was reliable.

*Sampling Protocol.* Intercept interviews were conducted at specified intervals and in diverse locations throughout the residence halls being studied (see Fig. 8.2 for a description). Once the interviewers entered the residence hall, they took positions in what seemed to be the most heavily traveled open area (e.g., a lounge, central hallway, by the door, etc.). To begin the interview administration, they approached the fifth (a number chosen at random) person they saw and asked him or her to participate in the research. Following this, they approached every third person and asked them to participate in the study. To ensure that students with various class schedules would have an equal opportunity to participate in the interview, administration occurred at three different time intervals: 9 a.m. to 2 p.m., 2 p.m. to 7 p.m., and 7 p.m. to midnight. Interviewers also followed standardized guidelines for approaching the target audience (contained in Fig. 8.2). Students were thoroughly trained prior to their involvement in the campaign and in data-collection efforts to ensure appropriate message dissemination and to avoid interviewer bias. (See Chapter 6 for a description of the training received by AHC students.)

It is extremely important to avoid bias in choosing the sample for your interviews. In other words, although it may seem easier to approach people who seem friendly, look like they would be willing to stop and talk with you, or are someone you know from previous work in the dorm, you should do everything that you can to prevent this from occurring. The best procedure for sampling from the target population of first-year students would be to interview a random sample of dorm residents. But, as you know, we are not permitted to knock on doors, so we are going to try to be as systematic as possible within the limitations we face.

In order to do this, the class will be divided into teams who will enter the dorms during randomly assigned time periods. These time periods have been chosen throughout the day and evening to reflect the fact that not all students enter and leave their residence halls at the same time. It is important that you visit the dorm you are assigned during the specified time period. If you cannot do this, please notify an instructor and get assigned a new time.

Once you enter your assigned residence hall, take a position in what seems to be the most heavily trafficked open area (in other words, a lounge, central hallway, by the door, etc.). Then count the first four people that you see in that area and do not approach them. You should approach the fifth person you see and ask him or her to participate in the research. Follow the instructions you have been given for approaching participants. Then approach every third person that you see and ask them to participate in the study. If two people pass you at the same time, only interview the person who fits the "every third person" criteria. If it seems awkward to you to only interview one person, you can let the other person fill out the survey, but make sure you mark it in some way so that it can be discarded later on.

This procedure may seem cumbersome to you, but it is very important to follow so that we can have some faith in the reliability of our data. It is always important to collect data in a systematic manner so that we can have confidence in the statistical analyses that we will perform.

**Figure 8.2.   Instructions to Intercept Interviewers.**

***Results.*** During one semester, results of the intercept interviews ($n$ = 127) indicated that 74% of the respondents were aware of the campaign. Sixty one percent of the students accurately completed the phrase, "According to the RU SURE Campaign, X out of 3 Rutgers students stop at 3 or fewer drinks" by indicating the number "2," and 55% ($n = 114$) correctly completed the phrase, "According to the RU SURE materials: X in 5 don't drink at all" by indicating the number "1." When asked what the message of the RU SURE Campaign was, 72% ($n = 148$) accurately responded that the message was that "everyone at [this university] doesn't drink dangerously, and you don't have to either." When asked how often they have seen or heard about the RU SURE Campaign, 35% ($n = 72$) reported they have heard about it "often," 27% ($n = 56$) "some," 18% ($n = 37$) "very often," 10% ($n = 21$) "not at all," and 9% ($n = 19$) "not very often." Less than 1% ($n = 1$) did not answer this question.

As discussed in detail in Chapter 5, the RU SURE Campaign had two key messages: "Two out of three Rutgers students stop at three or fewer drinks," and "one in five don't drink at all." The main point of the messages is to convey the idea that not everyone at Rutgers drinks dangerously. The intended implication for first-year students is that dangerous drinking is not the norm. In asking about retention and comprehension of campaign messages, the Intercept Interview Survey was designed to look for first-year students' accurate recall and comprehension.

When asked what the message of the RU SURE Campaign is, 72% ($n = 148$) responded accurately that the message was that "everyone at Rutgers doesn't drink dangerously, and you don't have to either," 13% ($n = 26$) responded that they did not know the message, 8% ($n = 16$) thought the message was that "Rutgers students should not drink alcohol," 6% ($n = 13$) thought the message was that "many students at Rutgers drink dangerously," and 2% ($n = 3$) reported knowing the campaign message.

To determine the most effective message channels, a question was included that asked students to indicate where they learned the statistics about drinking on campus. Table 8.4 summarizes the various media that students have attended to during several runs of the campaign. As can be seen from these data, print channels such as posters and flyers are more likely to catch students' attention and, thus, be worthy of investing campaign resources in developing. One reason for the appeal of these posters is the amount of effort that was expended in developing a message in the voice of the students (see Chapter 4 and 5 for more discussion of the necessity for obtaining student input in all phases of campaign design). T-shirts are also memorable carriers of the campaign message.

Because we were concerned about the credibility of the campaign message, students were queried about their perceptions of the effectiveness of the campaign message. When asked if they thought the RU SURE Campaign would influence students' drinking-related behavior, 43% ($n = 88$) thought it would, 51% ($n = 104$) reported that they did not think it would, and 7% ($n = 14$) did not respond to the question.

Table 8.4    Percentage of Students Who Learned About RU SURE
Campaign Message Through Various Media

| MEDIA | SPRING 2000 (N = 206) | FALL 2000 (N = 149) | FALL 2002 (N = 450) |
|---|---|---|---|
| Posters & flyers in residence halls | 70% | n/a | 63% |
| Posters & flyers on campus | 29% | 18% | 31% |
| T-shirt | 17% | 33% | 35% |
| Candy bar | 3% | 1% | 2% |
| Coffee mug | 2% | 0 | 4% |
| Knight Express (debit) Card | 1% | 0 | 2% |
| RU SURE Bingo night | 10% | 1% | 6% |
| Ad in student newspaper | 16% | 7% | 17% |
| Word of mouth | 11% | 19% | 17% |
| Other | 7% | 17% | 9% |

*Note:* Percentages add up to more than 100% because students were
instructed to check multiple media sources if applicable.

Follow-up, open-ended responses from students who indicated that
they thought the campaign *would* influence their drinking were categorized
into three major themes:

1.  Increases awareness (e.g., "allows people to know that not
    everyone drinks," "It makes you aware that the word of mouth
    by a certain group of people isn't the word of mouth for all
    33,500 students at [this university]," "constant reminders").
2.  Decreases peer pressure (e.g., "Many [students] drink because
    others are, and if they know how many don't drink excessively
    or don't drink at all, they might want to follow that behavior,"
    "Because students will understand that not everyone else
    drinks and they don't have to drink to fit in," "People who are
    intimidated by 'partying' will know it's not necessarily the
    norm").

3. Reinforcement for students who have made a healthy decision (e.g., "Because students may see the statistics and see that they are not a minority in not drinking," "It shows you aren't alone if you don't drink").

Follow-up, open-ended responses from students who indicated that they thought the campaign *would not* influence their drinking were categorized into five major themes:

1. Students don't change (e.g., "because people are going to drink no matter what," "By this point, there is not much a flyer or spokesperson can say that will stop someone from drinking," "People come to college with their ideals instilled, the posters won't change a thing").
2. Students don't attend to messages (e.g., "Most people don't pay attention to these types of campaigns," "No one really reads them [posters]").
3. Statistics are not credible (e.g., "because people lie on these surveys to make themselves look sober," "statistics don't seem true").
4. Students are not affected by peer pressure (e.g., "If people don't want to drink, they won't. If they want to, they will. Peer pressure is never really a factor").
5. Drinking is a way to have fun (e.g., "because students will always look for ways to 'have fun' and drinking is their solution," "People drink either because it's a good way of social gathering or because it feels good to be drunk").

## Core Surveys[1]

The Core Alcohol and Drug Survey (available from The Core Institute located at Southern Illinois University at Carbondale) has been used nationally since 1990 to "assess the nature, scope, and consequences of students' drug and alcohol use, as well as students' awareness of relevant policies"

---

[1]The administration of the Core Alcohol and Drug Survey each year is made possible, in part, by funding from the New Jersey Higher Education Consortium on Alcohol and Other Drug Prevention and Education supported by the New Jersey Department of Health and Senior Services. The Core Survey was not administered before the campaign was begun and is, thus, not included in the discussion of baseline data collection in Chapter 2.

(The Core Institute, 2003). This survey is an additional quantitative tool used to assess the effectiveness of the RU SURE Campaign and is administered each year in the spring semester. Table 8.5 presents a summary of the results of data from the Core Survey for the first five years of the RU SURE Campaign.

Because one of the major goals of the campaign was to decrease students' misperceptions of the drinking norms on campus it was important to assess the effectiveness of these efforts. The Core Survey provided data that support the contention that the RU SURE Campaign was effective in meeting this goal. As can be seen from Table 8.5, first-year students' misperceptions of others' high levels of drinking have decreased in the following ways: (a) students' perception of the percentage of students who drink dangerously (had five or more drinks in a row) decreased from 53.9% in 1999 to 46.4% in 2003 (a 13.9% difference) and (b) students' perception of the average number of alcoholic drinks they think others consume was reduced from 5.9 in 1999 to 5.0 in 2003 (a 15.3% decrease). In addition, examining data collected after the first year of the campaign revealed that the perceived norm for the frequency of other students' use of alcohol decreased from "three times a week" to "once a week."

Although the data reported in Table 8.5 reveal that the percentage of students who drink dangerously (have five or more drinks in a row) has not

Table 8.5   Summary of Core Survey Data for First-Year Students

|  | 1999 | 2000 | 2001 | 2002 | 2003 |
|---|---|---|---|---|---|
| Percentage of students who had five or more drinks in a row in the past 2 weeks | 42.6 | 54.1 | 46.4 | n/a | 42.7 |
| Percentage of students who thought other students had five or more drinks in a row in the past 2 weeks | 53.9 | 60.8 | 42.4 | n/a | 46.4 |
| Average number of alcoholic drinks consumed at parties and bars | 3.9 | 4.6 | 3.4 | n/a | 3.6 |
| Average number of alcoholic drinks they think others consumed at parties and bars | 5.9 | 5.9 | 4.4 | n/a | 5 |

decreased, the average number of alcoholic drinks students consume at parties and in bars has decreased. This result is not surprising since the RU SURE Campaign is not designed for high-risk drinkers. (Prevention and treatment efforts for high-risk drinkers are discussed in Chapter 12.) In addition, there is no measure of campaign awareness included in this survey. Thus, from these data it is not possible to determine if the students are aware of the campaign or not. Therefore, this survey should be seen as a measure of general campus climate (the culture of college drinking) and not necessarily as a specific measure of the campaign's effect on the target audience.

Additional examination of the Core data yields some other interesting results. For example, an analysis of the Core data comparing students' perceptions and behaviors in Spring 2000 (after the first year of the campaign) versus Spring 2001 indicate some of the effects of the campaign. Alcohol use for first-year students decreased in the following ways:

- The median frequency use of alcohol decreased from "once a week" to "twice a month."
- The actual norm for alcohol use decreased from "once a week" to "twice a month."
- Although males report a higher amount of alcohol consumption, both male and female students report a similar percentage decrease in the amount of alcohol they drank. Males' average number of alcoholic drinks decreased from 7.5 to 5.3 (a 29.3% reduction); females decreased from 3.5 to 2.5 (a 28.6% reduction).

## Personal Report of Student Perceptions[2]

As discussed in Chapter 2, the PRSP was developed by Rutgers researchers to assess students' alcohol attitudes, perceptions, and use (Lederman et al., 1998). Results of the administration of the PRSP in Spring 1998 are described in Chapter 2 and were used as baseline data. The PRSP was administered again in Spring 2000 to help assess the effectiveness of the RU SURE Campaign in influencing students' alcohol-related attitudes, perceptions, and behaviors.

One of the RU SURE Campaign messages is that two out of three Rutgers students stop at three or fewer drinks when they drink. In 2000, 60.6% of students reported that they had had three or fewer drinks on the last occasion in which they drank alcohol. Thus, their drinking behavior is

---

[2]The development and administration of the PRSP was funded, in part, by a grant from the Rutgers University Health Services.

consistent with campaign messages. In addition, 29.3% report that they have reduced their consumption of alcohol in the previous year.

The RU SURE Campaign is designed, in part, to communicate to students that not everyone on campus drinks dangerously. One component of this message is changing the culture of college drinking so that students do not feel that the social atmosphere on campus promotes drinking dangerously. The campaign has demonstrated some success in this effort. The percentage of students who believe that the social atmosphere on campus promotes drinking decreased from 48.3% in 1998 to 44.5% in 2000. Although this perception is far from ideal, it does demonstrate a trend in the desired direction.

The most startling finding from the 2000 PRSP was the increase in abstainers. In 1998, 18% of the students reported that they were "nondrinkers," whereas in 2000, 30% of the students claimed that they did not drink. We are somewhat suspicious of this finding, however. Focus groups and individual interviews conducted with students reveal that many students consider themselves to be "nondrinkers" if they consume very moderate quantities of alcohol occasionally (such as at weddings or parties). Thus, further research is needed to more accurately assess the true level of students on campus who refrain from drinking at all. This finding does provide evidence, however, that there is a need for understanding the language that students actually use in conceptualizing their drinking-related behavior.

## CONCLUSION

Evaluation is an important part of any prevention campaign. It is important to assess the perceptions of the target audience during the development of the campaign messages (formative evaluation), to track the progress of the campaign implementation (process evaluation), and to evaluate the effectiveness of the campaign messages in bringing about the desired results (outcome or summative evaluation). The RU SURE Campaign progressed through its design, development, and implementation while undergoing each of these evaluative processes. In this way, the campaign designers were able to develop a campaign that was consistent with students' values and attitudes while communicating the desired message about the misperception of dangerous drinking norms on campus. Thus, the success of the campaign (measured by outcome or summative evaluation) is due, in part, to a careful consideration of students' input during campaign design phases (assessed through formative evaluation) as well as successful implementation of the message dissemination strategies (tracked through process evaluation).

# 9

## UNANTICIPATED RESULTS

### THE IMPACT OF CAMPAIGN MESSAGES
### ON THE MESSENGERS[1]

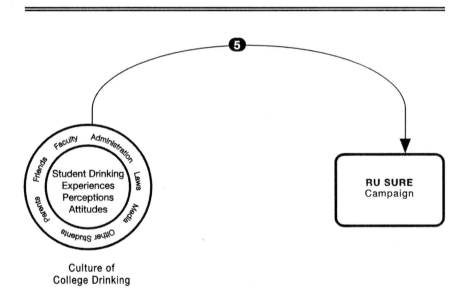

Figure 9.1.    Step 5 of the Conceptual Model.

[1]An earlier version of this chapter appeared, in part, in *Qualitative Research Reports* (Lederman, Stewart, & Golubow, 2002).

As illustrated in Fig. 9.1, the RU SURE Campaign was continuously evaluated and those evaluations led to further refinement of the campaign. One of the ways in which evaluation took place was to examine the impact of the campaign on the campaign workers themselves, to examine the impact of the messages on the messengers.

Perkins (1997) described the students who spread the misperceptions about college drinking to one another as the *carriers* of misperceptions. In changing the culture of college drinking at Rutgers, we have created a different kind of carrier. We call them the *messengers.* Students in AHC working on the campaign are the campaign messengers. They spread the campaign message, "You don't have to drink a lot to fit in at Rutgers," to their peers. They talk about it to first-year students. They even are challenged, in some of the interpersonal interactions described in Chapter 7, to talk about misperceptions with some of the very carriers themselves, some of those who believe that everyone drinks excessively and that the campaign message is not believable.

One student in AHC in Spring 2003, for example, told a story about leading the game, RU SURE Bingo, and having one of the people who played the game say to everyone after the game, "It's not true. Where'd they get those stats? Everyone that I know drinks a lot more." The AHC student began to answer him when another student in the audience stood up, quoting campaign statistics, "One in five don't drink," he said. "Do the math. There are five of us in this circle, and I don't drink. I'm the one in five!" The AHC student reported the incident when she came to "work" at AHC the following day. She added, "Some of these kids even help me to believe the message more."

Beyond the RU SURE Campaign's success in reducing misperceptions about the norms of dangerous drinking on campus among the target audience (discussed in Chapter 8 and illustrated in the example just given), there have also been effects on the students who worked on the campaign. These students consistently report positive effects as a result of working in AHC and creating and disseminating campaign messages (see Chapter 6 for a complete description of AHC). In effect, this means that the students served both as messengers for others and as influences on themselves and on one another.

Although this was not the intent of the campaign, it was a desirable additional outcome and led to some intriguing new questions. After we began to notice students in AHC talk about the impact of their experience on their own attitudes, we began to systematically collect quantitative data from students who next took the course and ran the campaign and, also, to design a purposive qualitative study for the end of the next semester in which the campaign was run. All AHC students completed pre- and postexperience questionnaires and also were invited to participate in group interviews about the RU SURE Campaign with trained interviewers. The method used with these participants is a variation on the focus group referred to as the debriefing interview (Lederman, 1992, 1995). This chapter presents the initial anecdotal findings and describes the quantitative and qualitative study that were undertaken to examine them further.

## ANECDOTAL EVIDENCE SUGGESTS IMPACT OF CAMPAIGN ON CAMPAIGN WORKERS

Each semester, the students who work in AHC comment about the effects of the RU SURE Campaign on them and how it changes them. They often remark on the ways in which they drink differently or think about drinking. They even comment on the ways in which they see their friends and others drinking, and how often they find themselves saying things to their friends about their drinking that they never would have said before taking the course and working on the campaign.

This reaction to participation in the campaign has been observed since students first began working in AHC. Students in AHC who implemented the RU SURE Campaign during the first two semesters it was run, provided anecdotal evidence of this impact when asked at the end of each of those semesters to complete an anonymous questionnaire that included the question, "How, if at all, have your attitudes changed as a result of working on the campaign?" Their responses fell into two different categories: (a) their perceptions of others as a result of working on the campaign and (b) their perceptions of themselves.

## Perceptions of Others

In terms of their perceptions of others, students responded on the questionnaire by reporting things like:

*I now know that everyone is not drinking and that many things that are the "norm" may actually be what the people around me are doing.*

*I've noticed more people don't drink that I thought were drinking.*

*I realize how many students do not drink. I also realize how much misperceptions had previously affected my beliefs.*

*Yes, I am definitely more observant of my peers in drinking situations.*

*I am aware that not everyone drinks on campus—something I really did not believe. I am much more aware of people drinking either not at all or just in small quantity.*

*I have noticed the number of people around me that do not drink.*

All of these responses have in common the changes in the perceptions of the AHC students in terms of the environmental reality in which they existed. Because data on other surveys at Rutgers indicated that students often perceived the environment to foster drinking (Lederman et al., 1998), working on the campaign clearly created a different sense of their reality for these students.

The second category into which AHC students' comments were divided was comments about themselves.

## Comments about Themselves

In these responses students reflected on their own drinking behaviors. They responded with statements like:

*Drinking has decreased drastically.*

*My drinking habits have been greatly reduced since the beginning of this course.*

*I do not drink dangerously anymore.*

*Yes, I am more conscious of my drinking behavior.*

*My attitudes toward my own drinking behavior have not fundamentally changed, but I am much more aware and pay more attention now—being more conscious of binge drinking.*

*This class has encouraged me to continue to practice abstinence from drinking.*

*This class has made me realize that I do drink a little too much.*

These responses were consistent with findings on the Intercept Interview Survey (Stewart & Lederman, 2003) that is used each semester as a postcourse survey. The Intercept Interview Survey is a short questionnaire created to assess students' drinking-related behaviors and perceptions. (See Chapter 8 for a detailed discussion of the instrument and its creation.) For example, during one semester, AHC students' dangerous drinking (defined as having five or more drinks in a row on one occasion) decreased by 26% from their reported drinking levels prior to taking the course.

## SYSTEMATIC EVALUATION IMPACT ON THE SECONDARY TARGET AUDIENCE

It was the anecdotal data as well as the responses to the Intercept Interview Survey that led to more systematic data collection as the campaign continued and new groups of students entered AHC. The impact on students of participating in the campaign design, development, implementation, and evaluation was measured quantitatively and qualitatively. At the beginning of AHC and at the end of the course, all students completed anonymous surveys in which they reported their drinking-related attitudes, behaviors, and perceptions. Data from these instruments gave some measure of students' self-reported attitudinal and behavioral changes. Additionally, to gain more insight into the impact of the course, the course ended with a set of group interviews with students who had participated in AHC.

### Survey Measures

At the beginning and ending of the course, AHC students completed the same surveys that were used to evaluate campaign effectiveness with the target audience (Intercept Interview Survey). Table 9.1 contains a summary of data from these surveys in response to two questions: (a) The last time you drank alcohol, how many drinks did you have? and (b) In the past 30 days, on those occasions when you drank alcohol, how many drinks did you have? These questions were asked specifically to determine the average number of drinks consumed during a typical month and the amount consumed on the last drinking occasion. As can be seen from these data, in most semesters, students' reported use of alcohol decreased during the semester that they participated in AHC.

**Table 9.1.  Changes in Reported Drinking by Students in Advanced Health Communication (mean number of drinks)**

| SEMESTER | The last time you drank alcohol, how many drinks did you have? | | In the past 30 days, on those occasions when you drank alcohol, how many drinks did you have? | |
|---|---|---|---|---|
|  | PRETEST | POSTTEST | PRETEST | POSTTEST |
| Fall 1999 (*N* = 15, 11) | 3.6 | 4.0 | n/a | n/a |
| Spring 2000 (*N* = 8, 16) | 4.9 | 4.4 | n/a | n/a |
| Fall 2001 (*N* = 15, 16) | 8.1 | 2.8 | 6.7 | 2.9 |
| Spring 2002 (*N* = 13) | 5.5 | n/a | 4.2 | n/a |
| Fall 2002 (*N* = 14, 15) | 5.1 | 4.9 | 4.9 | 4.5 |
| Spring 2003 (*N* = 24, 19) | 2.9 | 3.2 | 3.1 | 2.9 |
| Fall 2003 (*N* = 23) | 4.4 | n/a | 4.4 | n/a |

## Debriefing Interviews

At the end of the semester, group interviews were conducted with students who had participated in AHC. Initially it was thought that focus group techniques could be used. The focus group interview (Calder, 1977; Greenbaum, 1994; Herndon, 2001; Lederman, 1983b, 1990, 1995, 1999; Merton, Fiske, & Kendall, 1952; Morgan, 1988) is an in-depth, group interview in which participants are selected because they are a purposive, although not necessarily representative, sampling of a specific population.

The method is most effectively used when the research question necessitates finding out something about "what" people think and feel, "how" they act, and/or the "why" behind their behaviors. Members of focus groups are selected on criteria designed to assure that they share commonalities related to the topic and, therefore, can feel secure in discussing their thoughts or feelings with others like themselves. Participants do not know one another before the groups. The groups are strangers who meet, talk about a subject they have in common, and create bonds and synergy around that common denominator (Lederman, 1992). Because all of the participants in the groups conducted after AHC were students in the same class and were therefore not anonymous to one another, it became clear that traditional focus groups could not be used effectively (Herndon, 2001; Lederman, 1983b; Morgan, 1988).

Another type of group interview that has great potential as a source of qualitative data collection is the debriefing interview (Lederman, 1992, 1995; Pearson & Smith, 1986; Stewart, 1992; Tesch, 1977). The debriefing interview traces its roots historically to military campaigns and war games. Debriefing interviews took place after a mission or exercise when participants were brought together to describe what had occurred, to account for the actions that they had taken, and to develop new strategies as a result of the experience. In more contemporary times, debriefing interviews include debriefings of hostages and other crisis victims and the extensive use of debriefing techniques in classrooms as part of the post-hoc discussions of experiential learning activities (Stewart, 1992).

The debriefing interview is a stepwise interview following an experience in which the interviewer guides those who have been through the experience in a reflective discussion and analysis of that experience and its meanings (Lederman, 1995). It is a purposive and planned data collection method. It is a structured, post-hoc interview comprised of guided recall, reflection, and analysis. It can take place immediately following an experience or anytime thereafter. The interview technique is based on two assumptions. First, that the experience has had some meaning for the participants and second, that discussion of that experience can provide insight into its meaning and impact for the participants and for the interviewer. In a review of the literature on debriefing, Lederman (1992) found that the technique is used as a stepwise process with questions that address three phases: (a) reflection on the experience, (b) interpretation of the meanings of those reflections, and (c) applications/implications of the meanings.

The debriefing interview is distinguished from other group interviews in two ways. First, the single criterion for participant selection is that participants have information about the topic that comes from their own experience. Second, that the focus of the discussion is post hoc—on what has previously occurred (Lederman, 1995; Stewart, 1992). (For more about debriefing interviews, see Chapter 10.)

## A QUALITATIVE STUDY TO EXPLORE
## THE ANECDOTAL FINDINGS

### Procedures

Given the purposes of and criteria for conducting debriefing group interviews, they were selected as the technique for the group interviews of students in AHC. At the end of the course, students participated in these group interviews (Lederman, 1995) and filled out a short-essay response. The only selection criterion for the debriefing interview was that participants had taken the course and participated in the RU SURE Campaign implementation.

The debriefing group interviews were conducted to explore the participants' own experiences in addressing the subject of dangerous drinking on campus. The participants were divided into two groups. Graduate students who were trained by the authors conducted groups, using a debriefing guide created by a team of researchers including alcohol prevention specialists, communication researchers, and health educators. The debriefing guide began with a question that asked participants to recall their perceptions of the campaign and its impact on members of the target audience. The interview ended with a question to which participants were asked to provide individual written responses followed by semi-structured discussion. This question asked participants to reveal their perceptions of the impact of participation in the campaign on their own attitudes and behaviors. These questions were derived from the earlier data collection in which students had reported anecdotally about their experiences and changes in perceptions and behaviors.

All groups were taperecorded. Participants were informed that their identities would be kept in confidence. To accomplish this, specific names were removed from the summary transcripts of the tapes. To assure students that they could be candid without worrying about the impact on their grades, the course instructors did not conduct the interviews. Furthermore, the tapes of the interviews were not analyzed until after the course and course grading had been completed. Transcripts were analyzed using a constant comparison method (Strauss & Corbin, 1998) to identify emergent themes. These themes are the basis for the findings from the debriefing group interviews discussed in the next section.

## Findings

The themes that emerged are divided into two parts for discussion: (a) interview participants' perceptions of the campaign's impact on the target audience—impact on others and (b) interview participants' perceptions of how working on the campaign affected their own perceptions, attitudes, and behaviors—impact on self.

*Part 1: Impact on Others.* Some participants reported success in getting first-year students to understand the RU SURE Campaign message. These participants attributed their success to the experiential learning activities and artifacts that helped gain students' attention. Other factors contributing to their successful interactions with first-year students included their belief that communication majors could relate "on the same level" to the target audience because they were not professionals, teachers, or parents. Additionally, some participants stressed that the campaign message was not "anti-drinking" but "anti-dangerous drinking" which helped establish a realistic, trusting rapport with first-year students.

Several themes emerged regarding student drinking as perceived by the participants. These themes included first-year students' anxiety regarding assimilating or "fitting in" to campus life, peer pressure, level of self-esteem, and lack of prior education (e.g., in high school) about campus life/drinking before entering college. Most participants felt the RU SURE Campaign was effective in helping create more awareness about the misperceptions regarding college drinking. However, despite the campaign's perceived effectiveness in dispelling these misperceptions, several participants expressed reservations about the impact of the campaign on students' drinking behavior with comments such as "Hard to stop behavior, but bombardment of message may get them to think about their behavior with friends" and "Going into the dorms, the majority did get the message, but not sure how much behavioral change will occur."

These comments reveal the effective outcome that communication majors believe the RU SURE Campaign message had on heightening the awareness of first-year students about the social misconceptions of college drinking. They reported that this knowledge could, despite the contrary remarks by some participants, ultimately bring about a positive behavioral change and attitude towards drinking among students.

*Part 2: Impact on Self.*    At the conclusion of each debriefing interview the participants were asked to briefly write, in their own words, how the campaign and working on it had affected their own drinking-related perceptions and behaviors. This question generated detailed and heartfelt responses. For example, comments such as these were made illustrating a feeling of responsibility toward educating and being a role model for first-year students:

> *I had a crucial role to play in this campaign, and it was great to know that I could get out into the dorms and get this message out and also have complete knowledge about what I was talking about.*

Participants also wrote about how working directly on the RU SURE Campaign with the target audience dramatically affected their understanding of college drinking, as well as their own behavior during four years spent at college, as for example:

*It wasn't until this class that I noticed I was in a "bubble." All my friends were the drinkers and I didn't notice how many people didn't drink and accepted them for the first time as who they were.*

*So much of my own time and effort has been put into learning about the campaign, developing and refining activities, and inter-action with the students that I can't help but think about it in relation to my own drinking behaviors.*

Working on the RU SURE Campaign enabled individuals to take a closer look at the actual socialization process behind the myths surrounding college drinking. It is also clear that once participants started working directly with-in the campaign and interacting with a target audience to dispel mispercep-tions about levels of college drinking, it was difficult not to reflect on per-sonal drinking behaviors, self-images, social surroundings, and interperson-al relationships. Educating others and being peer role models also provided a sense of positive meaning and self-image or identity for several AHC members.

This data collection resulted in findings that indicated both quantita-tively and qualitatively that participation in the course, as well as design and implementation of the campaign, had an effect on students' perceptions and behaviors. Group interviews provided insight into why these changes were being reported. When participants were asked to anonymously write how this campaign has influenced them, one student wrote:

*I now know that everyone is not drinking and that many things that are the "norm" may actually be what the people around me are doing.*

Another student expressed it this way:

*I take note of people who drink and quantities. I feel more and more that drinking in excess is very unattractive and immature.*

In the debriefing group interview, one participant explained:

*When I first started on this campaign, I found it hard to believe the statistics because most of my "night life" revolves around the*

*bar scene or drinking. But when I actually started to pay atten-
tion to my surroundings, I realized that a lot of people did go to
a party or bar to socialize, not drink. A lot of people did stop at 3
or fewer [drinks], as the statistics showed.*

Working on the RU SURE Campaign enabled individuals to take a closer look at the actual socialization process behind the myths surrounding college drinking. Thus, the course met its educational goals by helping students
to learn about communication and health campaigns. It met additional goals
by allowing students to confront their own thinking and drinking.

## LESSONS LEARNED

Involving students in a dangerous-drinking prevention campaign apparent-
ly has an unanticipated benefit: the impact on students' own drinking-related perceptions and behaviors. By using survey instruments and the debriefing interview technique, it was possible to explore this impact. The surveys
marked some of the specific changes in their drinking behaviors and perceptions. The interviews allowed for more in-depth understanding about how
and why those changes occurred.

In the interviews, students were in groups with fellow students who
had gone through the experience of working for AHC together. As a consequence, they were debriefed together, allowing them to share their experiences with one another. The comfort of the group allowed the participants
to talk about their shared experiences and perceptions. Inclusion of individual, written responses allowed them the freedom and privacy to reveal
information about themselves. Students reported insights into the impact of
the campaign on the target audience and even more interestingly, on themselves. The messengers were affected by the messages. Perhaps the most
important finding was that the experience of disseminating messages to
other students and talking about the campaign to them was transformative
for AHC students.

Finally, one of the themes that came up in the group interviews was
about the ways the RU SURE Campaign affected students' behavior with
their friends and families. Students described themselves as talking about
the course and the campaign to roommates and significant others. They
said they felt appalled when they discovered how ignorant some of these
people were about drinking. As one student put it, "then I realized that
before working on the campaign I thought so, too. I guess I had a lot to
learn."

## CONCLUSION

The debriefing interview is most often used in classrooms to help students process experiential activities. This chapter described the use of debriefing interviews in their more historical usage: to learn from participants about experiences through their insights and in their own eyes. Using these interviews as a means of qualitative data collection is a source of otherwise potentially less accessible insights. As a consequence of these insights, we have been able to design ways to involve more students in the dissemination process of the RU SURE Campaign as a way of helping them to have the transformative experiences that many of the students in this study reported.

In prevention campaigns it is always important to examine the dosage necessary to get the message out. In the RU SURE Campaign we learned a great deal about the effects of continuous exposure to the message and examination of it from the campaign messengers. The message was solid. It was based on real evidence. The campaign workers compared the messages with their everyday experiences, in their social interactions, and the message became more believable to them. The impact on these campaign workers as they compared the message to what they experienced in their everyday interactions was a good example of the ways in which socially situated experiential learning takes place (Lederman & Stewart, 1998). These students experienced the campaign messages and believed them more as time went by and as they used their own experiences to test out the messages. It is our contention that the same thing happens over time to the target audience, so long as we get them the message and get it to them often enough and coming from sources they trust.

# 10

## THE RU SURE GAME OF CHOICES
## AND CONSEQUENCES

### A ONE-HOUR BRIEF INTERVENTION ALCOHOL
### DECISION-MAKING TOOL

As illustrated in Fig. 10.1, the RU SURE Campaign was continuously refined as a result of its evaluation (described in Chapter 9). Refinement included the creation of additional materials. This chapter describes in detail one of the interventions, the *RU SURE Game of Choices and Consequences*, that grew out of the campaign.

Fundamental to the approach of the entire RU SURE Campaign is the belief that it is necessary to understand the manner in which individuals or groups for whom prevention programs are being designed acquire information about substance use (Lederman et al., 2003; Stewart & Lederman, 2002). Equally important is the manner in which that information is integrated into the behavioral repertoire of individuals. In essence, the approach taken in the campaign is based in the belief that it is important to examine the relationship between information and behavior. Thus, as discussed in Chapter 3, the RU SURE Campaign is rooted in, and built on, fundamental principles of traditional learning theory and also informed by experiential learning theorists who posit that much of what we learn comes from our experiences and our reflections on those experiences (Dewey, 1929; Kolb, 1984; Lederman, 1991). This perspective underlies the SSEL model (Lederman & Stewart, 1998) that guides and informs all of the prevention efforts that we have undertaken at Rutgers. It is what distinguishes our campaigns from many other prevention efforts.

This chapter focuses on one specific prevention tool developed as an outcome of the evaluation of the implementation of the RU SURE Campaign to encourage structured, guided interactions about alcohol use

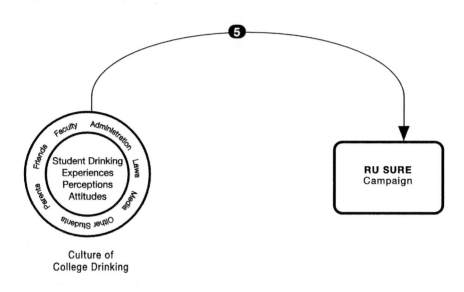

**Figure 10.1. Step 5 of the Conceptual Model.**

among college students. It is the *RU SURE Game of Choices and Consequences* (Lederman, Powell, Stewart, Goodhart, & Laitman, 2001), a 1-hour brief intervention comprised of a simulation of college students' alcohol-related decisions and guided, structured, reflective discussion of those decisions. The *RU SURE Game of Choices and Consequences* was created at Rutgers and is currently used at more than 50 other institutions as a tool in prevention efforts on campus.

## BACKGROUND

Over the last decade, and especially over the last several years, there has been massive growth in college prevention programs designed to reduce dangerous drinking (Milgram & Anderson, 2000). A thorough review of individually oriented interventions with adequate evaluation designs was conducted for the NIAAA (2002) task force on college drinking, which concluded that the most effective individually oriented practices to be implemented on campuses are brief motivational or skills-based interventions targeting high-risk students. A major advantage of brief interventions is that they are cost-effective and, thus, can reach large numbers of people. Therefore, even programs with small individual effects can have an overall large effect on society.

One form of brief intervention used at Rutgers as an outgrowth of the RU SURE Campaign and its findings is alcohol simulation games. Simulation games are working models of reality or some aspect of reality, designed so that participants in the simulation can discover for themselves their own behavioral choices and the consequences of those choices (Lederman, 1992; Tansey, 1971). They are potentially effective brief interventions for use in the prevention of alcohol abuse with a random selection of students, including but not exclusive to those who are high-risk drinkers. Like other brief motivational interventions, simulation interventions focus on helping students understand their decision-making processes and how to self-regulate their behaviors. This chapter describes one simulation of college drinking-related decisions, the *RU SURE Game of Choices and Consequences,* and its utility for both prevention efforts and for collection of behavioral data.

## BRIEF HISTORY OF SIMULATION GAMES

Simulation games have a long, interdisciplinary history, tracing as far back, depending on one's definition, to medieval times and the creation of the game of chess to teach warring strategies (Tansey, 1971). Simulation games are characterized as activities that have roles, rules, interactions among players, goals, and final outcomes (Lederman & Ruben, 1984). Thornton and Cleveland (1990) noted that the essential aspect of a game is interactivity and others agree that, despite cosmetic differences, simulations must have certain characteristics if they are to be effective (Thurman, 1993).

Although simulations and games have not been found to be more effective in terms of increased learning of cognitive content, they have consistently been shown to be superior to traditional forms of instruction in terms of affective and behavioral dimensions of learning (Lederman, 1992; Pintrich & Schrauben, 1992). The advantage of simulation games for learning is that they enhance motivation to learn (Bredemeier & Greenblat, 1981) as well as provide opportunities to encounter problems in ways analogous to the way they are encountered in real-world contexts.

For almost a decade the National Research Council's Committee on Techniques for the Enhancement of Human Performance has examined a wide variety of approaches that make strong claims for improving learning. Simulation games need to have validity and reliability in order to be effective; their validity is measured by their correspondence to the aspect of reality they are modeling (metaphorically or literally), and their reliability rests on their capacity to produce the same *processes and outcomes* regardless of the players. Although the evidence indicates that much is yet to be learned about the effectiveness of simulations since the time Pierfy (1977) reviewed them, it is clear that simulations with high validity and reliability (Ruben & Lederman, 1982) provide controlled opportunities for behavioral data generation, the analysis of which, when carefully designed to correspond with simulation-game variables, can be powerful. Thus, well-constructed simulation games, models of reality, can provide both learning experiences for those participating in them and opportunities to collect behavioral data from those participants.

Underlying the design and implementation of simulation games at Rutgers has been Lederman and Stewart's (1998) construct of socially situated experiential learning (SSEL) and the conceptual model that expresses the process of acquiring and interpreting social information received from peers and other sources within the context of their direct learning experiences. Communication as social interaction is one of the conceptual bases of the SSEL construct. Basically, mass communication messages (including formal lectures), which are generally conveyed through written or visual media and addressed "to whom it may concern," are viewed as functioning in society to set the agenda for conversation. It is through interpersonal communication, generally in the form of conversation, that the topics of mass communication (including campaign posters and slogans) are sifted for meaningfulness to the individual and eventually come to influence—or not influence—behavior. Thus, mass-mediated messages establish what topics are meaningful and interpersonal, usually unmediated, messages establish how individuals will act with regard to those topics.

On the college campus, interpersonally communicated messages provide opportunities for students to discuss issues of great personal concern (e.g., the role of alcohol in everyday life). Peer-to-peer interpersonal communication is the most persuasive mode in a situation where the topic being addressed, like alcohol use, is highly charged. For the most part, students do not perceive adults to be credible sources on alcohol issues—adults are seen as having an agenda foreign to the "having fun" and "exercising our rights" agenda of students.

To take advantage of these factors, we have designed simulation games that create interactive opportunities for interpersonal interaction that are structured within a "game" framework (games have roles, rules, interactions, outcomes) and "simulate"/model real-world alcohol and other drug decision-related behaviors.

# THE RU SURE GAME OF CHOICES AND CONSEQUENCES


As one of the outcomes of the continuous research at Rutgers to understand the culture of college drinking as seen through the eyes of college students, the *RU SURE Game of Choices and Consequences* (Lederman, Powell et al., 2001) was designed and implemented. The *RU SURE Game of Choices and Consequences* is a simulation game designed to provoke discussion and self-awareness about drinking-related behaviors and perceptions among college students. This simulation game grew out of an earlier one, *Imagine That!* (Lederman, 1991), that was based on research on alcohol use conducted at Rutgers from 1988 to 1991 (discussed in Chapter 2). *Imagine That!* was designed and produced in 1991 and is still currently in use at more than 275 colleges and universities across the United States and in Canada. *The RU SURE Game of Choices and Consequences* is based on research from the late 1990s through 2001, extending earlier research described in Chapter 2, and also using insights from that research to refine the simulation game.

The *RU SURE Game of Choices and Consequences* focuses on typical alcohol-related decisions and the potential for dangerous consequences related to those decisions. It reflects contemporary choices facing college students. While in many ways the choices have not changed over the 10 years since the earlier simulation game was designed, what has changed is the recognition that widely held myths and misperceptions about drinking often influence students' drinking-related decisions. The *RU SURE Game of Choices and Consequences* is designed to encourage discussion of individual behaviors as well as the choices that others make and comparisons with both to the actual norms on a campus.

The *RU SURE Game of Choices and Consequences* was designed initially as an instructional tool for students at Rutgers and other colleges and universities across the nation who may have to make alcohol-related choices on a daily basis that have the potential for long-term effects on their lives. It was designed to provide them with some insights into themselves and their fellow students and to reinforce for them that not everyone in college drinks dangerously and that they do not have to either. One of the things that reality-simulating games do is provide a safe place for students to talk about their experiences and the reasons for their choices. Thus, simulation games like the *RU SURE Game of Choices and Consequences* provide insight not only for the students playing the simulation game but also for the educators working with them as the participants talk through their perceptions. It is during the discussion after the simulation game (the debriefing session) that both students and educators are able to gain better under standing of the participants and their choices. Both the student and the teacher learn from the experiences about which students talk.

Another important use of simulation games is for behavioral data collection. The next sections of this chapter describe the construction, design, and implementation of the *RU SURE Game of Choices and Consequences* and how to use it as a prevention tool and/or a tool to collect behavioral data.

## USING THE SIMULATION GAME
## AS A 1-HOUR PREVENTION TOOL

The most frequent use of the *RU SURE Game of Choices and Consequences* at Rutgers and at other institutions across the country who have implemented the simulation game is as a prevention tool (the game kit can be ordered from the authors). The simulation game is based on more than a decade of qualitative research at Rutgers that provided data about the sorts of situations that were part of a college student's experiences. More than 2 years of data collection, design, and pilot testing went into the construction of this version of the simulation game and the materials used to play it.

### Brief Description of the Simulation Game

The *RU SURE Game of Choices and Consequences* was designed to be played and debriefed in a 1-hour time period. This simulation game explores the choices that college students face when introduced into social settings that involve alcohol and the impact of their perceptions of others' attitudes and behaviors. The simulation game simulates a "night out" and presents a series of scenarios in which players make choices about drinking-related behaviors. Players collect colored-coded chips each time they make a choice. At the end of play, each player has 10 colored chips and is given a Chip Score Sheet to provide an assessment of the degree of danger connected with these alcohol-related choices. The simulation game does not stress good or bad, right or wrong. It simply examines the consequences that can occur when individuals make personal choices, emphasizing that potentially unwanted consequences are more likely when more dangerous decisions are made. In short, the simulation game provides "a safe place for risky thoughts."

### Objectives

The objectives of the simulation game are as follows:

- To allow participants to make choices concerning familiar alcohol-related situations that they may encounter;

- To provide participants with an experience that enables them to learn about themselves and the choices that they make;
- To discuss choices and explain those related to alcohol;
- To allow players to compare their own choices with the choices others make;
- To compare players' choices in terms of drinking-related perceptions and behaviors to actual campus norms.

## How the Simulation Game is Played

Students are asked to play the simulation game as honestly as possible. They are asked to listen to a series of five scenarios in which they make decisions about choices they would make if these were real-life situations. It is important to remember that all of the scenarios and all of the decision options were extensively field-tested before they were incorporated into the simulation game in order to assure its validity and reliability.

Because of the extensive field-testing it is possible to run the simulation game with confidence that the options provided are realistic. When and if participants, for example, want further options, the facilitator can point out that in the game as in real life individuals do not always have the ideal options from which to choose and have to make decisions among those options available (e.g., in real life a person might prefer to drive home with a designated driver but if one is not available he or she has to choose from the other options).

Figure 10.2 presents one of the scenarios in the simulation game and the choices available to players.

At each decision point, participants receive red, green, and blue chips corresponding to the decisions they make. After individuals collect chips, they gather together to discuss their decisions with those who have picked the same color chips (made the same decision). After a short discussion period, each group selects a representative to speak for them. Representatives are given 2 minutes to publicly present their group's position and to try to persuade others to join them. Participants then have the opportunity to switch groups and side with the group that they feel most represents what they would do. If participants decide to change their decision, they move to the new group and take a chip that represents that option. Participants who remain with their original option also take another chip of the same color.

At the end of the decision-making phase, each participant will have 10 colored chips. Chips are recorded on a Chip Score Sheet. The higher the score, the higher the level of danger associated with the decisions the participants have made.

## SCENARIO

When you finally leave the party and go back to your dorm, you hear that your roommate is getting violently sick. Someone has seen them in the bathroom vomiting and has informed the preceptor. Worried, the preceptor notifies the other preceptors in the building and the RA so they can help find this person. They come to a group of you in the lounge and promise that if you tell them who and where this person is that the person who is sick will not get in any trouble. The preceptors and RA only want to make sure your friend is safe.

## DECISION

Do you:

BLUE       a. Ignore the preceptors and sit up with your friend all night to make sure he or she is okay?

RED        b. Trust the preceptors and allow them to take your friend to the health center?

GREEN      c. Put your sick roommate in your room and let him or her sleep it off?

**Figure 10.2.    Example scenario: RA, resident advisor.**

### Game Materials

In order to assure that participation in the simulation game adheres to its intended design, materials were created so that any trained facilitator could run it. Each of the materials is described briefly here.

The *Scenario Guide* provides both the scenarios to read to the participants and the corresponding decisions, chip colors, and rankings. It is written with specific instructions for its implementation and organization of participants for the play of the simulation game.

*Plastic Chips* are used to signify the choices participants make during each scenario. Bingo chips in the three colors are used throughout the simulation game, each representing a level of danger in terms of the consequences of the choice:

> **Green** = most potentially dangerous consequences
> **Blue** = moderately dangerous potential consequences
> **Red** = least potentially dangerous consequences

Participants are never told of the color coding of the chips. They interpret the meaning of the chips through their engagement in the simulation game and observations of others' decision making.

*Cue Cards* are used as a visual reminder of the choices that participants make. They are color coded in green, red, and blue. A cue card contains the key words of the scenario and is placed next to the color chips to which it corresponds. It is a reminder for players of the choice they made.

*Chip Score Sheets* are used after the decision-making phase to record how many chips of each color each participant collected. Once participants have completed the sheets they are used to discuss the meanings of the choices participants have made.

*Decision Charts* summarize each scenario and its three choices so that individuals can visually mark each decision that they made during the course of the simulation game. This tool is used for participants to reflect on the degrees of danger associated with each of their choices.

The *Alcohol Fact Sheet* provides the actual drinking norms on a campus for students to compare with what they did in the simulation game and what choices they saw others make. To make the simulation game most effective, the Alcohol Fact Sheet has to be of the actual norms on campus to use for participants to compare what happened in the simulation game with actual reported behavior on campus.

The *Debriefing Guide* describes debriefing and provides specific questions suggested for debriefing the simulation game. It is included so that participants' decision making is carefully discussed. The real learning is provoked by a debriefing that is the reflective, guided, post-hoc discussion of the simulation game.

## Debriefing

The *RU SURE Game of Choices and Consequences* is designed so that participants can learn about the behaviors, feelings, and thoughts they experience in typical situations involving decisions about alcohol. It is also used to provide individuals with a realistic sense of other people's choices and behaviors. Because a simulation game is a very powerful and demanding experience, debriefing is a critical part of interpreting the experience. To facilitate this learning, participants are led by the instructor/facilitator through a structured, post-hoc discussion comprised of guided recall, reflection, and analysis. It can take place either immediately after an experience or sometime later. This guided discussion is referred to as the *debriefing* (Lederman, 1983a, 1992).

Debriefing involves discussing the experiences in which the participants have engaged and guiding them through their reflections on and interpretations of those experiences (postexperience analysis). It is a learning process designed to facilitate analysis and internalization of an experience. The emphasis is on what happened — the application of the play of the simulation game to the reality that it is designed to simulate. A debriefing is generally conducted immediately after the decision-making phase, and it takes a question (facilitator) and answer (participants) format. It focuses on what the facilitator wants the participants to learn from their experiences in the simulation game. Debriefing should last approximately as long as the decision-making phase. Because the simulation game is designed to be completed within 1 hour, this means that the reading of the scenarios and selection of options should be completed in 30 minutes to allow 30 minutes for discussion.

During the debriefing, the person who leads the discussion takes the role of facilitator rather than teacher. As a facilitator, the individual asks questions to help the participants think reflectively about their thoughts, feelings, and behaviors during the simulation game for the purpose of learning about themselves through this process. The questions are designed to elicit thoughtful responses. During debriefing, the facilitator must be prepared to handle answers, questions, and other possible responses, even those that may not have been anticipated. The challenge is to be able to shift roles between expert and nonexpert. The facilitator is the expert about dangerous drinking and the actual norms on the campus; the facilitator is, however, a nonexpert about the feelings and experiences of the actual participants — they are the experts on those thoughts and feelings. Facilitation of the debriefing involves a complex set of behaviors including good question-asking skills, listening and interpreting, creating a nonjudgmental climate, and dealing with ambiguity (Lederman, 1983a).

There are three generic categories of questions that are used for debriefing: (a) descriptive questions that ask participants to describe what they did in the simulation game; (b) analytic questions that ask them what it felt like to participate; and (c) application questions that ask them how these experiences apply to their everyday lives (Lederman, 1992). In general, the questions are effective because they put the facilitator in the role of a nonexpert. Students are allowed to talk without feeling judged right or wrong. In addition, the questions that are posed need to be open and directive. These types of questions promote reflection on the experience and encourage discussion.

Lederman (1992) identified three primary questions on which most people frame debriefing: (a) what did participants do in the simulation game (behaviors); (b) what was it like to participate (feelings); (c) what can be learned for "real life" experiences (implications). Figure 10.3 presents a series of steps for debriefing the simulation game. The suggested questions are designed in a sequence that moves from descriptive to analytic to application. During a debriefing period, the answers that flow from these questions can conveniently be tied to the next question. However, it is important to note that *these questions need not be followed verbatim or in sequence.* It may be that a dynamic or discussion topic emerges in a discussion that the facilitator feels is important to concentrate on at that time.

## WHEN TO DEBRIEF

Once the Chip Score Sheet is completely filled out, the participants then add the number of chips they had for each color and multiply it by the number next to each color. The chips are then collected, and the decision charts are given out. Participants are then asked to circle the choices they made. (The same choice should get two circles.) Next, they are asked to assemble themselves in groups according to the number they got on their score sheet. There are three groups:

Blue:    10–14 points
Red:     15–25 points
Green:  26–30 points

## POSITIONING

The participants are assembled in their risk groups around the room. The debriefing begins immediately after they are grouped and seated according to their color as indicated by the score they received. Blue is positioned to the far left, Red to the far right, and Green in the middle. Participants do not move around at this point.

## SUGGESTED QUESTIONS

1.  Ask the participants to relax in their seats. Begin the discussion with a leading statement like "Let's talk about the game."
2.  Ask them the following questions one at a time:

    "Describe what happened in the course of the game."
    "What decisions did you make in the game?"
    "How real did these decisions seem to you?"

**Note:** If at any time during the simulation game the participants do not feel as if the choices that they were given were ample, begin a discussion about choices by asking:

> "Why didn't you like the choices you were given?"
> "Do you always have unlimited choices in situations in real life?"

3. Once you have talked to them about what it was like to participate in the simulation game, turn to the discussion of the Chip Score Sheet. Emphasize that there are no right or wrong answers and that it is not necessary to share the results on their individual sheets. Ask them:

> "What do you think the colors mean?"
> "Explain what it was like being part of that particular group to you and to your friends."

4. Following the general discussion about the Chip Score Sheet, begin to question the participants about how it feels to be labeled in a "degree of danger category." Delve into the implications of their actions.

5. Talk now about how this simulation game applies to everyday reality. Ask them:

> "Did the decisions you made seem realistic?"
> "Have you experienced similar personal experiences?"
> "How could what you experienced in the game change from hypothetical to real?"

6. Talk about actual drinking on campus. Count how many people are in each group. Now it is time to emphasize that the groups have to do with degree of danger. Note that most students are in the moderate group. Ask them:

> "In what ways do you think this is similar to the choices students actually make on campus?"
> "What do you think the actual number of students is who don't drink or who drink moderately?"

Talk about the actual statistics on campus and give them the Alcohol Fact Sheet. Say that this is something to think about as they reflect on the simulation and the decisions they made.

8. Finally, create closure to the experience for them. Ask them:

"Is there anything else we should talk about?"
"If you were going to say the most important thing you learned today what would you say?"

9. End the debriefing by thanking everyone. Ask them to reflect on the choices they made in the *RU SURE Game* when they are faced with the same types of decisions the next time that they go out.

**Figure 10.3.   How to Debrief the RU SURE Game.**

## Ethical Considerations of Debriefing

Debriefing helps participants in a simulation game internalize new learning in positive ways by helping participants "make sense of what has been taught or experienced, to operate on experience by organizing it, to emphasize some elements and not others, or to relate the experience to other events or ideas" (Raths, 1987, p. 27). Thus, the implicit ethic in this conceptualization is that debriefing is used to facilitate positive cognitive, behavioral, and/or affective change in participants (Stewart, 1992).

Debriefing can be conceptualized as a dialogue between the debriefer (or facilitator) and the participants in the simulation game. Johannesen (1990) contended that "the essential movement in dialogue, according to Buber, is turning toward, outgoing to, and reaching for the other. And a basic element in dialogue is 'seeing the other' or 'experiencing the other side'" (p. 59). In this way, dialogue is characterized by authenticity, inclusion, confirmation, presentness, spirit of mutual equality, and supportive climate.

The Hastings Center (cited in Jaksa & Pritchard, 1988) recommended four goals for teaching applied ethics that can be extended to the debriefing situation: stimulating the moral imagination, recognizing ethical issues, developing analytical skills, and tolerating disagreement. These goals can serve as a model for conceptualizing the debriefing process as applied ethics training.

The first goal, *stimulating the moral imagination*, means that debriefers should consider potential ethical problems before they occur so that they will be prepared to face them in the future. Jaksa and Pritchard (1988) referred to this as "preventive ethics," that is, "anticipating needs in such a way that one will not be faced with an ethical dilemma later" (p. 6). Preparation for debriefing should include this component. For example, participants in the *RU SURE Game of Choices and Consequences* may react to the scenarios by admitting incidents of under-age drinking. The debriefer should consider the ramifications of such self-disclosure before debriefing the activity and explain them to the participants so that they can make informed choices about their own self-disclosure during the debriefing.

The second goal, *recognizing ethical issues,* includes thinking about one's immediate responses and identifying unstated assumptions. Although such reflection is a common goal of debriefing, this process can be extended by encouraging participants to examine the moral dimension of the situation. As Jaksa and Pritchard (1988) noted: "It is important not only to evaluate one's immediate reactions to situations but also to recognize when moral assessment of a situation is called for" (p. 7). They also noted that "sometimes recognizing the ethical dimensions of a situation require the assistance of someone who is less involved in it" (p. 7). Thus, the debriefer, who is not closely involved in instances of student alcohol use, can guide participants through a discussion of the ethical basis for their behavior. For example, did they make decisions based on utilitarian principles (the greatest good for the greatest number) or based on a categorical imperative (do not treat others as merely a means to an end)?

The third goal is developing analytical skills. This involves the following:

> Examining fundamental ethical concepts such as justice, utility, rights, duties, self-respect, respect for others, dignity, autonomy, informed consent, and paternalism to see to what extent these concepts can be applied consistently and coherently in similar cases. Learning what kinds of arguments and justifications best support . . . moral assertions is also important. (Jaksa & Pritchard, 1988, p. 8)

The second goal may be more familiar to debriefers than this goal. Debriefers are familiar with helping participants examine the unstated assumptions guiding their behavior. In addition to this examination, however, it is important for debriefers to help participants develop their ethical analytical skills. This type of learning will enable participants to apply their newly developed knowledge in similar situations outside the simulation game. In other words, students may use the ethical judgments they have practiced or learned during the simulation game when confronting alcohol-related situations in their daily behavior.

The fourth goal is *tolerating disagreement.* Although participants in simulation games may not often use words such as "immoral" to describe the actions of other participants, they may make these judgments when faced with responding to others' actions. Participants need specific guidance in responding to these judgments. Debriefers trying to achieve this goal should demonstrate a willingness to engage in reflective conversation with others, but must avoid an overly accommodating attitude. Remarks such as "everyone's entitled to an opinion" are not useful in helping participants develop the ability to analyze their own behavior from an ethical perspective. Opinions are based on values, and these values need to be discussed in light of the assumptions on which they are based.

Thus, participants in simulation games have a clear ethical responsibility. Gouran (1982) lists five questions to analyze the degree of ethical responsibility in small groups that can serve as guides to effective participation in debriefing:

1. Did we show proper concern for those who will be affected by our decisions?
2. Did we explore the discussion question as responsibly as we were capable of doing?
3. Did we misrepresent any position or misuse any source of information?
4. Did we say or do anything that might have unnecessarily diminished any participant's sense of self-worth?
5. Was everyone in the group shown the respect due him or her?

These questions result in the creation of a learning community characterized by concern, responsibility, and respect. Following these guidelines encourages all participants in the *RU SURE Game of Choices and Consequences* to be aware of how their behavior affects others both in the simulation game and in their daily decisions concerning alcohol-related behaviors.

## Uses of the Simulation Game

As a prevention tool, this simulation game has been used in classrooms, in dorms, at college orientation programs, and as part of Alcohol Awareness Week activities. Each of these are briefly discussed.

Because the simulation game is designed to be completed in 1 hour, it lends itself to classroom use. In a classroom, it can be used either as an example of curriculum infusion or as a tool to be used in prevention education classes themselves. The simulation game has been used in large lecture classes at Rutgers in communication, in small classes of interpersonal communication and health communication, and by alcohol educators in health education classes. It has also been used in introduction to sociology and introduction to psychology courses. As curriculum infusion, the class instructor will have some purpose other than the subject of college drinking.

It might be to illustrate observational data collection (communication research, qualitative methods in sociology), interpersonal dynamics (interpersonal communication, communication theory), persuasion theory, health campaigns, or deviance (introduction to sociology). This is a partial list. It merely illustrates that the simulation game works as a vehicle within a classroom where the focus of the course is on the subject matter of college drinking (health education) or other social sciences (communication, public health, sociology, psychology).

The simulation game is also useable in dorms for student life or health education programming. Students from AHC (see Chapter 5) often run the simulation game as part of the interactive strategies that they use to generate interpersonal discussions of the RU SURE Campaign concepts. Health educators and student life staff have also found the simulation game useful when they make dorm presentations. It allows them to open up discussions of drinking rather than presenting lecture materials.

One use to which the simulation game has been put in recent years at Rutgers is at first-year orientation. Student peer educators have been trained by university health educators to run it. These students then facilitate the play of the simulation game and talk the first-year students through their experiences with it. Peer educators are supervised in this activity by health educators who are there to field any difficult situations that arise. In Fall 2003, the simulation game was run with 20 peer educators each facilitating groups of 50 to 100 students. When run for such large numbers of students, the simulation game becomes more food for thought than something that can be debriefed in depth. But it does get new students thinking, presents them with actual behaviors, and inoculates them from the myth that all Rutgers students drink dangerously.

Finally, health educators at Rutgers use the simulation game as an activity during Alcohol Awareness Week. It is a good discussion trigger. Students enjoy the simulation game and like participating in it. It creates discussions and interest in thinking about the subject.

Although the primary use to which the simulation game is put is prevention activities such as those discussed here, because of the behavioral data generated, the *RU SURE Game of Choices and Consequences* is also a useful data-collection tool.

## USING THE SIMULATION GAME TO COLLECT BEHAVIORAL DATA

Simulations and games are often described as behavior or data generating activities and the debriefing (or reflective processing) as the learning activity. The *RU SURE Game of Choices and Consequences*, like other reliable and valid simulation games, can be used as a source of this behavioral data. There are actually three sources of data from the play of the *RU SURE Game of Choices and Consequences*. First, there are behavioral records; second, there are observational data that can be collected; and finally, third, postexperience debriefing interviews that can be used to learn from the participants their own insights into the choices and decisions made during the simulation game.

## Behavioral Records

As participants take part in the *RU SURE Game of Choices and Consequences*, they collect colored chips for each of the decisions they make. At the end of the simulation game, participants are provided with the Chip Score Sheets, described earlier in the chapter, to record the chips they collected. They are also provided with Decision Charts on which to record which decisions they made regarding each of the five scenarios. Although these data are gathered at the end of the simulation game in order for participants to reflect on their behaviors, they also provide a record of the choices that participants have made. In running the simulation game at Rutgers, for example, over the past 5 years, almost invariably most students make the blue (moderate) and red (safe) choices throughout the simulation game. Even when running it with fraternity/sorority members, fewer participants choose the green (dangerous) chips than the blue or red. The simulation game has been used with several hundred entering first-year students to emphasize for them that they did not have to drink dangerously to be part of the culture at Rutgers, as mentioned earlier. The record of their choices provides us with some insight into the profile of the incoming class. In fact, using the simulation game periodically with large groups of students allows researchers to keep their fingers on the pulse of student drinking behaviors. If participants were to play the simulation game very differently from what most have done in the past, it would be a red flag for some systematic data collection to determine if drinking behaviors on campus were changing.

## Observational Data

Throughout the simulation game, participants are behaving. They do not simply sit in seats and fill out forms. They get up, walk around, make choices, and talk about those choices. They even have opportunities to change their minds and rethink their decisions. Watching what they do and listening to what they say can provide a source of rich qualitative data to be explored further. It is possible to create flowcharts to record participants' activities and to use the techniques that trained observers use to gather behavioral data for insight into a phenomenon (Lindlof, 1995). In a sense a simulation like the *RU SURE Game of Choices and Consequences* provides researchers with a setting that is a cross between a laboratory (in that there is structure within which controlled activity takes place) and "the field" (in the sense that "natural" behaviors occur as students make choices). It is a rich context in which to observe students interacting, caught up enough in the simulation game to really be themselves.

## Post-Experience Interviews

Finally, participants can be asked to participate in a post-experience interview. These interviews can be conducted any time after the completion of the simulation game, but are best done within the next week or two. One interviewing method that can be used with either individuals or groups is the *debriefing interview* (Lederman, 1995; Pearson & Smith, 1986). This debriefing is a stepwise interview following an experience in which the debriefer guides those who have been through the experience in a reflective discussion and analysis of that experience and its meanings. Because it is post hoc it shares the name "debriefing" with the instructional debriefing discussed in the prevention uses of the simulation game. The critical difference is that in instructional debriefing the purpose is to help participants learn. The goal is that they are taught to be more self-reflective and to think about their behaviors. In the debriefing interview the goal is quite different: It is for *the interviewer to learn from* the participants rather than the participants being guided in their own learning by a facilitator. A debriefing interview is a purposeful and planned activity. It is a structured, post-hoc interview comprised of guided recall, reflection, and analysis. It can take place either immediately after an experience or sometime later.

The distinguishing feature of the debriefing interview is that it is a postexperience interview. That is, debriefing interviews take place after something has occurred. The event can be an experience, an interview, or a critical incident. Whatever the actual event, the debriefing interview comes after it has occurred and has the purpose of using interview techniques for the interviewer to gather information about the experiences that the interviewees have previously had. In many ways the debriefing interview is like both an individual interview and a focus group interview. There are two features that differentiate the debriefing interview from either the individual or the focus group interview. The first is that the single criterion for participant selection is people whose information comes from their own experience. Thus, people in the interview do not have to have any other common characteristics. Second, the focus of the debriefing is on what has previously occurred. This means that the interview structure is to help the interviewees look back on and recall what they have already been through.

*The History of Debriefing Interviews.* Debriefing interviews were first used in military campaigns and war games (Pearson & Smith, 1986). Debriefing interviews took place after a mission or exercise when participants were brought together to describe what had occurred, to account for the actions that had taken place, and to develop new strategies as a result of the experience. In more contemporary times, the literature on the debriefing of ex-prisoners has come to include debriefings of hostages and other crisis victims (Lederman, 1992; Pearson & Smith, 1986). The purpose of debriefing prisoners of war or former hostages is to provide information about the experience and insight into it for those who had not been there.

*The Debriefing Interview: A Three-Phase Stepwise Process.* The debriefing interview is undertaken in a *stepwise* fashion. Its goal is to review *and* describe the experiences through which interviewees have come and to assess the implications of these experiences and the meanings attributed to them. The debriefing interview can be used either as an information-gathering interview in which the interviewer ascertains what has happened to those who have been through an experience (Lederman, Stewart, & Golubow, 2002) or it can be used with other interviewers, after they have conducted any kind of interview (individual, focus group, or debriefing), to help them understand more about what has been learned during the information-gathering interviews.

Like the information-gathering interview, the debriefing interview uses effective experience-guidance behaviors. Experience-guidance behaviors are the ways in which the debriefer guides the interviewees in reviewing their experiences—of leading them through the necessary reflection and self-reflection that will make sense of the experience for its application to real-life behavior and experiences. There are four basic behaviors required to guide people through the debriefing of their experiences: (a) tolerance for ambiguity; (b) formulation of significant questions and attention to the answers about behaviors; (c) good listening and interpreting skills; and (d) sensitivity to, and management of, group dynamics.

# CONCLUSION

In sum, the *RU SURE Game of Choices and Consequences* is a useful tool for prevention efforts. It is a way to communicate a message to students and to get them talking with one another about that message in a brief time. It can be used with 15 to more than 100 students at a time. It is also a source of rich behavioral data. The data generated in the play of the simulation game provide evidence for prevention specialists to continue to examine their perceptions of college students' experiences and realities.

# 11

## EXTENDING THE CAMPAIGN AND ITS SOCIALLY SITUATED EXPERIENTIAL LEARNING APPROACH TO OTHER CAMPUSES

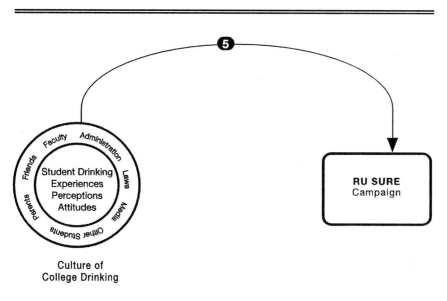

Figure 11.1.   Step 5 of the Conceptual Model.

As discussed in Chapter 8, the RU SURE Campaign was continuously evaluated and those evaluations led to further refinement of the campaign, as illustrated in Fig. 11.1. One of the ways in which this refinement manifested itself was in the analysis of the RU SURE Campaign, and the development of materials to disseminate it to other campuses. As a result, the RU SURE Campaign with its *Top Ten Misperceptions at Rutgers* media component has been implemented successfully since 1998 on the Rutgers–New Brunswick campus. It has also be adopted and adapted for use at other institutions.

Because Rutgers is part of the New Jersey Higher Education Consortium on Alcohol and Other Drug Prevention and Education, a statewide consortium, all campaign ideas and materials have been shared with other institutions in the consortium. We also provided guidance and mentoring when other institutions wanted to use any of the materials developed at Rutgers.

In addition, we have engaged in two specific mentoring projects in disseminating the campaign to other campuses. In 1998, we began a mentoring project with both Grand Valley State University in Michigan and with Rutgers University-Newark. In both instances, we made available the PRSP (Lederman et al., 1998), the *Top Ten Misperceptions at Rutgers* media campaign design, and all materials from the RU SURE Campaign, and pilot-testing of those materials. As a consequence, Rutgers–Newark volunteered to be a test site for all materials for the RU SURE Campaign, as a comparison with Rutgers–New Brunswick, where we are located. Grand Valley began Project Alert, a campus-wide project to address college drinking and, two years later, won funding from the U.S. Department of Education to run its projects and also collaborated with us in evaluating campaign effectiveness (Harper et al., 1999). Finally, the RU SURE Campaign has been presented locally and nationally at conferences of alcohol educators, communication scholars, and higher education administrators.

Much has been learned from implementing the campaign on the Rutgers campus as well as mentoring others who wanted to use the campaign or campaign products. The RU SURE Campaign model has been most successfully adopted when institutions translate the *Top Ten Misperceptions at Rutgers* media component into the language and culture of their own campus. (See Chapters 4 and 5 for detailed discussion of language use and campaign design.) The purpose of this chapter, therefore, is to provide a description of the most effective ways to replicate the *Top Ten Misperceptions at Rutgers* media component for another campus.

## BACKGROUND

Just as the construct of socially situated experiential learning and the five-step model into which it is incorporated are the foundation on which the

RU SURE Campaign and all its components are designed, the construct and model have important implications for the adaptation of the *Top Ten Misperceptions at Rutgers* media component of the campaign for use on another campus. Most importantly, the *Top Ten Misperceptions at Rutgers* media component of the campaign itself is simply a vehicle to provoke discussion and to intervene in students' social interactions with some food for thought about their perceptions of college drinking and the implications for them. It is the necessary but not sufficient component of the campaign. The campaign at Rutgers has six components (discussed in Chapter 5) and relies on the use of interpersonal strategies and curriculum infusion to create discussions about the mediated messages. The RU SURE Campaign is a communication approach to the use of social norms-mediated messages. From a communication perspective, meanings are socially constructed and messages need to be constructed based on the meanings that people bring to them through their social interactions.

Although social norms theory posits that exposure to accurate messages, in the proper dosage, is the basis for changing perceptions, Lederman and Stewart's (1998) SSEL Model argues that social norms marketing strategies are only one part of a three-legged stool for effective prevention. Social norms marketing needs to be taken together with an in-depth understanding of the socially situated nature of interpersonal and mediated communication as well as the role of experiential learning in college drinking. How and what students think about something, what they learn from their experiences, all prepare them to accept, reject, or react to social norms messages. In fact, as discussed in Chapter 3, the SSEL Model posits that different subgroups on campus who drink at differential levels will respond differently to campaign messages. Our data indicate that, for example, those who drink dangerously socialize with others who drink dangerously and are, therefore, *initially* more likely to use their own experiences to reject campaign messages (Burns et al., 1991; Yanovitzky, Stewart, & Lederman, in press). Therefore, it is incumbent on anyone who wants to take and adapt a successful campaign to make sure that students themselves are involved as messengers to create opportunities for social interactions around the campaign messages.

How to involve students depends on individual campuses as well as who is directing the campaign project. It is exceedingly advantageous to use a curriculum infusion plan as described in Chapter 5. We have found this particularly successful if the class can work throughout a given semester on the campaign as part of its learning experience. At Rutgers, the primary course in which we use curriculum infusion about alcohol-related issues is AHC. We have also used briefer curriculum infusion strategies in courses such as Social Marketing, Communication Theory, Communication Research, and Communication and Gender. Many other courses could be used to introduce the campaign as a student project.

Another effective way to involve students is through volunteer organizations or through service learning projects where the campaign can be the focus of the community service (Stewart & Shafer, 2002). For example, students could introduce a similar campaign into a local high school, talk about the campaign at events aimed at teenagers, or use the campaign as part of youth-mentoring activities. Finally, of course, the use of peer educators in conjunction with health educators is an excellent way to get students involved in a campaign. At Rutgers, our health educators teach courses each semester in health education, and students in those courses are available to work on the campaign.

It has been our experience that many students become intrigued enough with the campaign that they are interested in working on it for more than one semester. In 2002, for example, more than a 12 undergraduate students worked on independent study projects with us after they had been through the AHC course (see Chapter 6 for a detailed description of the course). These students mentored AHC students, ran additional data collection projects, designed new artifacts for the campaign (such as an RU SURE Calendar), or worked on data analysis and report writing. In each instance, based on the student's own career path, his or her interest in the campaign was channeled into an area of individual work that would also add to his or her own learning experience. In a recent anonymous course evaluation in AHC, one student who indicated "little prior interest" in the course subject matter responded to the open-ended question "What was the best part of the learning experience for you?" by writing, "I'd like to follow the campaign to see how it does in future semesters and if others continue the work we did."

As these examples illustrate, student campaign workers do more than provide free labor for the campaign. They do more than learn about the dynamics associated with successfully running a campaign. They obtain their own experiential learning. And perhaps even equally as important, they serve as a real channel to the voice of the students and to the campaign culture. Students are the ones, not the faculty or staff, who know what their peers consider to be "cool." They know what students like, and they know the language of students. All of these are invaluable assets that they bring to working on the campaign and to interacting with their peers.

## REPLICATING THE *TOP TEN MISPERCEPTIONS AT RUTGERS* MEDIA COMPONENT OF THE CAMPAIGN

When a campaign is successful it is tempting to take it and use it *as is* on another campus. We refer to this as the "Fast Food Approach to Alcohol Prevention." We may live in a culture where people from one end of the country to the other eat hamburgers and fries, but no two college campuses or cultures are identical. Who the students are, what they look like, where they come from, their educational experiences, their socialization all vary in both subtle and obvious ways. This idea is particularly important to remember for developing a campaign that is based on understanding socially constructed learning experiences, as is the RU SURE Campaign. Effective adaptations of already successful campaigns work well only when a careful analysis is undertaken to determine how well that campaign can be used elsewhere.

The process described in this chapter about the creation of the *Top Ten Misperceptions at Rutgers* media component of the campaign provides a roadmap for effective adaptation. But effectiveness includes using a similar process to that which was used in the creation of the *Top Ten Misperceptions at Rutgers* media component of the campaign initially. Most importantly, effective use of the campaign elsewhere demands collection of baseline data on the intended campus and assessment of a campaign theme, messages, and approach for your own target audience, modification of and testing of campaign materials, and development of strategies for implementation and evaluation. Each of these are discussed in detail.

## Adoption Begins with Needs Assessment: Gather Baseline Data

The needs assessment phase of the campaign is vital. It also takes time and the temptation is to skip it and get on with running the campaign, especially if one is using a campaign that is thought to be already successful. In campaigns such as the RU SURE Campaign with its social norms-based media component, however, it is not possible to begin without gathering baseline data. How can you know the percentage of students who drink dangerously if you do not gather baseline data? Or what their perceptions are of other students? Because the campaign assumes that most people *do not* drink dangerously, but that at the same time the perception is that they *do* drink excessively, it is vital to find out exactly what the statistics are on your campus at the time that the campaign is being adapted and adopted.

Some of these data may already exist in surveys collected by the institution's health services or institutional research unit. If some type of data is collected annually by the health services, the least labor-intensive way to collect baseline data for a campaign is to add questions about drinking behaviors and perceptions to the instrument that is used. If that is not possible, then surveys like the Core Survey (The Core Institute, 1996) or the PRSP (Lederman et al., 1998), the RU Sure Intercept Survey (Stewart & Lederman, 2003), or the College Experience Survey (Yanovitzky, Lederman, & Stewart, 2002) are available and contain the questions that need to be answered. An individualized instrument can be created but that is the most labor-intensive approach to collecting quantitative baseline data.

In addition to surveys to collect quantitative data, another way to collect important baseline data is to conduct focus groups (Lederman, Stewart, & Golubow, 2002). Focus group data do not substitute for quantitative data; they complement quantitative findings by providing insight into the reasons behind students' responses, the "whys" of their behaviors (Fabiano & Lederman, 2002). Focus group interviews can be used to discover drinking-related attitudes, behaviors, and perceptions, and to assess and test key messages. Each is discussed here.

*Discover Drinking-Related Attitudes, Behaviors, and Perceptions.* Fundamental to the RU SURE Campaign is the idea that students are learning from one another, in their social circles and through their own experiences, about the culture of college drinking. Furthermore, because the RU SURE Campaign uses social norms marketing, the campaign assumes repeated exposure to a campaign message. It is expected that students—especially those who drink at higher levels than the reported norm—will *not* believe the message initially. In fact, having initial disbelief is crucial to a social norms campaign because the campaign attempts to correct a long-established incorrect belief, encouraging students, over time, to reexamine their assumptions. Only after repeated exposure to the true norms are students expected to change their attitudes, perceptions, and behaviors. And this exposure has to include interpersonal interactions with other students who challenge the misperceptions held by their peers. Focus group interviews with students divided by drinking levels can provide deep insight into the thinking of their particular campus culture and that thinking becomes important to understand in terms of adapting the RU SURE Campaign to the campus.

*Assess and Test Key Messages.* Focus group interviews are also excellent vehicles for the assessment and testing of key messages. At Rutgers, for example, our quantitative data collection indicated that almost 75% of students stopped at four drinks or fewer and that about 65% stopped at three or fewer. One of the key messages of the RU SURE Campaign is the statistic on how many stop before they drink dangerously. The question was whether it was better to use the higher percentage (75%) or the fewer number of drinks (three). As discussed in Chapter 5, our focus groups indicated that four drinks sounded like "a lot" to many of the students, therefore, it was decided, based on their input, that the "two out of three stop at three or fewer" was a more powerful message than the "three out of four stop at four or fewer." It also would have been possible to say 21% of students don't drink at all, but the "one out of five" was selected for consistency in phrasing between the messages.

A third message was added to the two key messages: "We got the stats from you." Research indicated that students were impressed by the thought that the data had actually been collected on their own campus from them. The decision was made that wherever possible all materials disseminated for the *Top Ten Misperceptions at Rutgers* media component of the campaign would include these key messages. In adapting the campaign it is important to assess the campaign messages and modify them to fit the students on each campus.

Overall, then, it is important to develop the baseline data both quantitatively and qualitatively to get the best possible understanding of the campus culture. It is also important to find ways to tap into the culture periodically to see if the norms are changing and in what ways.

## Develop the Campaign Theme

As a result of the analysis of baseline data, it is possible to learn the extent to which the majority of students at your institution, including the target population, drink and whether or not it is excessive. It is also possible to find out what their perceptions are regarding others' drinking and whether these are misperceptions. If they are, then the RU SURE Campaign design will fit. The question is whether it is possible to use the same theme used at Rutgers that "Most students at Rutgers don't drink dangerously and you don't have to either." Although this may be the theme selected, it is not necessarily the phrasing that may be appropriate to use in campaign messages. Instead, the theme can be used to guide all decisions about messages and message construction. No message, verbal or nonverbal (e.g., the visuals that accompany words in ads), should be used unless it advances the campaign theme.

## Determine the Campaign Approach
## and Select Target Audience

Based on data collected from students about their preferences at Rutgers, it was decided to take a humorous approach to alerting them to alcohol-related misperceptions that might be influencing their drinking and drinking-related behaviors. The humor was the basis of creating the media component of the RU SURE Campaign, the *Top Ten Misperceptions at Rutgers*. In the *Top Ten Misperceptions at Rutgers*, humor was incorporated into the selection of items that would be included in lists of commonly held misperceptions about college life.

In order to adapt the campaign, baseline data should be used to analyze the extent to which this approach would work on a specific campus with that institution's students and how to execute it. It may be possible to use the *Top Ten Misperceptions at Rutgers'* humor as is or modify it slightly. An assessment of the campus will make the decision clear.

Finally, it is necessary to identify the target audience. Is it first-year students? Athletes? Fraternity and sorority members? Undergraduate women? Determination of the target audience influences all of the other decisions about adaptation of the campaign to the campus.

## Assess and Pilot-Test Messages and Media

During the design of the *Top Ten Misperceptions at Rutgers* media component of the RU SURE Campaign, all of the messages were continuously pilot-tested. We were determined to make sure that what we meant in our message was coming through to students. It is important to use the same process in adapting the campaign. Although the *Top Ten Misperceptions at Rutgers* media materials are available, the messages do not have to be created from scratch, but testing them with students from the actual target population is vital. For example, some items in the *Top Ten Misperceptions at Rutgers* list (see Fig. 5.3) may be unique to our university, such as "FAT CAT equals fat free and FDA approved." Because the Fat Cat is a sandwich available on the Rutgers campus, this statement is meaningless on other campuses. At Rutgers, the students get a real laugh out of this misperception, and it is one of the statements that makes them like our posters and "steal" them to hang on their dorm room walls. (The Fat Cat is a sandwich sold by street vendors at what are affectionately known by students as the "grease trucks." It is a cheeseburger, fries, and condiments put together in a large bun.)

## Use the Formula Created for the Top Ten Misperceptions

The concept of the *Top Ten Misperceptions at Rutgers* can be easily adapted to another campus if the same process we used at Rutgers is used. It is important to find commonly shared misperceptions about life on campus so that students can relate to them. This can be done with students in classes or with more formal focus groups. The right messages have been designed when students' responses become redundant. Qualitative researchers call this reaching *saturation.*

When it has been determined what students find humorous and what you believe can be used for the campaign you may have to filter out some messages that would be problematic for other campus constituencies such as faculty, administrators, or staff. After much experimentation with the formulation of the humorous messages and pilot-testing versions of them with target audience members and other audiences that are potentially affected by the messages, the formula we created at Rutgers can be used. As discussed in Chapter 5, here are four steps to the formula for creating a *Top Ten Misperceptions* list:

1. Create three alcohol misperceptions messages.
2. Create seven humorous statements to get students engaged in message processing.
3. Embed the three messages in a list of *Top Ten Misperceptions* with the seven humorous messages.
4. Follow the *Top Ten Misperceptions* with a norming message to give students accurate data. Mark each alcohol-related misperception with an asterisk. Below the list place an asterisk that explains the misperceptions about drinking with the normative message.

Many of the messages we used at Rutgers will work for other campuses because they are likely to be generic (e.g., "Used books are cheap"), but some are particularly unique to Rutgers (e.g., "There's always an empty seat on the bus"). Find the messages that are particularly unique to a given campus to guarantee attention to the campaign.

## Select Media and Create Logo

The goal of the *Top Ten Misperceptions at Rutgers* media component of the RU SURE Campaign is to deliver accurate messages about drinking through the continuous dissemination of norming messages. It is necessary to do a needs assessment of the target audience to find out what that they were most likely to pay attention to. For example, do they pay attention to ads in the campus newspaper (especially on certain days of the week), posters, flyers, or other artifacts? At Rutgers and the other campuses we have mentored, the two most popular artifacts that were created with the message were t-shirts and pens. But t-shirts are costly. The cost is justified by thinking of the t-shirt as a "walking bulletin board" for the campaign message, so it is important that the t-shirts have the logo and key messages on the front and the list of the *Top Ten Misperceptions* on the back. The messages that are printed on t-shirts can be distributed in various campus locations including in front of the library, in dormitories, and at various student events.

Along with the key campaign messages, a campaign needs a logo to visually embody the message. The RU SURE logo design consists of four beer mugs with the last one containing the message "RU SURE?" and an additional line—"Yes, 3 or fewer. We got the stats from you!" (see Fig. 5.4).

It is important to make sure that this logo will be effective on a specific campus in order to convey the intended message. For example, is it wise to use beer mugs in the logo? At Rutgers we found that students felt the design was appealing and understood the anti-dangerous drinking nature of the message. But it is not safe to assume that this would be true on all campuses. Testing this logo or creating and testing one that appeals to students is an important step in the successful adaptation of the campaign to each campus.

In a well-designed campaign, campaign materials are developed through a rigorous process, including multiple rounds of pilot–testing with students on the campus in which the campaign will be implemented. This type of pilot-testing should include students at all drinking levels. If this is not done with the target audience on the actual campus, some of the observed effects could be compromised by this lack of pilot testing. In addition, if photos are used in the posters, they need to be taken of students at the specific school, another factor that could detract from students' reactions to the campaign materials if not done carefully.

## Disseminate Messages

The media selected will be the channels through which there will be distribution of the messages: posters, newspaper ads, flyers, pens, computer disks, magnets, stickers, t-shirts with key messages, and so on. But this is only one part of the approach. The campaign is based in the use of interpersonal strategies. So the most powerful medium through which the message will be carried is the students' work on the campaign and their talk about campaign messages with their peers. To use the campaign most effectively it has to be more than a mediated campaign of posters, ads, and flyers. Enlisting students to work on the campaign and working with them to create social interactions and experiential activities where the message is carried is vital. (See Chapter 6 for a detailed discussion of this process at Rutgers.) Here are some suggested ways to disseminate the message:

- Interpersonally based activities in dorms
- Campus activities
- Posters and flyers, newspaper ads
- Distribution of artifacts including pens, computer disks, magnets, stickers, and t-shirts

*Dosage.* Fundamental to the social norms marketing aspect of the campaign is repeated exposure to a campaign message. It is expected that students—especially those who drink at higher levels than the reported norm—will *not* believe the message initially. In fact, having initial disbelief is fundamental to a social norms campaign because the campaign attempts to correct a long-established incorrect belief. Only after repeated exposure to the actual norms are students expected to reevaluate their beliefs. Thus, to draw conclusions about the potential overall effectiveness of the approach of social norms marketing from one exposure to a set of campaign materials borrowed from another campus is not sound.

## Collect Data to Evaluate

Successful evaluation efforts consist of three types of evaluations: formative, process, and outcome or summative evaluation (Witte et al., 2001). *Formative evaluation* consists of testing campaign messages as they are being developed in order to make sure that they are applicable to the target audience. As discussed in Chapter 5, the RU SURE Campaign was developed with continuous input from undergraduate Communication majors who were able to verify that the messages were "in the voice" of the students. *Process evaluation* involves collecting information during the campaign implementation that tracks the progress of the campaign and assures that the campaign is being conducted as designed. *Outcome evaluation* focuses on the effect a campaign has had on a target audience (Witte et al., 2001). See Chapter 8 for a complete discussion of the evaluation of the RU SURE Campaign.

## CONCLUSION

The *Top Ten Misperceptions at Rutgers* is the media component of the RU SURE Campaign used for disseminating prevention messages about dangerous drinking. The media campaign is designed to be used in conjunction with interpersonal interventions in which students can carry the campaign messages to their peers. It is based on Lederman and Stewart's (1998) SSEL Model. Although it was created specifically for Rutgers University, the process through which it was created and the lessons learned through its implementation, make it suitable for adaptation to other campuses. This chapter presented a step-by-step set of guidelines for use of the campaign. The emphasis is on the process. The most effective way to adopt the *Top Ten Misperceptions at Rutgers* is to *adapt* it. Careful consideration of the steps presented in this chapter will provide the basis for a successful adoption of the *Top Ten Misperceptions at Rutgers* component as well as any other aspects of the RU SURE Campaign selected to use on any campus.

# Part IV

## The Larger Context
## of Prevention

---

## Brief Overview

This book has focused on the development of the SSEL Model and the design, implementation, and evaluation of a health communication campaign based on this model. This section includes material from invited authors who provide additional contexts for this work. As discussed previously, the SSEL Model expands on the traditional social norms approach to prevention in a number of significant ways. But it is still important to understand social norms in a broader context, and some of these chapters provide insight into the theoretical foundation of the social norms approach and its use in prevention work. Because the SSEL Model is a communication perspective that incorporates social norms into an experiential learning framework, two of these chapters provide additional views of what the social norms approach is and how it have been incorporated in various prevention efforts. The other two chapters focus on prevention work in the context of an environmental approach to prevention and a narrative approach to understand dangerous drinking among a college population.

In Chapter 12, An Integrated Environmental Framework, Fern Walter Goodhart and Lisa Laitman, health educators and counselors at Rutgers, explain the university context in which the RU SURE Campaign and other socially situated experiential learning activities have been designed, implemented, and evaluated. Goodhart and Laitman worked in the design and implementation phases of the RU SURE Campaign, and it is through their work that the campaign has become institutionalized as part of the on-going array of approaches to reducing dangerous drinking at Rutgers. Their chapter describes the environmental approach used at Rutgers within which the

RU SURE Campaign has been embedded and the cultural context of Rutgers as an institution.

In Chapter 13, An Overview of Social Norms Approach, Alan Berkowitz, one of the two creators of social norms approach, provides a thorough review of the theoretical foundation of the social norms approach and its application to college campuses. Berkowitz reviews the literature on social norms and provides a thorough explanation and description of the approach.

Chapter 14, Managing Multicampus Campaigns Using a Social Norms Approach, by Linda Jeffrey and Pamela Negro, presents a case study in the use of the approach described by Berkowitz in a multicampus design that includes a number of colleges and universities in New Jersey. Their chapter describes how a large-scale attempt to change social norms was put in place on several campuses simultaneously and details the successes and challenges of this effort.

In Chapter 15, Brief Interventions and Individual Messages, by Patricia Fabiano, a case study of the use of social norms messages in one-on-one brief interventions is presented. Fabiano, an experienced preventionist and researcher, talks about how an interpersonal approach to students with problems with alcohol was undertaken using a social norms approach.

Finally, Chapter 16, by Thomas Workman, describes the approach of one-to-one interactions using a social norms framework. Workman works with the stories (narratives) told by college students, primarily fraternity men, of their drinking-related experiences and analyzes the impact of these stories on their attitudes and behaviors.

# 12

# AN INTEGRATED ENVIRONMENTAL FRAMEWORK

## EDUCATION, PREVENTION, INTERVENTION, TREATMENT, AND ENFORCEMENT

*Fern Walter Goodhart*

*Lisa Laitman*

Colleges and universities are complex communities that help shape the behavior of their members—especially their students (Goree & Szalay, 1996). As centers of learning, they are entrusted to create a community that nurtures intellectual and social development and to develop an environment where students study, live, work, and play in safety and harmony (Burns & Klawunn, 1997). There are many factors that affect this environment, including student behavior, cultural norms and assumptions, societal practices, and institutional and community policies and opportunities.

Rutgers University is also a complex institution with 51,000 students attending 1 of 29 schools or colleges spread across seven campuses in four cities. Fourteen of these colleges are for undergraduate students (including Schools of Engineering, Pharmacy, Nursing, and the arts), with their own deans of students and student life staff. Six of these are full undergraduate colleges (Camden Arts and Sciences, Cook, Douglass, Rutgers, Livingston, and Newark Arts and Sciences) with residence halls, commuter programs, and recreational facilities. Although part of the university overall, these undergraduate colleges also have their own identity and, therefore, have their own policies and expectations for their students.

Rutgers University is the eighth oldest degree-granting institution in the nation. It is known as a safe campus and not seen as a "party school" due, in part, to the fact that dangerous drinking on campus is below national norms (Lederman et al., 2003). In large measure, this is because for more than two decades the University has consistently addressed alcohol use among its students with a comprehensive five-pronged effort that includes education, prevention, intervention, treatment, and enforcement working together in what DeJong et al. (1998) refer to as the *environmental management approach*.

Education and learning are especially impaired by alcohol abuse and misuse (American Council on Education, 1988). Thus, in the early 1980s, Rutgers developed a comprehensive policy on the use of alcoholic beverages, and, in the last 5 years, under presidential mandate and the guidance of other senior administrators, has created additional university-wide blue ribbon panels to institutionalize prevention as a priority on campus. In addition, a coalition of health educators, counselors, student life staff, faculty, campus police, and community partners has been meeting regularly for at least 4 years to ensure the widespread involvement of key campus and community stakeholders including students, faculty members, parents, alumni, and community members in the program's design and implementation.

In the late 1990s, senior research faculty from the Department of Communication and senior professional staff from the University Health Services formed a collaboration to provide research-based additions to augment the Health Services' already active programs. To foster their goals of changing the culture of college drinking, the collaborators created the Communication and Health Issues Partnership for Education and Research in 1997 that soon became the CHI. In a collaborative effort led by Professors Linda Lederman and Lea Stewart, CHI created the RU SURE Campaign (see Chapter 4) designed with funding from the U.S. Department of Education Safe and Drug-Free Schools Program 1998 grant competition and recognized by the Department of Education in 2000 as a model program.

CHI conducts research and implements prevention programs to understand and change college drinking-related behavior at the university. With funding from the U.S. Department of Education (Safe and Drug-Free Schools Program), the New Jersey Higher Education Consortium on Alcohol and Other Drug Prevention and Education, and sources within the university, CHI has conducted surveys, curriculum infusion initiatives, prevention campaigns, and program evaluation. Periodic surveys on drinking behavior track trends in student alcohol use and perceptions. To contextualize this work, this chapter presents a discussion of the environmentally based 5-pronged approach at Rutgers.

# THE HISTORY OF ALCOHOL AWARENESS
# AT RUTGERS UNIVERSITY

## Setting Policy

In 1980, Edward J. Bloustein, then president of the university, charged a new university committee to craft a comprehensive report for considering alcohol use on campus. Chairing the committee was the director of the student health services, W. David Burns, also an associate vice president for student life policy and services. Several underlying values guided the committee's deliberations:

1. Create an environment that promotes knowledge and freedom, and rewards responsibility. If responsibility is to be developed, it must have a chance to be exercised.
2. Attempts to make behavior conscious and then modify it to improve a situation imply that an individual has the capacity to act responsibly using knowledge and awareness of consequences.
3. Policy enforcement comes from voluntary compliance by informed people with reasonable standards of behavior.

Several specific principles emerged from these ideals that continue to guide thinking about alcohol policy at Rutgers today:

1. Knowledge matters and can influence behavior (and so the Alcohol and Other Drug Education Program for Training was created).
2. Freedom is important, and if individuals are free they must have options and not be coerced (requiring strategies that reduce the pressure on students to conform to drinking misconceptions by providing alternatives to drinking—either by requiring that nonalcoholic choices are available or holding social activities that serve as alternatives to drinking).
3. Individuals taking responsibility for their own actions presents the best hope for overall responsibility and reduced undesirable consequences (recommending activities that do not have drinking as their purpose).
4. Individuals and groups may best obey those rules they believe are fair and had an opportunity to create (encouraging specific student groups to develop their own policies and regulate

themselves, such as in residence halls, student organizations, and fraternities/sororities).

5. Universities have an obligation to promote well-being, reduce danger, and limit liability, and provide reasonable care (resulting in restrictions on alcohol use in certain places, such as athletic facilities, and specific expectations of supervision and assumption of responsibility in others, such as student bartender training and conduct of student party planners as legal server-hosts).

6. An institution's integrity rests, in part, on reasonable enforcement of its rules (recommending both discipline procedures and the Alcohol and Other Drug Assistance Program for Students in order to prevent problems or rehabilitate students who violate the policies).

Other principles include expecting faculty and staff to follow the same rules as students, and expecting the university's activities to focus on including all students (and not have activities with alcohol, which would exclude some students based on the legal drinking age).

The Rutgers Board of Governors adopted a set of guidelines in 1984 for the responsible use of alcohol on campus, which remained in effect as of 2004. The goals of the policymakers were to have clear policies that promote both an educational environment with minimal misuse and abuse of alcohol and other drugs and reinforce a healthy, responsible, respectful community. This conforms to the American Council on Education (1988) advice that colleges and universities consider four areas for managing issues of alcohol on campus: policy (institutional issues), education (and prevention issues), enforcement (of laws and campus regulations), and assessment (surveillance and environmental issues).

In the 30 years since the Rutgers Board of Governors adopted these guidelines, an integrated approach to alcohol use has emerged. This five-pronged approach is the hallmark of the university's commitment to creating a safe learning environment. The prongs of the integrated approach are intervention, treatment, enforcement, education, and prevention. Each prong offers a comprehensive approach to supporting student development, campus safety, and the academic mission of the university. Each component is necessary, but insufficient without the others. In recent years, the U.S. Department of Education's Higher Education Center for Alcohol and Other Drug Prevention has recommended this type of approach and offers a good overview of what it calls an environmental management approach, with examples from other colleges and universities across the country (http://www.edc.org/hec). In the following sections of this chapter, each of the prongs of the Rutgers approach will be explained.

# RUTGERS' FIVE-PRONGED APPROACH: EDUCATION, PREVENTION, INTERVENTION, TREATMENT, AND ENFORCEMENT

## Education

Since the original policy that created the program in 1983, the Alcohol and Other Drug Education Program for Training (ADEPT) grew from a program where five students were trained as peer educators to deliver six programs and four exhibits and faculty and staff participated in a six-session workshop to a comprehensive environmental management program of awareness and education, training and advocacy, social norms and harm reduction, community-wide interventions, curriculum infusion, and surveillance.

After reviewing the literature and college programs nationally, the Higher Education Center (2002) concluded that colleges have had limited success by only addressing prevention, intervention, and treatment services designed for the individual. Health behavior is influenced by many factors in an ecological perspective: intra- and interpersonal, institutional and organizational, environment, community, and public policy (McLeroy, Bibeau, Steckler, & Glanz, 1988). Using multiple strategies to modify both behavior and distribution (supply) of alcohol has a greater combined effect than any strategy alone (ACE, 1988).

It was realized that our education and intervention strategies needed to go beyond the individual student to a more comprehensive approach involving the community, the institution, and the environment. At Rutgers, ADEPT activity addresses each of these spheres, grounded in research and based on health promotion theory, in collaboration with partners across the university and community. This approach is population-based, strategically considering our audience based on their roles and behavior for programs and messages, while creating policies in an institution and environment that support our goals.

The university expects students to demonstrate respect and regard for the rights, property, and persons of all individuals; to take responsibility for and be conscious of the consequences of their actions; and to act to reduce the risks of damage and harm to themselves and others (including that harm results from the use or abuse of alcohol and other drugs) (RUHS, 1990). Students learn these skills and values in many ways during their academic career.

Richard P. Keeling (2003) suggested that institutions start thinking about their education programs not with their assumptions about who students are, but by asking critical questions: "What role does alcohol and other drugs play in student's lives? What needs do they fulfill? What is the role of addiction?" As discussed in Chapter 2, research at Rutgers has provided health educators with the answers to many of these questions. For example, students report that they use alcohol and other drugs as follows:

- A social facilitator (also referred to as social lubrication and connectedness). For example, "It's easier to meet people when you're drinking."
- Social glue (also referred to as social affirmation and bonding), which serves to develop group identity.
- An excuse for irresponsible or unexpected behavior—blaming the alcohol rather than the behavior (from vandalism to sexual activity).
- A form of relaxation, a relief of stress and tension, adding excitement, or relieving boredom.

Students drink differently (different amounts, with different expectations and outcomes) and cannot be grouped together for, nor expected to respond to, the same educational programs. Thus, a targeted approach was developed to address students' needs in a comprehensive way.

At Rutgers, the educational programs have different audiences, each with their own goals and strategies. The overall goal is primary prevention, to avoid the unwanted, dangerous consequences of alcohol misuse and abuse. The strategies complement other services at the university in order to provide a comprehensive program to help students socialize at times and places appealing to them (such as late night activities), manage their stress, and find others to associate with or groups to belong to. Student life, residence life, leadership development, recreation services, community service programs, and other activities and services help meet these developmental and student needs.

Educational strategies to address intrapersonal factors increase awareness of alcohol, its effect on the body, laws and policies governing its use, and aim to encourage students to make informed decisions that reinforce health-promoting goals and accurate social norms. These activities include a range of health communication activities (such as exhibits, ads, posters, public service announcements, brochures, Web site pages, peer programs, patient education clinical messages) and messages, including the RU SURE Campaign (discussed in Chapter 4).

Educational strategies addressing interpersonal factors include social norms and misperceptions campaigns. ADEPT works with students (called Alcohol and Other Drug Awareness Generated by Students [ADAwGS]) to sustain a continuing conversation about these issues. These conversations often take the form of student-developed programs facilitated in residence halls, academic classrooms, and student groups. These programs include the following:

> *Drugburst*—An interactive game, modeled after the game *Outburst*, that provides general information about commonly used drugs on college campuses.
>
> *Alcohol: What it is, What it does*—A program comprised of a fact-based quiz and an activity that looks at values and consequences. Students experience the effects of alcohol without being impaired by using fatal-vision goggles ("beer goggles").
>
> *Marijuana Jeopardy*—A program providing information about marijuana in the fun and familiar format of TV's *Jeopardy*.
>
> *All About Club Drugs*—A program that begins with a mock rave, followed by facts about usage and effects of club drugs. A club drugs' paraphernalia quiz is used as a tool to discuss social, physical, and legal consequences of their use.
>
> *RU Up In Smoke?*—A program designed to provide students who want to stop smoking with a foundation to quit on their own by providing information about tobacco, strategies to quit, tips to maintain quit status, and other resources.

These programs offer scenarios, realistic situations that students may find (or already have found) themselves in, and consider the desired goal or outcome of these situations for themselves, possible choices and consequences of different decisions, and strategies to communicate their values and choices to peers in those situations. Information about student drinking, smoking, and drugging on campus are included as part of the student facilitation to enhance decision-making skills. In addition, peer programs on other subjects, from nutrition and sexual health to stress and body image, also incorporate messages about alcohol use and responsible choices.

These activities occur during orientation for incoming first-year students to expose them to information about alcohol, its effects, the policies and laws, and campus/community resources, and accurate social norms. ADAwGS, part of the student community, also serve as opinion leaders on campus in classrooms, libraries, and residence halls, and on campus alcohol/other drug policy committees, available to offer information, comment in different situations, and offer suggestions to friends and acquaintances for making healthy choices.

# Prevention

Regular surveillance activities indicate the behavior and trends of student drinking on campus and which student groups may be at greater risk for dangerous drinking. Historically, White male students ages 18–25 (and even more so, athletes and fraternity members) have shown a propensity as a group for higher rates of drinking than have nonwhite or nonfraternity or athletic student groups. In addition, first-year students, with newly found freedom from authority and still under the legal drinking age, are more at risk for experimenting by consuming alcohol more frequently and in larger amounts while learning their drinking limits.

Prevention programming includes training of gatekeepers (such as residence life staff, coaches and trainers, and fraternity leaders) regarding alcohol information, laws, how to recognize when a student may have a problem with alcohol, and how to make an effective referral to campus treatment programs. Upper class and graduate student residence life advisors are often in the dissonant position of enforcing the university alcohol policy while befriending students living in the residence halls and providing guidance and advice. Thus, one challenge is the consistent and humane enforcement of university and college policy while building trust and honesty in a student living community.

Another prevention strategy reaches many students with one intervention. This is the electronic birthday card sent to all students 2 weeks before their 21st birthday, with birthday greetings and messages encouraging safe celebration. This card is followed 1 week later with a brief, voluntary evaluation form to gauge the impact of the message on the student's celebratory behavior. Some students express appreciation for the birthday greeting and report either having no plans to drink or thinking ahead about their drinking, while a small proportion admit to ignoring the prevention message.

Prevention strategies also focus on first-year students, offering more peer programs and information about actual student behavior, decision making, and reinforcement for safe behavior. Overall, the alcohol education programs take into account the American College Health Association's (2001) standards for the practice of health promotion in higher education by employing a qualified alcohol educator who uses a collaborative process to develop a culturally competent alcohol education program consistent with the university's mission and informed by research, as well as complying with the Safe and Drug-Free Schools and Communities Act of 1994.

Institutionally, the university has several structures in place to address responsible alcohol use in the community. Once the 1981 alcohol policy committee issued its report, the university considered its recommendations and put many policies and programs in place. A raise in the legal drinking age in New Jersey from 18 to 21 years of age also changed the face of drinking on campus by eliminating pubs and increasing student drinking off campus or in solitary settings.

The alcohol policy was revisited in 1998 by a reconstituted President's Committee (chaired by Robert J. Pandina, Director of the Rutgers Center of Alcohol Studies), which continues today, to examine alcohol issues from the perspectives of health, safety, and academic and campus life. Although comparisons between Rutgers behavioral data and those for other colleges suggest that drinking prevalence is at or below expected levels of drinking, we strive to further reduce dangerous drinking and the unintended consequences of drinking in our community.

The undergraduate colleges take guidance from university policy and create guidelines to carry them out. Campus police have a program of awareness and enforcement. The university has asked academic departments to increase the number of classes scheduled on Thursday nights, Fridays, and even on weekends. Almost all social events on campus are alcohol-free. Faculty members are encouraged to notice student cues about problems related to drinking in student academic assignments and to make referral to campus treatment programs. Specific courses on campus focus on alcohol prevention or treatment. Public safety offers a free van service between 7 p.m. and 3 a.m. that goes across campus for safe rides (affectionately known by students as "the drunk bus").

Environmentally, Rutgers has looked at how accessible alcohol is around the campus by mapping the density of alcohol sales outlets (bars and liquor stores) within a 5-mile radius. In addition, Rutgers' staff investigated the ease and sources through which underage students obtain fake IDs (such as fake driver's licenses) and analyzed the content of the campus newspaper for the frequency and quantity of alcohol messages (e.g., number and column inches of ads and stories). Due, in part, to changes in state regulations, the number of advertisements for alcohol-related promotions in the student newspaper is decreasing.

Forming partnerships in the community helps reinforce a campus culture for reducing dangerous drinking. The university participates in the local campus community coalition, the Responsible Hospitality Resource Panel, comprised of store and tavern owners, educators, law enforcement officials, and other community members with a vested interest in the drinking behavior of college students. This group has worked well together, exploring some of the factors that drive accessibility and availability (such as bar hours, drink specials, use of kegs vs. cups), underage drinking (such as by putting police officers in liquor stores as undercover proprietors), and responsible drinking (such as "Night in the Bars," where teams of educators create fun learning situations in community bars between 10 p.m. and midnight).

## Intervention and Treatment

The Alcohol and Other Drug Assistance Program for Students (ADAPS) was established in 1983 based on a recommendation of the university's 1981 Alcohol Policy Committee report. The goal of ADAPS is to assist the university community in identifying and providing early intervention for alcohol and other drug problems among its student population. Rutgers University had been a leader in the development of one of the first faculty/staff employee assistance programs at a university. One of the goals of the employee assistance program (the University Personnel Counseling Service [UPCS]) is to provide assistance in recognizing alcohol and drug problems and to provide access to counseling and treatment.

ADAPS is based on an employee assistance model, but provides more individual and group alcohol/drug counseling to students on campus rather than referring them to community resources. ADAPS also developed interventions unique to the young adult college population regarding alcohol/drug abuse and dependence. This was groundbreaking work at the time because few, if any, models existed for treating this specific population. Much of the widespread knowledge and data that exists today about college student drinking or drug use was not available in 1983. National surveys regarding college alcohol use were rare. Intervention and treatment methods for the young adult college population were not well defined and fell somewhere between treatment for adolescent delinquents and the 30 to 50-year-old alcoholic treatment population. A few of the unique intervention methods developed are described in more detail in this chapter.

***Policy and Staff Training.*** Identifying high-risk students requires the development of a system for training front line staff in the areas where alcohol/drug problems are most likely to have consequences (Laitman, 1987). These areas include residence life, academic services, judicial affairs, health services, and mental health counseling services. Students with problems from alcohol/drug abuse will manifest these problems in nearly every part of their lives. When ADAPS first started, many professional and paraprofessional staff members were not trained to relate these problems to alcohol/drug abuse and were often providing superficial or temporary solutions to the larger problems brought on by substance abuse. Examples of this were as follows:

- Students appearing in health service clinics because of fights or accidents resulting from heavy alcohol use. ADAPS continues to train health care providers to ask appropriate questions as part of their medical assessment and help them develop the appropriate language and techniques to intervene and refer.

- Drinking or drug use that becomes excessive in the residence hall that often leads to problems that interfere with the quality of life of other residents and the social and academic success of the individual. Noise problems, vomiting in public residence hall bathrooms, and vandalism all affect other students. Students who are drinking or using drugs excessively often report missing classes, not studying adequately for exams, and losing academic motivation (Wechsler et al., 2002). Residence life policies that include referring these students for an assessment with an alcohol/drug counselor are critical in addressing residence life disruptions caused by excessive alcohol/drug use.

- Different studies estimate that alcohol/drug abuse is responsible for 30% to 60% of academic failures at universities. Yet when students are placed on "academic probation," a status incurred when a semester's grade point average or overall cumulative average falls below a certain standard set by the college, we know very little about why students are failing. Rutgers offers academic probation workshops for both first-year students who have been placed on probation after their first semester and for upper class students already on academic probation. As part of these workshops, ADAPS counselors include an alcohol/drug assessment to identify students with alcohol/drug problems and to offer intervention.

In psychological and mental health departments, students often present with depression, poor motivation, social problems, or poor family relationships. Such students need to be screened for alcohol/drug problems as possible contributing factors for these symptoms. In psychiatry, providers must be watchful for students seeking medication to deliberately abuse themselves or sell to others. Prescription drug abuse has risen dramatically among the adolescent population (SAMSHA, 2001).

To assure the timeliness and consistent enforcement of university policies on alcohol/drug issues, it is necessary to have both ADAPS and ADEPT staff involvement, as well as support and commitment at a high administrative level. Knowledge of the community resources, recognition of the availability and value of these support services, and judicial backing are all ways a university such as Rutgers continues to support the efforts of the alcohol/drug education and treatment programs.

*Identification of Students for Intervention.* The percentage of college students who meet the criteria outlined in the *Diagnostic and Statistical Manual of Mental Disorders-IV* for alcohol dependence, or other specific drug/poly-substance dependence, has been a debated topic among some college professionals. Some deny that college students meet the criteria for dependence and argue that college drinking is transitory (Brower, 2002), whereas others speculate that the percentage of college students who are alcohol/drug dependent is similar to that in the adult population.

A larger percentage of students meet the criteria for abuse and another percentage do not meet the criteria for either abuse or dependence yet have suffered negative consequences due to their use/abuse of alcohol/drugs. In 1983, there was little recognition in the alcohol/drug treatment community of effective interventions for young people who did not meet the criteria for dependence. Since the 1980s, a variety of approaches have been shown to be effective for students in this category.

One of the choices of these interventions is abstinence. Other approaches include harm reduction models (which focus on reducing alcohol consumption levels in order to reduce the negative consequences associated with abuse), the Brief Intervention Model and other approaches that help students connect the facts about their use with negative consequences (Dimeff, Baer, Kvilahan, & Marlett, 1999; Walters, 2000).

One dilemma in working with students' alcohol/drug use is that the highest risk students are often the least likely to seek help on their own. Students often live in an environment that is very close and noisy, where out-of-control behavior often results from substance abuse. Mandating alcohol/drug abuse intervention in these situations is an important part of institutional commitment and policy.

For some students who are able to make responsible choices about their own alcohol use, education and prevention strategies are sufficient. For students whose use results in undesirable or other negative consequences, policy calls for a personal approach of referral and treatment.

At Rutgers, emphasis is placed on a comprehensive approach. High-risk students respond to different strategies than low-risk students, and students with alcohol/drug dependencies respond to even different strategies. A "one-size-fits-all" approach to the prevention and treatment of alcohol/drug use in the college population fails to address the variety of student use patterns and problems. As a result of data indicating increases in smoking since the mid-1990s, ADAPS staff also incorporated tobacco use and dependence issues in its treatment and intervention with the college population.

*Treatment of Alcohol/Drug Problems.*   In a comprehensive model of addressing alcohol/drug and nicotine use in the college population, students who are often overlooked are those who are addicted and need treatment and those who are in recovery from an addiction. Since 1983, as part of its mission, ADAPS has provided on-campus recovery support for students in recovery. Although many of the students come to ADAPS and are diagnosed with addictions, some are students who come to college or transfer to Rutgers already in recovery. In fact, at one time the Rutgers University Health Services housed the first inpatient/intensive outpatient alcohol/drug treatment program for college students (1988–1993), a collaboration between the Health Services and the Clinical Division of the Rutgers Center of Alcohol Studies.

Currently, ADAPS offers outpatient individual and group counseling services. When students are in need of such higher levels of care as detoxification, inpatient rehabilitation, or intensive outpatient care, they are referred to community services. However, the vast number of these students do well with the outpatient level of services offered by ADAPS and maintain their academic status through the often stressful early transitions of recovery.

In 1988, Rutgers became the first university in the country to offer Recovery Housing as part of its on-campus housing as an option for undergraduate students. In its present location, Recovery Housing provides housing to 23 students who live together in an environment that supports them in their recovery. The ADAPS staff screens and selects residents based on their commitment to maintaining their abstinence and recovery. The house is maintained by the university and is part of the regular housing system. It does not differ in cost from other residence halls. In order to protect the privacy of individuals, there are no signs that identify the house as a Recovery House and the location is not advertised. The ADAPS staff conducts onsite house meetings with the residents once a month, and students are part of decision making in the residence. Students with less than 1 year of recovery are required to participate in individual counseling with ADAPS and be in an Early Recovery Group for support. Counseling is optional for students with more than 1 year but many do take advantage of these services.

In addition to the treatment provided to students with addictions, the ADAPS staff also provides nonabstinence models of counseling students with alcohol/drug problems. Many of these counseling perspectives have a goal of assisting to reduce harm to the individual. College students with family histories of addiction are at high risk, but many are uncomfortable with alcohol use. These students look for help in learning to be comfortable with use (not abuse) and being around other students in normal college social situations. Other students have experienced negative consequences due to episodic abuse, and we work in a short-term counseling model to help them make changes in their drinking patterns. The Brief Intervention Model (Dimeff et al., 1999) is an effective method that uses a two-session intervention to reduce the amount that students drink. (See Chapter 15 for an example of another brief intervention tool.)

## Enforcement

The role of enforcement in a comprehensive model cannot be underestimated. From an environmental perspective, enforcement of alcohol regulations by the residence life staff and enforcement of state and federal laws by campus and community law enforcement are necessary in order to make the residence halls and campus community safe and comfortable for all students. Law enforcement members are an integral part of many campus alcohol discussions and an active participant on campus and community coalitions, including the Alcohol Policy and Implementation Committees.

When the drinking age in New Jersey was raised to 21 in 1984, it created new challenges for enforcement on college campuses. Students saw attempts to enforce the 21-year drinking age as "interfering" with their liberty and expectations of drinking as integral to the social life of a college student as perpetuated by the media and alumni. Administrators and college staff were concerned with health, safety, and liability issues. The ability of a college to control student drinking is often called to question if there is an alcohol-related death on campus. We have seen this in some of the high profile alcohol deaths at all too many colleges in the last few years. Finding common ground to meet with students on these issues of enforcement continues to be a challenge on campus.

## CONCLUSION

Dealing with alcohol-related issues on a contemporary college campus is a complex issue that requires the involvement of a variety of stakeholders including university staff, faculty, police, administrators, and, perhaps most importantly, students. Since the early 1980s, Rutgers has served as a model for institutions attempting to integrate the educational support services available to students who have difficulties with alcohol—either in terms of violating university alcohol policies or suffering from substance abuse problems. Rutgers' five-pronged approach of education, prevention, intervention, treatment, and enforcement provides a comprehensive model for dealing with alcohol issues. It is clear in following this model that no single approach to dealing with alcohol problems can be successful. The magnitude of the challenges faced by institutions of higher education today requires the commitment of university resources designed to provide learning experiences for students combined with enforcement of alcohol regulations as well as clinical treatment/counseling when necessary.

# 13

## AN OVERVIEW OF THE SOCIAL NORMS APPROACH

*Alan D. Berkowitz*

"Social norms" is a theory- and evidence-based approach to addressing health issues that has gained increasing attention. Social norms interventions have been successful in reducing alcohol and tobacco use in college and high school populations, and have promise as an intervention to address violence and social justice issues. As a result of these successes, practitioners in the field of social norms have received national recognition for their work and social norms programs have received a number of best practice awards from federal agencies. Currently, social norms interventions are being funded by the U.S. Department of Education, the Department of Justice, the Centers for Disease Control, state health departments, private foundations, and, in some cases, the beverage industry. In addition, four large outcome studies funded by the NIAAA are currently underway that will provide additional data on the effectiveness of this approach. This chapter provides an overview of the theory of social norms, a brief history, reviews relevant research, presents evidence of successful outcomes, and concludes with a discussion of challenges and emerging issues.

## THE THEORY OF SOCIAL NORMS

Social norms theory describes situations in which individuals incorrectly perceive the attitudes and/or behaviors of peers and other community members to be different from their own when, in fact, they are not. This phenomenon has been called "pluralistic ignorance" (D. Miller & McFarland, 1991; Toch & Klofas, 1984). These misperceptions occur in relation to problem or risk behaviors (which are usually overestimated) and in relation to healthy or protective behaviors (which are usually underestimated). One of the effects of pluralistic ignorance is to cause individuals to change their own behavior to approximate the misperceived norm. This, in turn, can cause the expression or rationalization of problem behavior and the inhibition or suppression of healthy behavior. This pattern has been well documented for alcohol, smoking, illegal drug use, and a variety of other health behaviors and attitudes, including prejudice. In the case of ATOD use, perceiving the norm to be more permissive than it really is can facilitate increased use and provide a rationalization for problem users to justify their own abuse. At the aggregate level, the effect of pluralistic ignorance is to make invisible the majority support for healthy norms. The literature on social norms and the supporting research has been thoroughly reviewed by Berkowitz (2003b) and Perkins (2002a, 2003a). Most of the research conclusions in this chapter are based on the evidence presented in these literature reviews.

College student use of alcohol can provide an example. There is extensive research suggesting that most college students overestimate the alcohol use of their peers (i.e., there is pluralistic ignorance with respect to alcohol use). This overestimation results in most moderate or light drinkers consuming more than they would otherwise and may also encourage nonusers to begin drinking. Heavy alcohol users are even more likely than other students to believe in this misperception and use it to justify their heavy drinking. This latter case is an instance of "false consensus" (i.e., falsely believing that others are similar when they are not). The extent to which alcohol use is misperceived has been strongly correlated with heavy drinking in many studies. Similar patterns have been documented for tobacco use.

False consensus and pluralistic ignorance are mutually reinforcing and self-perpetuating. In other words, the majority is silent because it thinks it is a minority, and the minority is vocal because it believes that it represents the majority. Providing accurate normative feedback is one way to break this cycle, which can otherwise create a self-fulfilling prophecy (i.e., everyone drinks more because everyone thinks that everyone drinks more).

Social norms theory predicts that interventions to correct misperceptions by revealing the actual, healthier norm will have a beneficial effect on most individuals, who will either reduce their participation in potentially problematic behavior or be encouraged to engage in protective, healthy behaviors. Thus, information about healthy drinking norms and attitudes will encourage most individuals to drink less or not at all (which is more consistent with their underlying values and intentions) and also challenge the reasoning that abusers use to justify their drinking.

All individuals who misperceive contribute to the climate that allows problem behavior to occur, whether or not they engage in the behavior. Perkins (1997) coined the term *carriers of the misperception* to describe these individuals. Thus, social norms interventions attempt to correct the misperceptions of all community members whether they actually engage in the problem behavior or not.

Social norms theory can also be extended to situations in which individuals refrain from confronting the problem behavior of others. Thus, individuals who underestimate the extent of peer discomfort with problem behavior may refrain from expressing their own discomfort with that behavior. If the actual discomfort level of peers is revealed, these individuals may be more willing to confront the perpetrator(s) of the behavior. Recent research on homophobia, for example, suggests that most college students underestimate the extent to which their peers are intolerant of homophobic remarks (Bowen & Bourgeois, 2001; Dubuque, Ciano-Boyce, & Shelley-Sireci, 2002) and may be willing to confront these remarks when made aware that peers also feel uncomfortable (Berkowitz 2002a, 2003a). Similarly, men underestimate other men's discomfort with sexist comments about women and are more willing to confront perpetrators when they believe that other men feel the same way (Fabiano, Perkins, Berkowitz, Linkenbach, & Stark, 2003).

The term *social norms* as used here must be distinguished from public health approaches that attempt to change social norms. In this chapter, the term *social norms approach* refers to the correction of misperceptions of social norms (when the majority of a population already behaves in a healthy manner and/or has healthy attitudes) rather than attempts to change norms that are unhealthy or problematic. Thus, the goal is to reveal and enhance already existing healthy norms that have been underestimated and weakened. Although there may also be social and public health issues for which actual norms need to be changed, this is not what is meant by the use of the term *social norms* here. Because both meanings of *social norms* are widely used and have different connotations they must be carefully distinguished because they refer to different phenomenon and presuppose different models of change.

The assumptions of social norms theory are presented in Table 13.1.

The social norms approach integrates a variety of concepts and phenomena that have been well documented in the social science literature. For example, the social psychological phenomena of *pluralistic ignorance* and *false consensus* have been extensively studied and provide a coherent explanation of why individuals act differently from how they feel (in the case of pluralistic ignorance) or rely on a self-serving bias like false consensus to justify problem behavior. Social norms interventions can also be understood in terms of cognitive dissonance theory, another well-established framework within the social science literature. Providing accurate information about

## Table 13.1 Assumptions of Social Norms Theory

1. Actions are often based on misinformation about or misperceptions of others' attitudes and/or behavior.
2. When misperceptions are defined or perceived as real, they have real consequences.
3. Individuals passively accept misperceptions rather than actively intervene to change them, hiding from others their true perceptions, feelings or beliefs.
4. The effects of misperceptions are self-perpetuating, because they discourage the expression of opinions and actions that are falsely believed to be nonconforming, while encouraging problem behaviors that are falsely believed to be normative.
5. Appropriate information about the actual norm will encourage individuals to express those beliefs that are consistent with the true, healthier norm, and inhibit problem behaviors that are inconsistent with it.
6. Individuals who do not personally engage in the problematic behavior may contribute to the problem by the way in which they talk about the behavior. Misperceptions thus function to strengthen beliefs and values that the "carriers of the misperception" do not themselves hold and contribute to the climate that encourages problem behavior.
7. For a norm to be perpetuated it is not necessary for the majority to believe it, but only for the majority to believe that the majority believes it.

*Note:* From Berkowitz (2003a). (Portions of this table are adapted from D. Miller & McFarland, 1991 and Toch & Klofas, 1984.)

norms creates cognitive dissonance by informing those who are "in the misperception" that what they believe is atypical (i.e., that those who are pluralistically ignorant are in the majority and that those who are in false consensus are in the minority). Introducing cognitive dissonance can catalyze a process of change if information about the true norm is introduced in a way that is believable and credible. Social norms relies on indirect methods of persuasion that provide accurate information about what people think or do without telling them what they should do. The information provided helps the recipient to act differently without feeling that this change is being imposed from without. This methodology is consistent with a variety of social psychological approaches to change that have been empirically supported (Kilmartin, 2003).

## A HISTORY OF THE SOCIAL NORMS APPROACH

The social norms approach was first suggested by myself and H. Wesley Perkins based on research conducted at Hobart and William Smith Colleges in the 1980's (Berkowitz & Perkins, 1987; Perkins & Berkowitz, 1986), although it was initially referred to by different names. It has since been implemented at all levels of prevention: primary or universal with entire campus or community populations, secondary or selective with particular subpopulations (such as fraternity/sorority members and athletes), and tertiary or indicated with individuals. These approaches use a variety of methodologies to provide normative feedback as a way of correcting misperceptions that influence behavior.

The first social norms intervention was initiated in 1989 by Michael Haines at Northern Illinois University (NIU; Haines, 1996; Haines & Barker, 2003; Haines & Spear, 1996). Haines expanded on the theory of social norms by applying standard social marketing techniques to present the actual healthy norms for drinking to students through specially designed media. This approach has been called "social norms marketing" (SNM) to distinguish it from traditional social marketing, which does not contain information about actual norms. The social norms marketing campaign at NIU is an excellent example of universal prevention, because it reached the entire population of a community. It has been in existence since 1989 and has produced significant increases in the proportion of students who abstain (from 9% in 1989 to 19% in 1998), and in the proportion of students who drink moderately (from 46% in 1989 to 56% in 1998) and a decrease in the proportion of students who drink heavily (from 45% in 1989 to 25% in 1998), as reported by Haines and Barker (2003).

The NIU intervention was followed by campaigns with equally impressive results at the University of Arizona (Glider, Midyett, Mills-Novoa, Johannessen, & Collins, 2001; Johannessen et al., 1999; Johannessen & Gilder, 2003), Western Washington University (Fabiano, 2003), Hobart and William Smith Colleges (Perkins & Craig, 2002, 2003a), Rowan University (Jeffrey et al., 2003), and later at dozens of institutions of higher education around the United States and in a number of high schools as well. On these campuses, reductions in high-risk drinking of 20% or more were achieved within 1 to 2 years of initiating a media campaign. Since then, successful social norms marketing campaigns have been conducted for tobacco (Haines, Barker, & Rice, 2003; Hancock, Abhold, Gascoigne, & Altekruse, 2002; Hancock & Henry, 2003; Linkenbach & Perkins, 2003a), in a statewide media campaign (Linkenbach, 2003), and with promising results for sexual assault (Bruce, 2002; White, Williams, & Cho, 2003). Other social norms marketing campaigns have focused on particular groups of students (such as athletes or fraternity/sorority members) rather than on an entire campus population. The Web sites of the National Social Norms Resource Center (http://www.socialnorm.org) and the Higher Education Center (http://www.edc.org/hec) contain numerous examples of successful social norms campaigns and the media used to present actual norms.

Concurrent with the development of social norms marketing campaigns, targeted social norms interventions utilizing interactive workshops in small groups were being developed. This approach was conceived in the late 1980's by Jeanne Far and John Miller at Washington State University. They developed a protocol for providing normative feedback to groups in an interactive talk show format (Far, 2001; Far & Miller, 2003). The Small Group Norms Model (SGNM) was offered to a variety of student groups, including sororities and fraternities, athletic teams, first-year students in orientation seminars and residence halls, and students in academic classes. Far and Miller's research suggests that this methodology is more effective in preexisting groups where group norms are relevant to the individual, rather than in ad hoc groups such as classes and some living units. They reported significant reductions in student misperceptions of drinking frequency and quantity that were correlated with actual decreases in drinking among fraternity/sorority members, athletes, and in the general campus population (Far & Miller, 2003) as a result of SGNM.

A third type of normative intervention is to provide feedback to a single individual. The initial research on using normative feedback as an indicated or tertiary intervention was conducted by Alan Marlatt and his colleagues at the University of Washington and Gina Agostinelli and William Miller at the University of New Mexico using motivational interviewing and stages of change theory as a framework. They have developed standardized protocols for providing individual feedback that can be administered by trained clinicians, peers, and/or in interactive computer sessions. One of these, the Alcohol Skills Training Program (ASTP), has been extensively researched with well-documented effectiveness (Dimeff et al., 1999; Marlatt & Baer, 1997), confirming that providing normative feedback to individuals is an essential ingredient contributing to the success of individual interventions. A recent study suggests that providing individualized normative feedback by itself, without the other components of ASTP, may be equally effective (Neighbors & Lewis, 2003, Neighbors, Larimer, & Lewis, in press.

## RESEARCH ON SOCIAL NORMS

### Documentation of Misperceptions

Misperceptions have been documented in more then 45 studies published in refereed journals (see Berkowitz, 2003b, for a detailed list of these studies). Alcohol-use misperceptions have been found in studies with small samples of college students from an individual campus, in larger surveys of individual campus populations, in multiple campus studies analyzing data from The Core Survey (http://www.siu.edu/~coreinst/) and the College Alcohol Study (http://www.hsph.Harvard.edu/cas/), and among middle and high school students and young adults not in college. Some of these studies are also discussed in recent reviews by Perkins (2002a, 2003a).

Misperceptions of alcohol use are held by all members of campus communities including undergraduate and graduate students, faculty and staff, students and student leaders. Researchers have also reported misperceptions for driving while intoxicated (DWI) and riding with someone who is intoxicated (RWID).

Other studies have reported misperceptions for cigarette smoking and for marijuana and other illegal drug use. In addition to alcohol, tobacco, and other drugs, misperceptions have been documented for homophobia, attitudes about sexual assault, gambling, and eating behaviors in studies reviewed by Berkowitz (2003a).

Misperceptions are formed when individuals observe a minority of individuals whose behavior is salient to them engaging in highly visible problem behavior (such as public drunkenness or smoking) and remember it more than responsible behavior that is more common but less striking (Perkins, 1997). These misperceptions are assumed to be normative and are spread in public conversation by all community members (Perkins, 1997).

Misperceptions have been found among fraternity members, athletes, student leaders, among students of different religious backgrounds, and may vary by gender. In addition there are more than 15 studies of pluralistic ignorance documenting misperceptions for topics such as White's attitudes toward desegregation, gang behavior, and student radicalism (see D. Miller & McFarland, 1991, and Toch & Klofas, 1984 for reviews of this literature).

Table 13.2 contains a summary of studies documenting misperceptions, listed by topic and population.

## Table 13.2 Misperceptions Documented in Published Studies by Topic, Setting, and Population

### ALCOHOL

| | |
|---|---|
| Agostinelli et al. (1995) | Individual college campus |
| Baer (1994) | |
| Baer & Carney (1993) | |
| Baer et al. (1991) | |
| Barnett et al. (1996) | |
| Bourgeios & Bowen (2001) | |
| Carter & Kahnweiler (2000) | |
| Clapp & McDonnell (2000) | |
| Fabiano (2003) | |
| Far & Miller (2003) | |
| Glider et al. (2001) | |
| Haines & Barker (2003) | |
| Haines & Spear (1996) | |
| Jeffrey et al. (2003) | |
| Johannessen & Glider (2003) | |
| Larimer, Irvine, Kilmer, & Marlatt (1997) | |
| Page et al. (1999) | |
| Peeler et al. (2000) | |
| Perkins (1985) | |
| Perkins (1987) | |
| Perkins & Berkowitz (1986) | |
| Perkins & Craig (2003a) | |
| Prentice & Miller (1993) | |
| Schroeder & Prentice (1998) | |
| Sher et al. (2001) | |
| Steffian (1999) | |
| Thombs (1999) | |
| Thombs (2000) | |
| Thombs et al. (1997) | |
| Werch et al. (2000) | |
| | |
| Agostinelli & Miller (1994) | Multiple college campuses |
| Perkins et al. (1999) | |
| Pollard, Freeman, Ziegler, Hersman, & Gross (2000) | |
| Perkins & Wechsler (1996) | |

| | |
|---|---|
| Beck & Trieman (1996) | Middle and/or high school |
| Botvin, Griffin, Diaz, & Ifill-Williams (2001) | students |
| D'Amico et al. (2001) | |
| Haines et al. (2003) | |
| Hansen & Graham (1991) | |
| Linkenbach & Perkins (2003b) | |
| Perkins & Craig (2003b) | |
| Thombs et al. (1997) | |

## TOBACCO

| | |
|---|---|
| Haines et al. (2003) | Middle and/or high school |
| Hansen & Graham (1991) | students |
| Linkenbach & Perkins (2003a) | |
| Perkins & Craig (2003b) | |
| Sussman et al. (1988) | |
| | |
| Hancock & Henry (2003) | College students |
| Hancock et al. (2002) | |

## ILLEGAL DRUG USE

| | |
|---|---|
| Hansen & Graham (1991) | High school students |
| Perkins & Craig (2003b) | |
| | |
| Perkins (1985) | College students |
| Perkins et al. (1999) | |
| Pollard et al. (2000) | |
| Wolfson (2000) | |

## OTHER BEHAVIORS

| | |
|---|---|
| Bigsby (2002) | Bullying |
| Bowen & Bourgeios (2001) | Homophobia |
| Bruce (2002) | Sexual assault |
| Dubuque et al. (2002) | Homophobia |
| Hancock (2002) | Prayer |
| Kusch (2002) | Eating disorders |
| Larimer & Neighbors (2003) | Gambling |

**Table 13.2    Misperceptions Documented in Published Studies
by Topic, Setting, and Population** *(Continued)*

| | |
|---|---|
| Linkenbach, Perkins, & DeJong (2003) | Parenting behaviors |
| Thombs (1999) | Driving while intoxicated |
| Thombs et al. (1997) | Driving while intoxicated |
| Wenzel (2001) | Income tax compliance |
| White et al. (2003) | Sexual assault |

SPECIFIC POPULATIONS

| | |
|---|---|
| Baer (1994) | Fraternity members |
| Baer et al. (1991) | |
| Carter & Kahnweiler (2000) | |
| Far & Miller (2003) | |
| Larimer et al. (1997) | |
| Sher et al. (2001) | |
| Trockel et al. (2003) | |
| | |
| Berkowitz & Perkins (1986b) | Resident advisors |
| Korcuska & Thombs (2003) | Men and women |
| | (gender differences) |
| Lewis & Neighbors (in press) | Men and women |
| | (gender differences) |
| Thombs (2000) | Athletes |

## Which Norms Are Salient?

Individuals have friends, are members of groups, may live in residence halls, and are part of a larger community. Each of these overlapping groups has norms that may be similar or different, and some or all of these norms may exert an influence on an individual's behavior. Thus, one critical issue is to evaluate the relative strength of these different norms. For example, on most campuses students have a general idea of the average student and are influenced by this campus norm (Perkins, 2003b) even when the norms of friends and more immediate groups are more influential. In other cases, group identity may supplant campus or community identity, especially if the community is very heterogeneous or diffuse (e.g., on a commuter campus).

Misperceptions increase as social distance increases, with most individuals perceiving that friends drink more than they do and that students in general drink more than their friends (see Berkowitz, 2003a, for a summary of this research). Among college students, others in a living unit are thought to drink more than friends but less than students in general, and students who live together tend to develop similar patterns of misperceptions over time (Bourgeois & Bowen, 2001). Misperceptions, thus, tend to increase as social distance from the misperceiver increases, but social groups that are "closer" are more influential in shaping behavior. This leads to the question of whether closer local norms of a group or more distant global campus norms should be addressed in designing an intervention. In most cases both can be addressed together through a combination of primary and secondary prevention strategies such as small group norms interventions and campus-wide social norms media campaigns. Selecting the most relevant and salient norms for a particular intervention and the appropriate strategy for changing those norms should be an integral part of planning a social norms intervention.

## Do Misperceptions Predict Behavior?

There are at least 15 published studies in which misperceptions are positively correlated with drinking behavior or predict how individuals drink.

In a study by Perkins and Wechsler (1996), perceptions of campus drinking climate explained more of the variance in drinking behavior than any other variable. Similarly, Clapp and McDonnell (2000) found that perceptions of campus norms predicted drinking behavior and indirectly influenced drinking-related problems. In a number of other studies, misperceptions predicted alcohol use and/or problem use (Beck & Trieman, 1996; Korcuska & Thombs, 2003; Perkins, 1985, 1987; Thombs et al., 1997; Trockel, Williams, & Reis, 2003). Similarly, Page, Scanlan, and Gilbert (1999) found that overestimations of other's "binge drinking" were directly correlated with one's own rates of "binge drinking." In other studies examining drinking behavior over time, perceptions of drinking norms at time one predicted drinking behavior at time two (Prentice & Miller, 1993; Sher, Bartholow, & Nanda, 2001; Steffian, 1999).

In studies of high school and middle school populations, perceptions of norms have accurately predicted behavior change at a later point in time

(Botvin, Griffin, Diaz, & Ifill-Williams, 2001; D'Amico et al., 2001; Marks, Graham, & Hansen, 1992). Finally, Thombs (1999) tested four different models of DWI or RWID and found that misperceptions for DWI and RWID had the greatest predictive value in explaining both DWI and RWID.

These studies are listed in Table 13.3.

In summary, a substantial body of research suggests that misperceptions exist, that misperceptions are associated with increased drinking or other problems, and that problem behavior is often best predicted by misperceptions of attitudes and/or behaviors. This includes correlational studies, longitudinal studies, and outcome studies with experimental and control groups.

---

**Table 13.3    Studies in Which Misperceptions Predict Behavior**

MISPERCEPTIONS ARE CORRELATED WITH DRINKING BEHAVIOR

Beck & Trieman (1996)
Clapp & McDonnell (2000)
Korcuska & Thombs (2003)
Marks et al. (1992)
Page et al. (1999)
Perkins (1985)
Perkins (1987)
Perkins & Wechsler (1996)
Thombs et al. (1997)
Trockel et al. (2003)

PERCEPTIONS OF DRINKING NORMS AT TIME 1
PREDICT BEHAVIOR AT TIME 2

Botvin et al. (2001)
D'Amico et al. (2001)
Prentice & Miller (1993)
Sher et al. (2001)
Steffian (1999)

---

# SUCCESSFUL INTERVENTIONS UTILIZING
# THE SOCIAL NORMS APPROACH

As mentioned earlier, social norms theory can be used to develop interventions that focus on three levels of prevention specified as universal, selective, and indicated (Berkowitz, 1997). *Universal prevention* is directed at all members of a population without identifying those at risk of abuse. *Selective prevention* is directed at members of a group that is at risk for a behavior. *Indicated prevention* is directed at particular individuals who already display signs of the problem. Interventions at all three levels of prevention can be combined and intersected to create a comprehensive program that is theoretically based and has mutually reinforcing program elements. Interventions in each of these categories are reviewed here.

## Universal Prevention:
## Social Norms Marketing Campaigns

A number of campuses have successfully reduced drinking by developing campus-wide electronic and/or print media campaigns that promote accurate, healthy norms for drinking and non-use. These include Western Washington University (Fabiano, 2003), the University of Arizona (Glider et al., 2001, Johannessen & Glider, 2003; Johannessen et al., 1999), NIU (Haines, 1996; Haines & Barker, 2003; Haines & Spear, 1996), Hobart and William Smith Colleges (Perkins & Craig, 2002, 2003a), and Rowan University (Jeffrey et al., 2003). These campaigns use social marketing techniques to deliver messages about social norms. At these schools, a reduction of 20% or more in high-risk drinking rates occurred within 2 years of initiating a social norms marketing campaign and, in one case, resulted in reductions of more than 40% after 4 years. Haines et al. (2003) reported similar results for both tobacco and alcohol in social norms marketing campaigns conducted in two midwestern midwestern high schools. In all of these campaigns, positive changes in behavior were associated with correction of misperceptions over time. In contrast, efforts in past years using other approaches to drug prevention did not result in any behavior change.

The Web site of the National Social Norms Center (http:// www.social-norm.org) presents data from these and other schools. Monographs developed by Haines (1996), Johannesen et al. (1999), and Perkins and Craig (2002) and chapters by Fabiano (2003) and Linkenbach (2003) outline the stages of developing a social norms marketing campaign, offer guidelines for creating effective media, and present evaluation data in support of the effectiveness of social norms marketing campaigns.

Perkins and Craig (2002) conducted the most thorough and comprehensive evaluation of a campus social norms marketing campaign. Their intervention combined a standard poster campaign with electronic media, an interactive Web site, class projects that developed parts of the campaign, and teacher training for curriculum infusion. It was begun in 1996 at a college with higher than average alcohol use. Multiple evaluations that were conducted determined that (a) increases in drinking that normally occur during the first year in college were reduced by 21%; (b) previous weeks' high-risk drinking decreased from 56% to 46%; and (c) alcohol-related arrests decreased each year over a 4-year time period. Corresponding reductions were also found in misperceptions of use, heavy drinking at a party, and negative consequences associated with alcohol use. Surveys conducted at three time periods over a 5-year period indicated successive linear decreases in all of these measures over time.

More recently, social norms marketing campaigns have been successful in reducing smoking prevalence and delaying smoking onset. For example, in a seven county campaign directed at 12- to 17-year-olds in Montana, only 10% of nonsmokers initiated smoking following the campaign, whereas 17% in the control counties began smoking—a 41% difference in the proportion of teens initiating smoking in the intervention counties as compared with those in the rest of the state (Linkenbach & Perkins, 2003a). Another study at the University of Wisconsin-Oskosh reported a 29% decrease in smoking rates as a result of a multicomponent intervention, whereas rates at a control campus remained unchanged (Hancock et al., 2002). Finally, at Virginia Commonwealth University cigarette use remained stable as perceptions became more accurate while the number of cigarettes smoked per month at a control campus increased (Hancock et al., 2002; Hancock & Henry, 2003). These tobacco studies provide strong support for the effectiveness of social norms campaigns for smoking, and their use of control groups strengthens the scientific literature in support of the model. Hancock et al. (2002) discussed the differences between smoking and alcohol use behaviors that need to be considered when designing a social norms marketing campaign for smoking.

Table 13.4 provides a summary of these social norms marketing campaigns.

In summary, these interventions using social norms marketing provide strong evidence that the social norms approach can be effectively applied as a universal prevention strategy for alcohol to reduce high-risk drinking and promote moderate use, and for smoking to reduce smoking prevalence and delay its onset.

## Table 13.4  Outcomes of Social Norms Marketing Campaigns

| SCHOOL AND STUDY | DESCRIPTION | OUTCOMES |
|---|---|---|
| *Alcohol* | | |
| Northern Illinois University (Haines, 1996; Haines & Barker, 2003; Haines & Spear, 1996) 45% | 1989–1998, cluster sampling, yearly $n$ from 550 to 1,052 | From 1989 to 1998 decrease in 6+ drinks when partying from to 25%, increase in 1 to 5 drinks when partying from 46% to 56% and increase in abstainers from 9% to 19% |
| University of Arizona (Glider et al., 2001; Johannessen & Glider, 2003; Johannessen et al., 1999) | 1995–1998, $n = 300$ each year | From 1995 to 1998 decrease in heavy drinking (> 5) of 29%, 30-day use rate decrease from 74% to 65%,  plus decreased negative consequences |
| Western Washington University (Fabiano, 2003) | 1997–1998 $n = 489$ and 1,127 | No change in drinking from 1992 to 1997. From 1997 to 1998 decrease in 5+ drinks weekend night from 34% to 27%, and increase in 1 to 2 drinks from 34% to 49%, plus decreased negative consequences |
| Hobart and William Smith Colleges (Perkins & Craig, 2002, 2003a) | 1996–1998 $n = 156, 274$ | 21% decrease in 5+ drinks in a row, 20% increase in abstaining 14% decrease in average drinks at a party |
| | 1995–2000 $n = 232, 326$ | 19% decrease in average drinks at a party, 18% decrease in days drinking last 2 weeks, 24% decrease in average drinks at a party, 50% increase in rarely or never experience negative conse-quences, 46% decrease in liquor law violation arrests |
| Rowan University (Jeffrey et al., 2003) | 1998-2001 $n = 483, 453$ | Decrease in 5+ drinks at a party from 40% to 30%, 5+ drinks in a row in last 2 weeks from 48% to 37% |
| Two midwestern high schools (Haines et al. 2003) | 1999–2001 $n = 317 - 380$ | Decrease in 5+ drinks in a row in last 2 weeks from 27% to 19%, Decrease in got drunk in last 30 |

days from 32% to 26%
## Table 13.4   Outcomes of Social Norms Marketing Campaigns
*(Continued)*

| SCHOOL AND STUDY | DESCRIPTION | OUTCOMES |
|---|---|---|
| *Tobacco* | | |
| Virginia Commonwealth (VCU) (Hancock & Henry, 2003; Hancock et al., 2002) | Fall 1999 Ten weeks apart *n* = 371 VCU, *N* = 163 control (matched samples) | Mean number of days smoked/ month and mean number of cigarettes/day stable at VCU and increases at control school |
| University of Wisconsin-Oskosh (Hancock et al., 2002) | 2000–2001 Intervention campus *n* = 437, 621 Control campus *N* = 774, 678 | 29% decrease in smoking rates No change in control group |
| Montana Youth (Statewide) (Linkenbach & Perkins, 2003a) | 2000–2001 229 intervention counties and 258 control counties | In control group, 17% of adolescents initiate smoking, whereas only 10% of intervention sample does = 41% lower rate of smoking initiation |
| Two midwestern high schools (Haines et al. 2003) | 1999–2001 n = 317 – 380 | Decrease in number of cigarettes smoked in last 30 days from 27% to 19% |

*Note.* In all of these campaigns, alcohol and/or tobacco use remained unchanged in years prior to the social norms campaign. In addition, at the end of the evaluation period, decreases in alcohol and/or smoking were associated with decreases in the degree of misperception of these behaviors.

# Selective Prevention:
## Targeted Social Norms Interventions

Targeted interventions focus on members of a particular group, such as first-year students, fraternity and sorority members, athletes, or members of an academic class. In most of these campaigns, information about the actual norms for the group are provided in small interactive group discussions, workshops, or academic classes. Because of their smaller size and more manageable format, many of these interventions have been evaluated using control groups.

Successful targeted small-group norms interventions have been reported by Schroeder and Prentice (1998), and by Barnett, Far, Maus, and Miller (1996), Far and Miller (2003), and Peeler, Far, Miller, and Brigham (2000) using the SGNM. Steffian (1999) compared a small-group norms approach for alcohol abuse prevention with a traditional alcohol education program and found that "changes in normative perception were among the strongest contributors to a function discriminating between those who decreased their drinking and those who did not" (p. 1).

Social norms messages have also been integrated into interactive peer theater performances, with significant reductions in the frequency of use, DWI, and regretted behavior, and corresponding increases in protective behaviors in comparison with a control group (Cimini, Page, & Trujillo, 2002).

Other selective interventions have utilized more focused media campaigns directed at a particular group of students in combination with other strategies. For example, the University of Virginia designed a targeted social norms marketing campaign for first-year students. Over a period of 3 years, the number of drinks per week for first-year students decreased from 3 drinks a week to 1, the median number of drinks per week for first-year fraternity men was reduced from 15 to 7, and the percentage of abstainers rose from 35% to 49% (Bauerle, 2003; Bauerle, Burwell, & Turner, 2002).

At Rochester Institute of Technology a social norms marketing campaign was developed for deaf and hard-of-hearing students to reduce the incidence of sexual assault (White et al., 2003). The tailored campaign was successful in changing attitudes and perceptions, and resulted in fewer sexual assaults.

These examples provide strong support for the effectiveness of selective social norms interventions directed at particular groups of at-risk students when used alone or in combination with other strategies. Targeted social norms interventions such as these appear to be more effective when the normative data are tailored to the group in question and when they are presented in more extended, interactive formats.

## Indicated Prevention
## (Individualized Social Norms Interventions)

Normative data about drinking can be presented to high-risk drinkers and abusers as part of individual counseling interventions. Because abusers tend to adhere strongly to misperceptions that serve to rationalize their abuse, providing individualized normative feedback is a nonjudgmental way to create cognitive dissonance in heavy drinkers and catalyze change. Alan Marlatt and his colleagues at the University of Washington (Dimeff et al., 1999) developed the Alcohol Skills Training Program (ASTP), an eight-session motivational interviewing approach based on stages of change theory to provide heavy drinkers with nonjudgmental feedback about their drinking indicating that it is much more extreme than that of peers on a variety of measures. ASTP has been condensed into both a 1-hour intervention (BASICS) and a correspondence course in which subjects use a manual. All three interventions have been successful in reducing drinking at follow-ups as long as 1 to 2 years (Dimeff et al., 1999; Larimer & Cronce, 2002), including with high-risk drinkers (Murphy et al., 2001).

Agostinelli, Brown, and Miller (1995) were able to produce similar reductions in drinking by mailing participants personalized graphic feedback following their completion of a mailed survey. Similar results were found in a larger population study in which a normative feedback pamphlet was mailed to more than 6,000 households, with respondents in households receiving normative feedback reporting significantly lower alcohol use than controls (Cunningham, Wild, Bondy, & Lin, 2001).

High-risk drinkers and smokers have also been influenced by campus-wide media campaigns. Thus, in studies mentioned previously, Perkins and Craig (2002) reported fourfold reductions in the typical increase in high-risk drinking among first-year students and a 21% reduction in weekly heavy drinking, and a University of Wisconsin campaign resulted in a 29% decrease in smoking rates in 1 year. As noted earlier, social norms interventions at Washington State University (Far & Miller, 2003) and the University of Virginia (Bauerle et al., 2002) have also been successful in reducing high-risk drinking.

In summary, norms corrections interventions with heavy drinkers are theoretically sound and can be effective both in individual contexts as part of a motivational interviewing strategy or as part of campus-wide media campaigns.

## EMERGING CHALLENGES AND ISSUES

As noted earlier, interest in the social norms approach is growing, research continues to validate the theory, and new applications are being developed in a variety of areas. With this growth and expansion and the enthusiasm that accompanies it are a number of challenges. In particular, it is important to learn from unsuccessful interventions along with the numerous and growing examples of success. These failed interventions can be very instructive and serve to articulate, refine, clarify, and expand the model. Because most of these failures may be due to lack of fidelity to the model, it is important to consider the following challenges:

## Developing the Necessary Infrastructure to Support a Social Norms Campaign ("Readiness")

The theory of social norms makes intuitive sense to many prevention specialists in contrast to other approaches which may have failed to produce results. Yet, although the theory is elegant, implementation is difficult and requires a significant amount of "readiness" or preparation to ensure that an infrastructure is available that can deliver a quality intervention. Johannessen and Dude (2003) reviewed elements of readiness that include the following:

1. Training key stakeholders and staff in the model.
2. Creating support and discussion in the larger community.
3. Revising policies that may foster misperceptions.
4. Collecting and analyzing data.
5. Training and supporting project staff to implement the model properly.

## Deciding Which Messages Are Appropriate and Relevant for Which Audience (Salience)

In relatively homogeneous communities, all members may feel a part of the community and react positively to a community norms-based message. Many social norms marketing campaigns adopt this format with slogans such as "most of us" or "students at our university . . ." However, in a very heterogeneous community students may not identify with messages like these unless they are carefully constructed to have broad appeal. Some students may identify more with particular identities such as participation in a sport or affinity group and be better reached through these channels. Thus, which messages are salient to which groups is an important consideration in social norms campaigns.

## Creating Credible Messages in Terms of Message, Source, and Explanation of Data (Believability)

Social norms messages contradict widely held beliefs and introduce cognitive dissonance by suggesting that the truth is different from what is popularly thought. Ideally, these messages will stimulate a process of self-reflection and re-examination of what is normative. However, when a message is not believed and easily rejected, a campaign is compromised. This can be due to a variety of factors, including when the source of the message is not trusted, the presentation of the message is not appealing, or data that is questioned is not explained thoughtfully. Granfield (2002) has provided a case study of a social norms campaign in which issues of believability initially undermined the campaign. Another impediment to message believability occurs when competing messages from the campus and community utilize scare tactics or an exclusive focus on negative behavior, making it appear that substance abuse is rampant on campus.

## Making Sure That Program Evaluations Are Thorough and Reveal Any Successes (Evaluation)

Kilmer and Cronce (2003) suggested that inadequate evaluation of social norms campaigns may lead to the incorrect conclusion that they have not been successful when, in fact, positive changes have been overlooked (i.e., a Type II error has occurred). Thus, although the overall percentage of students who drink less than a certain amount may remain unchanged, beneficial changes can occur within this group (e.g., students may drink less per occasion or with less negative consequences). Positive changes may also be overlooked when the experimental group's behavior is unchanged, whereas the rates in a potential control group may have increased. Similarly, some groups may be positively affected, whereas others are not, and these changes among particular groups of students can be overlooked when data are aggregated. Finally, methodological difficulties in evaluation design may obscure positive changes.

## Responding to Critics

The social norms approach has met with criticism from some individuals. Berkowitz (2002b), DeJong (2003), Perkins (2003b), and Rice (2002) provided detailed responses to a variety of criticisms. They suggested that critics may be holding the social norms approach to a higher standard of evidence and implementation than other approaches, and that many of the complaints are based on misunderstandings or lack of familiarity with the research. Among the issues they raise include the fact that many of the failed interventions reported in the literature are one's that were poorly implemented, and that many of the theoretical criticisms of social norms are based on a misunderstanding of the theory or its central concepts. Finally, when the lack of rigorous scientific proof for social norms is pointed out, critics often fail to mention that similar proof is lacking for other drug prevention efforts.

## Issues of Replicability

Social norms campaigns are context specific. Thus, a particular message or style of media presentation may be appealing in one community and not in another. In addition, the best means of disseminating information may differ among groups or communities. Because of this context issue, attempts to replicate social norms interventions independent of a specific context may fail. Similarly, when a social norms intervention is adapted to a different health issue, the intervention must be tailored to the culture of the new problem (Berkowitz, 2003a).

## Combining Social Norms With Other Approaches to Drug Prevention

There is currently no consensus regarding whether the social norms approach is effective when combined with other drug prevention strategies—particularly other forms of environmental management. At a minimum, other strategies and methodologies that foster fear and call undue attention to extreme behavior should be minimized because they will undermine social norms efforts and have not been found to be effective. Some experts argue that social norms and other environmental management strategies can be effectively combined, whereas others argue that the desired changes can be created through social norms alone. In the absence of definitive research, it is important that any strategies that are combined are done so in a way that is mutually reinforcing and compatible.

In summary, as the social norms approach has evolved a variety of issues and concerns have surfaced at the same time as new successes are reported. It is important to consider to what extent an intervention is faithful to the model when evaluating it and to address the factors noted above.

## CONCLUSION

The social norms approach has met with considerable success in preventing alcohol and tobacco use and abuse since it was proposed more than 15 years ago by H. Wesley Perkins and myself. Successful social norms programs have been developed for universal, secondary, and indicated prevention, and applications have been tested for a variety of other issues. The social norms approach provides an excellent example of how theory- and research-driven interventions can be designed, implemented, and evaluated to address health problems. Finally, it represents a paradigm shift in which the underlying health of a community is emphasized and enhanced, in contrast with traditional fear-based messages that focus exclusively on the problem.

# 14

## MANAGING MULTICAMPUS CAMPAIGNS USING A SOCIAL NORMS APPROACH

*Linda R. Jeffrey*
*Pamela Negro*

In 1987 a New Jersey college professor called an administrator at a nearby campus to ask if his institution would like to join a new consortium of higher education institutions to address campus alcohol and other drug problems. "We don't have drug problems on our campus," he asserted. "You don't?" the consortium organizer asked. "But I thought your campus was on 'cocaine alley'— Route 295—where the cocaine moves from Washington D.C. to New York City." "You're right. It comes right by us, and just keeps on going. We have no drug problems here."

In the late 1980s the U.S. Department of Education supported a national effort to establish statewide and regional consortia to address campus problems with alcohol and other drug abuse. As part of this national initiative, and through the support of the New Jersey Department of Health and Senior Services, Division of Addiction Services, the New Jersey Higher Education Consortium (NJ consortium) on Alcohol and Other Drug Prevention and Education was founded. It was hoped that NJ Consortium meetings, events, and projects would provide opportunities for college administrators, professional staff, and faculty to share ideas and strategies to increase the effectiveness of campus prevention programs.

The original focus of the consortium was to raise New Jersey campus consciousness about the negative consequences of student alcohol abuse and to change the "campus climate" about excessive drinking. In that era, college administrators feared the creation of public relations problems if campus alcohol abuse was acknowledged. The response of the New Jersey administrator quoted here indeed was not an anomaly. It was believed at that time that the prudent and responsible administrative response was denial. The first task of the NJ Consortium was to open a statewide dialogue concerning the widespread negative impact of campus alcohol abuse. The messages of these early prevention efforts were not infrequently based on scare tactics. The drinking student was implicitly condemned. The negative spin on the early prevention work stemmed in part from the professional background of a number of the founding consortium members who had joined the ranks of academia after a career in alcohol/other drug treatment. These individuals did not wish to see students follow in the steps of the adult clients that they had treated in drug rehabilitation centers, and their fear for the students permeated the messages first communicated by the NJ Consortium. Just as they had battled the denial of their drug-abusing clients, they felt it was their responsibility to fight the institutional denial so ubiquitous in higher education. Outcome evaluation was not emphasized, in part because it was not a substantive part of the grant-funding process of that period and also because knowledge of survey methods and statistical analysis was not common among the alcohol/other drug campus educators, counselors, and program staff.

In the early 1990s the NJ Consortium sponsored five statewide student conferences on campus alcohol abuse prevention, supported the establishment of peer education programs across the state, and produced a volume of course syllabi integrating alcohol and other drug information into the general curriculum. Consortium subgrants supported prevention projects in 2- and 4-year institutions across the state. Efforts were made to link the prevention efforts of colleges with their local prevention municipal alliances. Consistent with the increasing willingness of national higher education leaders, such as the then University of Wisconsin Chancellor Donna Shalala, to identify alcohol abuse as a central campus problem, NJ higher education administrators, staff, faculty, and students increased their understanding of the impact of alcohol abuse on campus life. It was a fond hope and belief that increasing awareness and educating campus personnel and students about the negative effects of alcohol abuse would lead to a transformation of the campus climate about drinking.

Survey research results from 1992 by consortium members Peter Myers and Victor Stolberg captures the alarmed concern of New Jersey collegiate prevention staff when they considered the status of campus alcohol abuse at that time. They reported the results of FIPSE (Fund for the Improvement of

Postsecondary Education) surveys conducted at 15 New Jersey institutions, involving 5,750 students. Their findings included the following:

- Heavy drinking (five or more drinks at one sitting during the previous 2-week period) was reported by 42.7% of caucasian students, 25.2% of Hispanic students, and 15.7% African-American students.
- 20% of the students surveyed reported having a memory loss due to drinking or drug use at least once during the previous year.
- 29.9% reported engaging in behaviors after alcohol or other drug use that they later regretted.
- 17% reported getting into an argument or a fight after alcohol or other drug use.
- 22.7% reported driving a car under the influence, yet less than 1% reported having been arrested for DWI/driving under the influence.
- 24% reported missing a class after alcohol or other drug use.
- 17.5% reported performing poorly on a test or project as a result of alcohol or other drug use.

The NJ Consortium viewed its role as lone "voices in the wilderness" trying to call attention to widespread fatalistic acceptance of the inevitability of collegiate excessive drinking. It was assumed that just as the alcoholic must be confronted with his or her denial, the enabling higher education community must be made to see the dangers lurking in the tacit acceptance of excessive drinking. Energy was directed to prevention efforts such alcohol awareness weeks and "alcohol-free" events that, ironically, defined themselves in relation to the dysfunctional behavior they were meant to decrease. We were blissfully unaware that in defining 1 week of the year as "alcohol-free," we were implicitly defining the other 51 weeks as "alcohol-full." A great deal of faith was placed in the intrinsic value of "good people doing good things" even if those valiant efforts did not yield measurable changes in student drinking attitudes or behaviors.

Although student drinking attitudes and behaviors did not undergo substantial changes between 1990 and 1995, the climate of grant funding did and, fueled by an increasing demand by funding agencies for measurable outcomes in funded prevention projects, the NJ Consortium reviewed its progress or lack thereof with increasing concern. Those individuals who had been on board for a decade were experiencing a midlife crisis of sorts that a great deal of prevention organizing had after all yielded very little social change.

Survey research results documented the lack of outcome effectiveness of many well-intentioned and exhausting efforts. For example, in 1996 the NJ Consortium administered the FIPSE Core Survey to 4,232 students at 10 New Jersey colleges (six 4-year institutions and four 2-year community colleges). Surveys were distributed in classes, through mailings, and in person at campus events including registration. The survey results included the following:

| KEY ALCOHOL USE FINDINGS FROM 1996 SURVEY | 2-YEAR COLLEGES (2,096 STUDENTS) | 4-YEAR COLLEGES (2,136 STUDENTS) |
|---|---|---|
| Percent of students who used alcohol in the past 30 days | 60% | 71% |
| Percent of underage (younger than 21) students who used alcohol at least once in previous 30 days | 59% | 69% |
| Percent of students who engaged in heavy drinking (5 or more drinks at a sitting in the previous 2 weeks) | 32% | 46% |

Consistent with national patterns, the rate of "binge drinking" was higher at 4-year than 2-year institutions. It was noteworthy, however, that the heavy drinking rate reported for both New Jersey 2-year and 4-year institutions exceeded by several points reported national college heavy drinking rates for comparable types of institutions at that time. The national reported rate for 4-year institutions was 44% and 29% for 2-year institutions. These results were from a state with an organized and viable consortium of prevention specialists who were actively trying to decrease student drinking through education, peer education, and curriculum infusion. Why had all our good efforts yielded such poor results?

Survey results indicated that in 1996 New Jersey students believed that alcohol use was normative weekly behavior on campus:

| 1996 FIPSE SURVEY | 2-YEAR INSTITUTIONS | 4-YEAR INSTITUTIONS |
|---|---|---|
| Percent of students who believe the average student on campus uses alcohol once a week or more often | 86% | 95% |

Some members of the NJ Consortium greeted the 1996 survey results with the same fatalistic resignation that they had been fighting in others for a decade. Ten years after the establishment of the consortium and its investment in alcohol education, despite prevention efforts by college personnel across the state and increasing public acknowledgment of the effects of campus alcohol abuse, rates of excessive drinking continued to be high at New Jersey campuses. Perhaps excessive drinking was, after all, best understood as a rite of passage and as an inevitable part of adolescent freedom from parental supervision, simply a "normal" part of growing up.

The NJ Consortium came to terms with the fact that although years of investment in prevention by college staff had yielded a plethora of prevention initiatives, including the development of peer education programs, statewide student conferences, and education media campaigns, collegiate prevention efforts were having little impact on campus alcohol abuse. Aware of the personal and institutional damage that alcohol abuse can wreak, we were not willing to concede the inevitability of campus excessive drinking. A new approach was needed.

## THE SOCIAL NORMS APPROACH

Under the leadership of Dr. Alfred Frech, chair of the NJ Consortium and network coordinator for New Jersey and Delaware, the NJ Consortium began a search for a better approach. True to our identities as academics, consortium members gathered research about promising approaches pursued on campuses across the country. For a period of time, the consortium meetings transformed into a study group in which we shared information, discussed the possibilities of various approaches, and sought consultation with state and national prevention leaders. For example, working with the Higher Education Center, we organized workshops for consortium members about social marketing. We studied approaches detailed in *Promising Practices: Campus Alcohol Strategies* (Anderson & Milgram, 1997), a compendium co-edited by Dr. Gail Milgram from Rutgers University, including an emerging approach variously called a "Social Influence Campaign" at NIU and "Norms Correction Efforts" at Washington State University. At first, we did not understand what the students were allegedly misperceiving; after all, hadn't we ourselves accepted that "everyone was drinking" on our campuses? However, our attention was captured by statements such as the Washington State University assertion that "a general decrease in heavy drinking on the campus is noted" (p. 3.2.17). Was it possible that college prevention staff at other campuses were succeeding in decreasing what we were beginning to think were intractable levels of campus risky, dangerous, and excessive drinking?

In 1996 and 1997, Dr. Wes Perkins, a pioneer in the social norms approach, made multiple trips to meet with the NJ Consortium as we considered the possibilities of this "new" way of thinking about the social context of student drinking. Although it soon became evident that the social norms approach is derived from classic social psychological principles about the place of perceived group norms in the determination of individual behavior (Asch, 1952; Berkowitz & Perkins, 1986a; Sherif, 1972), its application to collegiate alcohol prevention required a significant cognitive shift in our understanding of the place of denial, distortion, and misperception in the construction of group life on college campuses. Up to this point, we had tacitly assumed that the existence of moderate drinkers and abstainers was irrelevant to an understanding of campus drinking. After all, those students weren't the problem, and, we believed, they were the healthy *minority*. As prevention educators we needed, we thought, to be focusing on the unhealthy *majority*. Some consortium members viewed themselves as lonely prophets on their campuses and as among the very few willing to raise the problem of student alcohol abuse despite potential public relations problems for their campuses. To focus on students embracing healthy decisions felt inauthentic, dishonest, and disloyal to our students' best interests. We believed our own scare tactics—a crunched up car on the quad was believed to be a better representation of student life than Dr. Perkins' assertion that the majority of students were not drinking as much as their fellow students thought they were. Ironically, we felt an obligation to be true to our own misperception of student drinking out of a concern for the students we felt were endangered by risky drinking.

There were other barriers to a fair consideration of the social norms approach. Just as therapists sometimes become comfortable with a therapeutic approach, and may wish to use that approach even if research indicates it is ineffective with particular problems or circumstances or groups, so too do prevention educators become accustomed to a particular strategy regardless of its applicability or efficacy. Change and growth are difficult. Complacency is energy efficient. There were some individuals who greeted with outright hostility the decrease in attention given to their favorite prevention approach as the NJ Consortium explored the possibilities of the social norms approach.

## Consortia and Change

There is safety in numbers. What would not be possible alone, we can do together. In its early years the NJ Consortium offered support for institutions that wished to address their campus alcohol abuse problems. Recognition that alcohol abuse is a general collegiate community problem, and not the aberration of a single campus, made it safer for campuses to lessen their institutional denial. In the late 1990s, the consortium provided a context for its members to think more deeply about the group psychology at the heart of campus drinking patterns. The task of the consortium, however, radically transformed with its adoption of the social norms approach. The need for a new stage of consciousness raising was recognized when it became increasingly clear that public impressions and, indeed, our own impressions of student drinking might themselves be a part of the problem.

The social norms approach sheds light on many dark corners of campus alcohol abuse, especially the unthinking ways in which well-intentioned or at least oblivious faculty and staff inadvertently support a climate of campus drinking. It is axiomatic that individuals seek acceptance and belongingness through conformity to what they perceive as the behavioral norms in their environment. When, after all, was the last time that college administrators, staff, or faculty wore shoes to class that did not match? College students, seeking peer acceptance and approval, act the way that they think college students are supposed to act and the way that they think other college students are acting. Applied to the problem of excessive drinking on campus, social norms theory predicts that high rates of excessive drinking will be found on campuses where students believe that excessive drinking is the normal pattern of student drinking, where excessive drinking is an expected and accepted behavior by the majority of students, and where students who do not excessively drink have less status and acceptance than those who do. If students believe that excessive drinking is the normal, accepted, and expected pattern of student drinking, then they risk being perceived as abnormal (odd, unacceptable, out of step), if they do not drink to excess. Before the advent of the social norms approach, we collegiate prevention educators were blind to the *perceived* social costs we were asking of students when we advocated that they pursue an alcohol-free social life. Without an educational campaign, for that truly is what a social norms campaign is, to decrease student misperceptions about college drinking norms at their institution, how marginal and lame alcohol-free activities must seem to the average moderate drinking student.

## Perception vs. Reality

It was the experience of the NJ Consortium that one of the most difficult concepts for collegiate prevention educators to accept in the social norms approach is that it is the *perceived* rather than the *actual* group norm that affects the actions of individuals. The social norms approach holds that it is the widely shared social impression of the group behavioral norm, not necessarily the actual behaviors displayed, that governs individual behavior. The perception of the norm is the guiding force that determines behavior. If the perception of the norm is changed, motivation to change behavior is increased.

As we considered the social norms approach, the NJ Consortium members observed that indeed many college students do have the impression that excessive drinking is normative behavior. They misperceive ( i.e., overestimate) the amount of drinking taking place in their campus community. They believe that most students attending their institution routinely excessively drink. They are not alone in this misperception. Faculty who often think of themselves as so very separate from students, as living in a different world than students, frequently fully participate in this cognitively constructed reality. Messengers of the shared misperception abound and include professors who make comments such as, "Yes, I know that Thursday nights are party night here, but don't let your hangover keep you from turning in your papers Friday," and residence hall assistants who say, "We all know that everyone will be going drinking after exams, but try to keep it a little quieter when you come in." We observed that outgoing senior class presidents also frequently carry the misperception, making all too predictable allusions in their graduation speeches to drinking escapades as the essence of their collegiate experiences. The carriers of the misperception indirectly suggest that excessive drinking is to be expected, benignly tolerated, and even encouraged as a form of experimentation necessary for adult individuation and separation from the norms of the parental nest. In other words, there is a general endorsement of the misperception that "everybody is doing it" and, by implication, that it is permissible to do it, and that to belong, to be a "real" college student, one must conform and drink to excess. Perhaps, we thought, this is the source of the "inevitable" feel of excessive college drinking.

For many students, perceived student social norms clearly carry more weight than codified institutional alcohol policies or our well-intentioned health messages about the risks of excessive drinking. Institutional social norms in the form of policies do not represent the behavioral standards of the peer group. Although most students do not wish to be expelled from the institution, it is the esteem and acceptance of their peers that most seek, not the approval of institutional authorities.

The social norms approach taught us about the students that we were ignoring (i.e., the moderate drinkers and abstainers). Because the overestimation of the extent and centrality of campus drinking functions to increase excessive drinking rates, more moderate student drinkers may drink more than they wish to do in search of peer acceptance. The misperception of campus drinking rates increases the probability that students will drink, and drink excessively, because that is the expected campus behavior, and some may even come to believe that one is not fully involved in campus life unless one is "partying" (i.e., drinking to get drunk).

## Misperceptions and Social Change

The social power of misperceived norms holds great promise for the creation of environmental change. Researchers and practitioners (Fabiano, McKinney, Hyun, Mertz, & Rhoads, 1999; Haines & Spear, 1996; Johannessen et al., 1999; Perkins, 2003a; Perkins & Berkowitz, 1986; Perkins et al., 1999; Perkins & Wechsler, 1996) have found that when students are provided with information about the actual norms of moderation on their campus (as opposed to the perceived norm) through a media campaign and related strategies, the self-reported rates of student excessive drinking decline. Informed, more students may feel empowered to refuse to drink or to drink less without the fear of peer rejection. The repertoire of students' behavioral options is enlarged when their perception of the drinking norm changes. To alter the perceptual environment, a social norms campaign builds on the norms of moderation and safety.

## LAUNCHING A MULTICAMPUS SOCIAL NORMS PROJECT

Working closely with and funded by the NJ Department of Health and Senior Services, Division of Addiction Services, the consortium launched a multicampus social norms project in Fall 1998. This project is now entering its sixth year. Fourteen institutions have implemented social norms projects. We have found that the social norms approach, so simple only at first glance, requires careful, comprehensive, and consistent implementation. As a consortium we have shared lessons learned on other campuses, liberally borrowed each other's media ideas, and have enjoyed the whimsical possibilities of the social norms approach that we could not embrace when we were committed to a fear-based health orientation. The consortium has also been exploring the application of the social norms approach to tobacco use. We offer lessons learned about implementing a consortium-based, multicampus social norms project.

## Collection of Baseline Data

One of the strongest features of the social norms approach is its reliance on empirical measurement. Empirical outcome assessment is integral at every step of a social norms campaign. Both quantitative and qualitative assessment are useful to the development, implementation, and evaluation of project effectiveness. The emphasis on assessment makes the social norms approach attractive to funding agencies, particularly in times of fiscal constraint. It introduces accountability into the field of prevention in a way that motivates effort, revision, and creative thinking.

The first step in a social norms project is the systematic collection of baseline data about alcohol use patterns. In the NJ Consortium Social Norms Project, in the spring semester of 1998, baseline survey data were collected from 5,011 students at 13 New Jersey 2-year and 4-year colleges and universities. Six 2-year and seven 4-year institutions participated. Ten of the institutions participating were publicly funded. In the 2-year colleges, surveys were distributed to students in introductory classes in the humanities, social and natural sciences. In the 4-year institutions, the surveys were distributed to students in a range of both introductory and upper level courses in the humanities, social and natural sciences. Selection of courses was counterbalanced for the time of day courses were offered. Administration procedures were standardized across colleges. *The Campus Survey of Alcohol and Other Drug Norms* asks students to report their own behavior and attitudes and to estimate the typical behavior and attitudes of various categories of other students.

Assessment problems encountered included the wide variability across institutions of staff available to assist in the collection of data, differing levels of willingness by institutions to allow surveying on campus, and differing opinions across institutions about the appropriateness of the collection of empirical data on campus, particularly about alcohol use. The institutions participating in the NJ Consortium range from large research universities to small community colleges. Some consortium members are alcohol/other drug specialists with a staff of subordinates to help them implement their prevention efforts. Other consortium members have no assistance and wear many hats in addition to their alcohol prevention responsibilities. It is only too easy for rivalries and resentments to surface or for individuals to lose sight of insights that they may gain from others working at institutions unlike their own. In the NJ Consortium, we have tried to create a shared context in which we can learn from experiences at institutions both like and unlike our own. We have also endeavored to understand college drinking in its consistency across New Jersey.

## New Jersey Collegiate Drinking Patterns

In 1998, 40% of the New Jersey college students surveyed reported "binge drinking" in the 2 weeks prior to their completing the survey. On average, students reported consuming 3.7 alcoholic drinks at parties and bars. (A drink is defined as a bottle of beer, a glass of wine, a wine cooler, a shot glass of liquor, or a mixed drink.) However, at their last social drinking occasion, students reported consuming an average of 4.5 drinks. Students reported drinking more at off-campus parties and fraternity social functions than at bars, athletic events, or sorority social functions.

Average self-reported consumption rates for male students when drinking at parties and bars was 4.9 drinks while females on average reported consuming 2.9 drinks. Fraternity members reported drinking 5.9 drinks on average, whereas sorority members reported an average rate of 3.6 drinks. Male students reported drinking on average twice a month, whereas female students reported drinking on average once a month. Almost 14% of the students surveyed reported abstaining from alcohol. An additional almost 16% of the students surveyed indicated that they would have preferred to drink less at their last social drinking occasion.

Students reported that they believed that occasionally getting drunk is okay as long as it doesn't interfere with academics or other responsibilities. Less than half of the students indicated that they generally know of and support their campus's rules and regulations regarding alcohol and other drugs. Almost 10% indicated that they generally know of, but oppose, these rules.

*Perceived Norms vs. Actual Norms.* Although the students surveyed had a median frequency of alcohol use of twice a month, they perceived the typical frequency of alcohol use by their friends and by students in general on their campus as once a week. They thought students drink twice as often as those students self-report, and they consistently overestimated the frequency of alcohol use and consumption levels (number of drinks) of all campus constituencies. Their responses revealed that they believed that other students drank a great more and more often than other students reported they did.

**Frequency of Alcohol Consumption**

PERCEIVED NORMS
VS.
ACTUAL NORMS

New Jersey college students overestimated the frequency of alcohol use by other students by factors ranging from 2 to 6 times their actual rates.

Students significantly overestimated campus drinking rates.

| 1998 Campus Survey of Alcohol and Other Drug  Norms Results | Perceived Norm (Median Perception) | Actual Norm (Median Personal Use) |
|---|---|---|
| Males | Three Times/Week | Twice/Month |
| Females | Once/Week | Once/Month |
| On-campus students | Once/Week | Twice/Month |
| Off-campus students | Once/Week | Twice/Month |
| Fraternity members | Three Times/Week | Once/Week |
| Sorority members | Three Times/Week | Once/Week |
| Intercollegiate athletes | Once/Week | Twice/Month |

### Amount of Alcohol Consumption

PERCEIVED NORMS
VS.
ACTUAL NORMS

> Students misperceived the drinking rate of every category of student. They reported the misperception that all students drank at least 5 or more drinks at the last social occasion.

Students overestimated the amount of alcohol consumed by other students. The overestimation ranged from one to slightly more than three drinks more than the students reported drinking. The greatest overestimation concerned the amount perceived consumed by sorority members. Students overestimated the consumption rate of sorority members by a factor of almost 2.

| 1998 Campus Survey of Alcohol and Other Drug Norms Results | Perceived Norm | Actual Norm Self-Reported Use (Overestimation) |
|---|---|---|
| Males | 7.5 drinks | 4.9 drinks (2.6) |
| Females | 5.0 drinks | 2.9 drinks (2.1) |
| On-campus students | 6.2 drinks | 3.8 drinks (2.4) |
| Off-campus students | 6.l drinks | 3.6 drinks (2.5) |
| Fraternity members | 8.5 drinks | 5.9 drinks (2.6) |
| Sorority members | 6.8 drinks | 3.6 drinks (3.2) |
| Intercollegiate athletes | 5.6 drinks | 4.6 drinks (l.0) |

Male students, fraternity and sorority members, and athletes were perceived by students as drinking often and a lot. Although the group drinking means of these types of students were higher than those of other kinds of students, these students themselves did not report to be drinking as much as they were perceived to be. Indeed, the perceived rates of drinking for some types of students would be impossibly high to sustain. For example, male students were perceived to consume almost eight drinks at one social occasion three times a week. This pattern of consumption would be impossible for most people, but particularly for those with an academic workload. The actual self-reported rate for males was five drinks at a sitting twice a month. This constitutes two bouts of excessive drinking each month and is an unacceptably high rate of alcohol use, but it is not as extreme as the *perceived* rate for males.

*Student Misperceptions of College Drinking Norms.* Although self-reported excessive drinking rates of 40% to 45% are alarming and present an unacceptably high risk to student safety, it has been observed that no matter how high the self-reported rate of binge drinking, *the perceived rate of binge drinking* is always higher. College students typically have the false perception that excessive drinking is normative behavior, and in most institutions students believe that the majority of students at their college engage in episodic excessive drinking. For example, this overestimation of drinking is evident in 1998 data collected at six institutions located in the three regions of New Jersey. Although the rates of self-reported binge drinking ranged

| Type of Institution | Perceived Norm for Binge Drinking at Their Institution (1998) | Actual Reported Norm for Binge Drinking at Their Institution (1998) (Overestimation) | |
|---|---|---|---|
| 4-year northern New Jersey state institution | 53.8% | 39.3% | (14.5) |
| 4-year southern New Jersey state institution | 63.4% | 47.9% | (15.5) |
| 4-year central New Jersey state institution | 55.2% | 45.7% | (9.5) |
| 2-year northern New Jersey community college | 56.4% | 31.5% | (24.9) |
| 2-year southern New Jersey community college | 48.8% | 37.2% | (11.7) |
| 2-year central New Jersey community college | 54.3% | 39.3% | (15.0) |

from approximately 32% to 48%, the perceived rate of drinking by students at their institutions ranged from about 49% to about 63%.

The institution with the highest misperception rate of the six schools was a northern New Jersey community college in which the binge drinking rate was misperceived to be almost 25 percentage points higher than the rate actually reported. Interestingly, the institution with the highest reported rate of binge drinking (47.9%) also had the highest perceived rate (63.4%).

## Media Campaigns

In the Fall 1998 semester, selected institutions launched social norms media campaigns designed to correct student misperceptions of college drinking norms. The media campaigns were based on survey results from *The Campus Survey of Alcohol and Other Drug Norms* and concentrated on informing the students of the actual as opposed to misperceived drinking norms on their campus.

One of the most appealing characteristics of the social norms approach to decreasing excessive drinking is that it provides a fruitful context for creativity. Campus prevention staff employed a variety of media outlets and associated activities to inform the students about actual drinking rates. Media campaign elements included widely circulated posters, flyers, buttons, newspaper announcements, and radio spots. Contests were held in which prizes were given to those who could accurately state the campus moderate drinking rate (i.e., the majority of students drink moderately). Rewards were given to students who had the media campaign posters hung in their residence hall rooms. Letters to the editors of campus newspapers about the percentage of students making healthy choices were written. At one campus, the media campaign director distributed buttons stating the campus moderate drinking rate and then randomly gave cash awards to students wearing the button as she encountered them on campus. The buttons quickly became a highly valued campus item, and soon students were seeking out the campus alcohol/drug prevention program office to obtain a button. Students at that campus quickly became aware not only of the campus moderate drinking rate, but also that their college had an alcohol/other drug prevention program office, where the office was located, and who the director was. Most importantly, student conversation about moderation and safety was facilitated.

Guerilla theater techniques were incorporated into some campaigns to inform students about moderate drinking norms; roaming student actors gave rewards to students who could accurately state the moderate drinking rate. Computer screen savers became a bulletin board for publicizing the moderate drinking rates on campuses.

Circulating information is important in the creation of a campus conversation, particularly among students. Statistics reported in the campaigns became the focus of discussion in student government meetings, in campus literary magazines, and in classrooms. Some students who often drank excessively sometimes found it impossible to believe that other students do not themselves drink excessively. Student skepticism is an essential component in creating the cognitive dissonance necessary for perceptual change.

Media ideas and materials were shared at consortium meetings, and collected into a compendium. Copies of the compendium and a monograph concerning the social norms approach were distributed to the presidents of the New Jersey colleges and universities.

*Media Messages.* The social norms approach assumes that misperceptions fuel negative behaviors. The goal of a social norms campaign is to communicate healthy norms, i.e., that the majority of students are moderate and safe drinkers, and thereby alter the perceptual environment of the students. When the NJ Consortium was founded in the late 1980s, the goal of consciousness raising was to decrease institutional denial and to increase awareness of the risks and dangers of alcohol use. With the advent of the social norms approach, the goal of information sharing transformed to highlighting and promoting healthy, protective, normative student behaviors.

For those socialized in earlier prevention approaches, the transition to the social norms approach was not without its challenges. The development of media messages communicating that the majority of students make healthy choices required collegiate prevention specialists to stop taking an adversarial approach (e.g., the war on drugs) toward campus excessive drinkers. Social norms is not about publishing accurate data about the actual levels of excessive drinking, but rather is about communicating moderate norms. It is very easy to fall into the trap of communicating a scare tactic rather than promoting information about moderate norms.

*Dosage.* The social norms message of moderation has to be communicated frequently and consistently. Posters, for example, have to be monitored and rotated to ensure that they are continuing to be seen. In the institution achieving the largest decrease in misperception, the percentage of students reporting that they had seen or heard media messages concerning campus drinking rates increased from 2% to 27% over five semesters.

*Message Testing.* Media concepts are not static. They have to be "market tested" to determine if they appeal to and accurately communicate the normative message to the target population. Focus group and intercept testing are critically important. Both ongoing evaluation and midpoint revision of the campaign is integral to the success of a social norms campaign.

## Coordination of Program Elements

Old habits die hard. Alcohol-free events such as nonalcoholic happy hours continue to be popular campus prevention events on New Jersey campuses. For these events not to undercut the social norms campaigns, it is essential that the campaign not become linked in students' minds with anti-alcohol, pro-abstinence efforts. Alcohol-free activities should focus on sociability and fun, and not on the alcohol-free nature of the events.

## Outcome Measurement

Multiyear implementations of social norms campaigns resocialize college prevention specialists to measure and revise continually. The effectiveness of media strategies is tested and documented. Media channels are not simply assumed to be useful or effective. The meaning of outcome measurement is fundamentally transformed in the social norms approach. If a message or media channel does not produce an effective outcome (i.e., it doesn't work) that is helpful information rather than a simplistic measure of program failure.

## FINDING THE "TIPPING POINT": TRANSFORMING CAMPUS CLIMATE

> Expecting that one person or one department is going to affect the culture of an entire institution is misguided. You need allies. You need collaboration.
>
> (Robert Ariosto, vice president for student affairs, Central Connecticut State University, New Britain, CT, quoted in *Building Long-Term Support,* Higher Education Center for Alcohol and Other Drug Prevention, p. 3)

*New Yorker* writer Malcolm Gladwell (2000) recently posed the intriguing question: "Why do major changes in our society so often happen suddenly and unexpectedly?" He pointed out in his book, *The Tipping Point,* that ideas, behavior, messages, and products often spread like outbreaks of infectious disease. Social epidemics begin in the minds and interactions of a few people, but take off when they reach their critical mass, which he terms the "Tipping Point." Tracing the contagiousness of behavior, he also observes that little changes can somehow have big effects and that change happens not gradually but follows the laws of geometric progression. He provides typologies of the kinds of people who play critical roles in social change processes of this kind (i.e., connectors, mavens, and salesmen) and the nature of ideas that are memorable and change producing ("the Stickiness Factor"). Gladwell's critique of social change offers the possibility of successful outcomes for the social norms approach and suggests strategies for conveying the media messages that may lead to rapid behavioral change.

Most helpful in Gladwell's analysis of social epidemics, however, are his observations that ideas are not inevitable, that rapid change does occur, and that there are identifiable variables underlying that change. It is possible to devise a strategy for change.

The most defeating idea in campus life is the belief that ubiquitous excessive drinking is inescapable, the widespread myth that campus life has always been and always will be organized around alcohol abuse. This is not only historically inaccurate, but is a distortion of the experience of most college students. Moreover, defeatism in the face of campus excessive drinking does not take into account the multitude of examples surrounding us of organized, collaborative social change and transformation.

In the field of drug prevention, there is one undeniable success story — the transformation of general social attitudes toward smoking. Those of us in collegiate alcohol abuse prevention must take inspiration from our antismoking colleagues who have launched a social revolution in one generation. Despite the best efforts of tobacco companies to sustain the 1940s view of smoking as the essence of sophisticated adulthood, smoking is now seen as an unattractive, unhealthy, and déclassé habit. The image of the romantic hero and heroine sharing a cigarette in the last scene of the movie has been replaced with visions of pathetically addicted smokers huddled over their cigarettes outside the doors of public buildings. It is the smokers who now have to question their behavior. Who would have thought this possible 20 years ago?

What the antismoking activists have accomplished in the transformation of smoking norms, we can do with college drinking norms. There were always more nonsmokers than smokers. There were always people who did not enjoy the secondhand effects of smoking. The antismoking movement empowered nonsmokers to assert that their behavior was both better and normal, which in turn, empowered smokers to examine their behavior and make their own decisions about smoking.

The fundamental feature of excessive drinking in New Jersey colleges is that it is non-normative. Most students do not engage in excessive drinking. Most students make healthy decisions and are seriously pursuing their educations and preparing for their futures. The members of the NJ Consortium are working together as allies to empower students to make their own decisions about drinking. Just as the antismoking activists did not work in isolation, we in New Jersey higher education can cooperate in doing what we do best, providing accurate information and knowledge to our college communities, through the social norms approach.

# 15

# A CASE STUDY IN USING A SOCIAL NORMS APPROACH WITHIN A BRIEF INTERVENTION FOR IDENTIFIED HIGH-RISK STUDENTS

*Patricia Fabiano*

The prevention field's enthusiasm for the social norms media approach to reducing alcohol consumption and its related negative consequences on college campuses is well founded (Perkins, 2002a). To reach various student audiences, practitioners use a combination of advertisements in student newspapers, posters, flyers, promotional items, bulletin boards, direct mailings, and campus radio and television announcements. Some also incorporate the use of electronic media strategies and curriculum infusion approaches modeled after the social norms work conducted at Hobart and William Smith Colleges (Perkins & Craig, 2002).

Social norms-based social marketing projects, like those conducted at NIU, University of Arizona, Western Washington University (WWU), and dozens of other institutions of higher education (Perkins, 2002a) have produced heartening results suggesting that this relatively low-cost strategy has considerable promise as part of a comprehensive campus approach to prevention. NIU conducted the first applied experiment using the approach in a college student population and laid out an extended time frame for assessing impact. The NIU project publicized actual norms to change perceptions using print media and co-curricular activities. It subsequently documented a dramatic and continuing 44% decline in heavy drinking among students over a 10-year period (Haines, 1996; Haines & Barker, 2002). University of Arizona replicated the NIU print media strategy with further development of media intervention methods and coordinated the strategy with coalition-building initiatives with the university, documenting a significant 28% reduction in heavy frequent drinking over a 5-year period (Johannessen et al., 1999; Johannessen & Glider, 2002). At WWU, a similar print media campaign was conducted, with the addition of social norms delivery through a large peer educator program and, for students already manifesting an alcohol problem, delivery through an alcohol screening and brief intervention program. A significant reduction in high-risk drinking of 20% over 3 years was achieved as a result (Fabiano, 2003).

Most social norms projects rely on media campaigns to communicate accurate drinking norms. These media campaigns are universal prevention strategies; that is, they are directed at *all* members of the population, in this case, all students at a particular college or university. Because "college students" are not a monolithic category, but rather a highly diverse group of people with vastly different levels of involvement with alcohol, universal prevention efforts may not be equally effective for everyone. Although social norms marketing may remain the central intervention for campuses wishing to reach large target audiences with positive, empowering information about healthy alcohol behaviors, other social norms delivery strategies may have increased efficacy with specific student populations.

Researchers at WWU set out to explore whether the social norms approach could be tailored to meet the needs of varying student populations by designing a number of social norms delivery approaches that target different audiences of students at WWU (Fabiano, 2003). This chapter focuses on how researchers at WWU created and implemented an indicated prevention infusion of the social norms model at WWU for a specific student population, that is, a risk-reduction intervention for students who have already developed signs and symptoms of alcohol-related problems.

## THE *WWU* ENVIRONMENT AND PERCEPTIONS OF THE FREQUENCY OF PEER ALCOHOL USE

Prior to introducing alcohol interventions using the social norms approach in Fall 1997, a moderate alcohol-use culture already existed at WWU—a culture similar to other institutions of higher education in the western United States that consistently report less frequent heavy drinking than schools in the eastern, central, or southern regions of the country (Presley, Meilman, & Cashin, 1996). WWU could be characterized as a campus where most students drank moderately or not at all, with some students engaging in episodic heavy drinking.

The fact that WWU has never had affiliation with Greek organizations may contribute to this culture of moderation as these organizations historically have been linked to heavier drinking than non-Greeks (Meilman, Leichliter, & Presley, 1999; Wechsler, Kuh, & Davenport, 1996). Furthermore, although no quantitative data have been collected to explain this difference, WWU students themselves have reported in focus groups that "Western is a serious academic place; people can't afford to get bombed every day here like at other places" (Hyun, Snyder, Harwick, & Fabiano 1998). As one of the six state-funded institutions of higher education in Washington, WWU has taken special pride in the quality of liberal arts programs required of all of its approximately 12,000 students. Academic reputation is repeatedly cited as the number one reason cited by entering students for choosing WWU, supporting the theme suggested in the student focus groups—that a relationship exists between a strong academic focus and moderation in alcohol use among most students.

Markedly different from other schools that have implemented social norms interventions, more than 20% of WWU students consistently reported no alcohol consumption at all. However, among students who drank—the population with potential risk of alcohol related problems—those who reported low-to-moderate use and those who reported high use prior to the social norms intervention remained statistically the same (Fabiano et al., 1999).

Regardless of whether students reported no alcohol use, moderate use, or heavy frequent use, the one characteristic all students in the 1997 Lifestyles Survey administration sample shared was their overestimation of how frequently their peers drank. The pattern of exaggerated perception that emerged from this survey administration paralleled research on other campuses that was beginning to show that college students generally misperceived the frequency and amount of drinking among their peers to be much higher than the actual norm or actual level of consumption (Perkins & Berkowitz, 1986).

The social norms mass media campaign that began at WWU in Fall 1997 focused on correcting this misperception with the general student body. The initial intervention was modeled on templates developed at NIU (Haines & Barker, 2002) and University of Arizona (Johannessen & Glider, 2002) and profited from the many lessons learned on these and other projects (Haines, 1996; Johannessen et al., 1999).

To measure the effect of the social norms media approach, the Lifestyles Survey on alcohol usage among WWU students was re-administered in May 1998 to a randomly selected sample of 2,500 students. The three most important findings from the 1998 survey administration as compared with previous administrations were reductions in students' self-report of misperceptions of peer drinking norms, frequent heavy drinking, and alcohol-related negative consequences. These reductions indicated to researchers at WWU that the accuracy of students' awareness of WWU alcohol norms had increased after introducing our social norms mass media intervention.

## HIGH-RISK DRINKERS

Because we saw such remarkable success applying social norms marketing techniques to the overall student population, we theorized that we could have similar success by tailoring the social norms approach to meet the needs of a specific student population: high-risk drinkers. High-risk drinkers are already experiencing at least some manifestations of alcohol-related problems (Institute of Medicine, 1990; Modeste, 1996). At WWU, high-risk student drinkers are identified as those who have been sanctioned for infringement of campus alcohol policies, deemed eligible for diversion by the local municipal court following charges of being a minor in possession, or self-referred because of personal concerns about alcohol use. These students enter WWU's alcohol screening and brief intervention program through mandated referrals from the residence hall staff, the university judicial officer, the local municipal court, the liquor control board agents, and, in some cases, voluntarily.

A vast literature documents why institutions of higher education are concerned about the impact of high-risk drinking on students' lives. Frequent heavy consumption of alcohol is implicated in a significant number of behavioral, health, and academic problems experienced by college students (Perkins, 2002b). Although the vast majority of college students "outgrow" high-risk drinking and alcohol-related problems, they are nonetheless vulnerable to a myriad of harmful consequences until they do so (Dimeff et al., 1999). Therefore, WWU, like other institutions of higher education, has sought effective models for reducing the physical, emotional, social, and academic harm experienced by this significant subpopulation of college students and assists them to move safely and successfully through this risky developmental period.

Prior to the development of the alcohol screening and brief intervention program at WWU, efforts to intervene effectively with high-risk drinkers took many different forms from a traditional counseling model to an "alcohol education school" approach. With the exception of a client satisfaction instrument that assessed students' perceptions of the treatment process, no data were collected that measured outcomes—that is, actual changes in students' knowledge, attitudes, beliefs, or behavior regarding alcohol use.

WWU's current and central intervention for high-risk student drinkers is a promising new cognitive-behavioral skills training and motivational enhancement strategy called the Alcohol Skills Training Program (ASTP), which was adopted and adapted from the University of Washington's Addictive Behaviors Research Center. Although the ASTP intervention alone generated encouraging results in reducing negative consequences to high-risk drinkers, the success of the social norms mass media campaign in 1998 prompted researchers to speculate whether personalized social norms comparisons (between "most WWU students" and "individual high-risk drinkers") could be a significant enhancement to the favorable potential of the brief ASTP intervention. Subsequently, accurate normative data regarding WWU students' alcohol use and consequences became a significant part of the three-page Personalized Feedback Profile developed for each student completing ASTP.

## INFUSION OF SOCIAL NORMS INTO BRIEF INTERVENTIONS

Students who enter the ASTP complete an intake assessment that measures the following:

1. Frequency and quantity of student's drinking.
2. Negative consequences resulting from student's alcohol use over the past 6 months.
3. Student's use of other psychoactive substances in the past 6 months.
4. Student's sexual behaviors, including risky sex behaviors involving alcohol and other drug use.
5. Student's alcohol outcome expectancies.
6. Student's interest in changing and degree of readiness to change drinking.
7. Symptoms of psychological distress.
8. Indices of alcohol dependence (Dimeff et al., 1999). These data are used to develop a three-page Personalized Feedback Profile, which provides (a) nonjudgmental information on personal drinking patterns and consequences and (b) moderation tips on reducing risks for alcohol-related harm.

WWU's intake assessment also measures sanctioned students' perceptions of other students' (a) frequency and quantity of drinking, (b) average blood alcohol, (c) range of alcohol-related negative consequences, (d) amount of money spent on alcohol, and (e) amount of calories consumed from alcohol. These data provide an intensive and individualized strategy for confidentially assisting students to compare their own drinking and alcohol-related consequences to WWU norms within the context of a motivational interview.

## MOTIVATIONAL INTERVIEWS

The overarching task of the prevention specialist in motivational interviewing is to actively develop and bolster a student's interest and motivation to change his or her behavior in a particular direction (W. Miller & Rollnick, 2002). Motivational interviewing is best conceptualized as movement along a continuum identified by researchers Prochaska and DiClemente (1984) as "stages of change." Using this framework for thinking about the change process, students move from precontemplation (a stage in which the person is unaware or underaware of risks or problems), to contemplation (a stage in which the person begins to feel ambivalence and recognize that some hazards or problems exist), to preparation (a stage that combines intention with behavior), to action (a stage in which the person modifies his or her behavior in order to overcome the problem), and finally to maintenance (the stage where efforts are made to support and maintain the behavioral gains that have been made). Just as motivational interviewing has been successfully applied to health behavior change in areas like blood pressure management, smoking cessation, weight loss, and exercise, ASTP uses motivational interviewing to help students work through their ambivalence about changing their behavior and to facilitate their movement along a continuum from high-risk drinking to lower risk drinking or abstinence.

Dozens of studies from many different countries document the effectiveness of brief interventions that use motivational interviewing to reduce heavy or problematic drinking (W. Miller, 2000). Following the Institute of Medicine's (1990) recommendations to broaden the base of interventions for alcohol problems to include interventions for targeting high-risk groups like college student drinkers, ASTP meets each student on his or her own terms by using a brief motivational intervention to encourage moderate, less risky use of alcohol if the student chooses to drink. Students who are assessed as alcohol dependent, who have been advised by a physician not to drink, or who have medical conditions in which use of alcohol may be contraindicated are encouraged to abstain from alcohol use, to seek a medical consultation, or to accept referral to an abstinence-based program. At WWU, the use of a Personalized Feedback Profile within the context of a brief motivational interview presents a student with the opportunity to compare his or her own drinking with that of other students.

## WWU'S BRIEF MOTIVATIONAL INTERVENTION

From a motivational interviewing perspective, the primary objective in working with students who have no desire to change their behavior (i.e., precontemplators) is to assist them through a change process that decreases defensiveness and increases motivation to begin thinking about the connections between alcohol use and unwanted consequences (Prochaska & DiClemente, 1984). WWU's risk reduction specialists use comparisons of individual use patterns with WWU norms to introduce ambivalence into the student's thinking. Once ambivalence is adequately addressed, the primary task shifts from comparing normative drinking profiles to assisting students to determine the best route for change.

Heavy-drinking students typically reacted with more surprise and concern to the normative feedback than to any other part of the data presented in the Personalized Feedback Profile. Some challenged the accuracy of the norms used in the graphic comparisons, reasoning that most college students would intentionally underestimate the amount of alcohol they drank when completing a questionnaire for university researchers. A range of common student objections included comments such as, "They [the other students] are lying," "No one tells the truth on those surveys," and "That's not what the people I know would say" (Hyun et al., 1998).

In these circumstances, prevention specialists typically respond in the nondefensive manner recommended by Dimeff and her associates (1999), that is, by telling students that although some "may attempt to falsify their report, the data from our studies are consistent with national figures" (p. 105). Another nonjudgmental approach to student disagreement about the veracity of the normative data consists of explaining the "peer-selection" process. Numerous studies have shown that persons choose to associate with peers who are similar to themselves and whose lifestyle resembles their own (Jacob & Leonard, 1991; Kandel & Andrews, 1987). Students who are already drinking heavily while in high school often select college living arrangements where heavy drinking is a social norm (Baer, Kivlahan, & Marlatt, 1995). One outcome of this socialization/selection process is that students often arrive at a "false consensus." They perceive their drinking as falling well within the typical range of college student consumption even when it is well above the average (Baer et al., 1991).

The comparisons between a student's Personalized Feedback Profile and actual campus drinking norms provide the introduction to the next stage of motivational interviewing: training in moderation skills and general lifestyle behaviors that may increase health protective behaviors and reduce alcohol-related negative consequences in the student's life. In some cases, the gap evidenced by the differences between the campus norms and a student's

Personalized Feedback Profile create an opportunity to talk with the student about possible needs for medical consultation or other outside treatment services.

The 446 mandated students who completed risk-reduction services in 1998–1999 were assessed at the completion of the intervention and at a 3-month follow-up. Of these 446 students, 196 or 44% completed and returned the voluntary follow-up assessment. Although the return rate was lower than hoped for and presented some threat to the validity of comparing pre- and posttest scores, it was consistent with previous response rates to follow-up surveys with mandated students at WWU. No additional analyses were conducted between those who responded to the follow-up survey and those who did not. To measure the impact of the intervention on alcohol use and consequences, researchers used paired sample $t$ tests to analyze the responses of participants who had completed both the baseline intake assessment and the follow-up surveys.

## RESULTS

From these analyses, researchers observed changes from baseline to follow-up in several key alcohol-related behaviors. The population-based data that describe *all* WWU students follows each result in order to show differences between mandated students and the "average" student.

1.   Students reported significant decreases in *typical* number of drinks consumed from an intake average of four drinks per typical occasion to a follow-up average of three drinks ($p < 0.001$). Most WWU students drink zero, one, two or at the most three drinks on a typical occasion.
2.   Students reported significant decreases in *peak* number of drinks consumed from an intake average of five drinks per typical peak occasion to a follow-up average of four drinks ($p < 0.001$). Most WWU students drink four drinks on peak occasions.
3.   Students reported significant decreases in the amount of time they spent drinking from an intake average of 4 hours per drinking occasion to a follow-up average of 3 hours per occasion ($p < 0.012$). Among WWU students who drink, most spend an average of 2 to 2.5 hours per drinking occasion.
4.   Students reported significant decreases in the number of drinking occasions per month from an intake average of three and a half times per month to a follow-up average of three times

($p$ < 0.001). Most WWU students reported drinking two to three times per month.

5. Students reported a statistically nonsignificant 10% decrease in overall negative alcohol-related consequences from an average of 10 negative consequences per heavy drinking occasion at intake (e.g., hangovers, unable to remember, fighting with a friend, unable to study, etc.) to 9 negative consequences per occasion at follow-up.

## DISCUSSION OF THE INFUSION OF SOCIAL NORMS DATA INTO BRIEF MOTIVATIONAL INTERVENTIONS

Researchers at WWU tentatively concluded that the infusion of personalized social norms comparisons into the alcohol screening and intervention for sanctioned students could be a significant enhancement within the already robust brief intervention using motivational interviewing. A limitation to this observation is the fact that the specific effects of the personalized social norms feedback cannot be differentiated from the treatment effects of other feedback categories (e.g., alcohol expectancies, family history, readiness to change, and moderation tips) in the Personalized Feedback Profile. However, these preliminary results at WWU are consistent with findings from studies showing the effect of brief interventions using individualized feedback (Baer et al., 1995; Marlatt et al., 1998) and studies showing the effect of modifying contextual variables like drinking norms (Baer et al., 1991; Perkins & Berkowitz, 1986) on reducing high-risk drinking and alcohol problems in the college student population. Additionally, recent research adds evidence for the efficacy of personalized normative feedback incorporated as an intervention component with ASTP. Neighbors and Lewis (2003) found that computerized feedback that communicated *only* personalized normative data (i.e., details about the student's own drinking, their perceptions of typical student drinking, and actual typical student drinking)—in the absence of any other information or components—was sufficient to reduce normative misperceptions and consequent heavy drinking among college students for up to 6 months.

## CONCLUSION AND IMPLICATIONS

The task of preventing alcohol-related problems in college students is by no means an easy one, as anyone who has attempted interventions for this widespread problem knows. Efforts to prevent alcohol-related problems in college students can take many different forms and can focus on very different audiences at various levels of drinking alcohol—from delaying the first drink in abstainers to preventing more serious problems from occurring in students who already drink heavily and may be experiencing at least minimal problems as a result. No single approach, however successful it is in reducing alcohol-related problems among college students, can be relied on to eliminate the problem entirely.

The social norms media approach holds great promise as a universal prevention component of effective comprehensive campus programs (NIAAA, 2002). A growing number of studies offer substantial evidence demonstrating the positive effect of the social norms mass media approach to reducing harmful misperceptions and, in turn, harmful behaviors among college student populations (Perkins, 2002b). Similarly, an extensive literature documents the indicated prevention effectiveness of ASTP—cognitive-behavior skills training within the framework of brief motivational interventions—in decreasing the alcohol-related harm in the lives of students who have chosen to drink and may, as a result, experience negative physical, emotional, social, or academic consequences.

The infusion of accurate normative data into brief motivational interventions like ASTP at WWU holds promise for campus leaders seeking to broaden the base of effective outcomes for those students at greatest risk. Theoretically, personalized normative feedback may be a more effective intervention for high-risk student drinkers than campus-wide social norms marketing because it is individually tailored and more likely to be personally meaningful to the individual. While future research is needed to determine the efficacy of increased normative feedback within the brief motivational intervention, the use of the social norms data in individualized feedback to high-risk student drinkers holds promise for producing notable improvements in patterns of alcohol consumption and consequences among this critical subpopulation of college student drinkers.

# 16

## DRINKING STORIES AS LEARNING TOOLS

### SOCIALLY SITUATED EXPERIENTIAL LEARNING AND POPULAR CULTURE

*Thomas A. Workman*

In 2002, a national television advertising campaign for a major beer producer mirrored a well-established behavior within the drinking culture to sell its product. The series featured friends telling each other stories about everyday blunders and foibles while they sat drinking the product. The tag line for the advertisements suggested that the product was made for such times when, among friends, we can laugh at the odd circumstances of life, or more accurately, sit and drink as others laugh about them as they are retold.

In 2003, the campaign's storylines made a significant change from innocent moments of embarrassment to behaviors that most of us would identify as sophomoric pranks or foolish stunts usually accomplished in a state of intoxication. In one advertisement, for example, a young man attempts to determine what, exactly, an electronic dog fence feels like by wearing the dog collar himself and walking through the boundary while friends look on, laughing. The "dog collar experiment" mirrors many of the stories that I have collected over the years in my study of the collegiate drinking culture. But the advertisement isn't about the experience; the central action of the ad is the retelling of the story to other friends as they sit around the patio enjoying the beer product. A young woman comments, "I'd never do that," although by the end of the commercial (and the story), she laughs as the collar is being placed around her neck.

The advertising campaign serves as the perfect illustration of the interaction between various forms of cultural discourse; the advertising is informed by the cultural practice of storytelling while the storytelling in the commercial reifies the practices of real life. Cultural theory suggests that an audience finds resonance in the context of the ad from their own lives (Williamson, 1978), while also being instructed in social norms and practices by the advertisement (Jhally, 1990). Like the proverbial chicken and egg debate, it becomes difficult, if not impossible to determine which form of cultural meaning production comes first. What we do know, however, is that together these forms of discourse produce a set of meanings that concretize social practices.

This form of "intertextual" meaning-making points to the role of popular culture in producing what Lederman and Stewart (1998) deem socially situated experiential learning, a construct that explains the acquisition and interpretation of social information around alcohol consumption for young adults (see Chapter 3 for a discussion of the development of this model). In this chapter, I argue that SSEL can be better informed by an understanding of the ways in which meanings are reproduced within Western popular culture, and I offer an analysis of personal and commercial narratives as an explanation of the process. I suggest that the "drinking story," told in both personal and commercial settings, plays a critical role in the reproduction of meanings for alcohol consumption in the United States, particularly for young adults. The analysis supports both the theory of socially constructed learning about alcohol use, as well as the need for prevention specialists to intervene in both the acquisition and the interpretation of meaning for young adults. I begin by laying a foundation from popular cultural theory to explain the uncritical reproduction of meaning within culture. I then examine the "dog collar" advertisement, among other narratives in popular culture, against drinking stories collected from college undergraduates in focus groups to explain the relationship between popular culture and personal enactments of meaning. Finally, I return to the role of social norms campaigns and environmental management as tools of intervention in the formation of meanings around alcohol consumption within the college drinking culture.

## CULTURAL THEORY AND SOCIALLY SITUATED EXPERIENTIAL LEARNING

Researchers investigating cultural practices do so from a set of epistemological assumptions concerning the intersection among symbols, signs, structures and meanings and the formation of rituals, practices and lifestyles that make up a "culture." Cultural research is "the study of relations between elements in a whole way of life" (Hall, 1996, p. 34). Williams (1965) described such study as "the attempt to discover the nature of the organization which is the complex of these relationships" (p. 63).

Lederman (1993) offered a definition of the culture of college drinking as "the shared images, behaviors, attitudes and perceptions that create a culturally-specific sense that drinking heavily in college is an inherent and inevitable part of the college years" (p. 243). An important aspect of this definition is the relationship between interpretation and enactment. Culture is "*both* the meanings and values which arise amongst distinctive social groups and classes, on the basis of their historical conditions and relationships, through which they 'handle' and respond to the conditions of existence; *and* as the lived traditions and practices through which those 'understandings' are expressed and in which they are embodied" (Hall, 1996, p. 38). In other words, meaning-making leads to personal enactment, whereas enactment adds meaning.

As such, SSEL rests on the assumption that the culture of college drinking is learned through a set of drinking-related experiences and the shared stories of experiences. Popular culture plays a critical role in such learning; popular culture texts create beliefs, attitudes, and perceptions of reality while also framing the actual experience of reality. Ultimately, popular culture becomes the background in which we perceive and make sense of our experiences. The texts of popular songs, advertisements, television shows, even greeting cards and cartoons become an interpretative frame that we use to make sense of the things we experience daily (Storey, 1993).

Although definitions of "popular" remain contested among cultural theorists, most equate "popular" culture with the products of mass production, engaged widely by those "consumers" for whom it was produced (Brooker, 1999; Storey, 1993). Fiske (1989b) defined popular culture as "the active process of generating and circulating meanings and pleasures within a social system" (p. 23). Such meanings "necessarily produce a social identity for the people involved" (Fiske, 1998a, p. 1).

This definition allows the vital connection of popular meaning-making as "pleasure" (Fiske, 1989a, 1989b) and implies an economic and political framework. Two thoughts emerge here: First, particularly in what is titled a "consumer society" (Jameson, 1998), the ultimate function of American culture is the consumption of pleasure. Second, there is also pleasure in the engagement or resistance of cultural meanings, in developing "our own way" of doing things (Fiske, 1989b).

Intertextuality, or the interaction between forms of popular discourse, becomes an integral part of the meaning-making process, for it is impossible to point at a producer of any one condition or metaphor of practice in order to identify signification. Storey (1993) explained:

> Connotations are therefore not simply produced by the makers of the image, but activated from an already existing cultural repertoire. In other words, the image both draws from the cultural repertoire and at the same time adds to it. Moreover, the cultural repertoire does not form an homogeneous block. Myth is continually confronted by counter-myth. (p. 80)

Articulation to the capitalist ideology is perhaps the most important theoretical construct in the study of American popular culture for, as Johnson (1996) asserted, "In our societies, many forms of cultural production also take the form of capitalist commodities" (p. 83). Most critiques of capitalist popular culture implicate the "producer" as signifying the consumption of a product in such a way that what is consumed is the signification itself, embodied through the consumption of the product (Jhally, 1990). It is essential, therefore, to explore the theoretical foundations of capitalism as a key articulation within U.S. popular culture. "Whatever popular culture is," Storey (1993) wrote, "what is certain is that its raw materials are those which are commercially provided" (p. 12).

Baudrillard (1988) wrote, "We have reached the point where 'consumption' has grasped the whole of life" (p. 33). The result, argued Peter Sacks (1996), is that Generation X (and, some would argue, Generation Y as well) are part of a culture marked by "hyperconsumerism" and entitlement. He wrote, "Increasingly, the postmodern person is relinquishing his responsibility to others and the larger society; she has an expectation of immediate gratification without necessarily having to work for it; and he's a 'victim' of the system if his gratification is thwarted or isn't immediate" (p. 156).

This is not to say that every reading of cultural practice is *conscious* of this function, but that an aspect of social function is embedded within the interpretations of cultural practices. Through the idea of function, we can better see how advertising has had such profound impact utilizing "lifestyle" frameworks which employ social position or social function as the ultimate commodity (Leiss, Klein, & Jhally, 1997). In other words, engaging the messages of popular culture serves as a way for a young adult—or the rest of us—to form a social identity.

Two basic premises emerge from this body of theory that inform the construct of socially situated experiential learning. First, all texts within the web of culture serve as *mirrors* and *cues* for human behavior and, as such, are imbedded with meanings of functionality that come from a host of messages, particularly those from commercial texts which commodify the functions themselves. As a *mirror*, these texts reflect the meanings of other related texts; they reify meanings that resonate in other places. They confirm engagement as "normal" by offering, even if only in imagination, a reflection of an activity seen by others as "normal" within a certain context. However, any one of these texts also serve as *cues* to interpretation, informing behavior by offering a function for a certain interpretation, forming a set of "rules" for the enactment of the behavior, and providing a legitimization of a specific interpretation. The interpretation of the practice serves as the key instructor of the route to social position; enactment provides a map for others to follow.

A typical collegiate drinking ritual illustrates this principle best. Students gathering to drink often begin their consumption by relating the humorous stories of overconsumption at previous social gatherings. The stories do more than provide the entertainment for the gathering; they offer a mirror on the many representations of overconsumption within the culture (found in film, television, greeting cards, commercials, other drinking stories, and drinking events) and they inform the excessive drinking performances that are to take place during the current gathering, providing a cue for how consumption "should" be enacted on this particular occasion to achieve the function of the practice.

Second, because they function as sources of identity confirmation, the mirrors and cues that instruct and normalize drinking behaviors are accepted by the culture without critical reflection. This idea is best explained through Bourdieu's (1984) "habitus" theory, where life-style is enacted as "conditions of existence" (p. 171). Bourdieu defined *habitus* as "an objective relationship between two objectivities, (which) enables an intelligible and necessary relation to be established between practices and a situation, *the meaning of which is produced by the habitus* through categories of perception and appreciation that are *themselves produced by an observable social condition*" (p. 101, italics added). It is a structure that is lived, created through class economics, relationships, social spaces, and the practices bound within them. Using the metaphor within the term, habitus is a "life-environment" in which meaning reproduces itself as a lifestyle without conscious thought; a habitus is a conceptual space—bounded by a set of class conditions—in which a lifestyle (and all practices therein) can be lived.

Returning to the context of college drinking, habitus theory suggests that the drinker uncritically discovers the context and rules of consumption through watching the enactment of consumption by others. But Bourdieu extended this one step further, suggesting that the enactment is given its own logic which "seals" the meaning as appropriate and "right." Bourdieu (1984) wrote: "All the practices and products of a given agent are objectively harmonized among themselves, without any deliberate pursuit of coherence, and objectively orchestrated, without any conscious concertation, with those of all members of the same class" (pp. 172-173). Once established as logical, criticisms of the behavior feel out of place. A resistance to critical reflection is developed, and uncritical reproduction is born.

Giddens (1984) also believes that practices are not "directly accessible to the consciousness of actors" (p. 4). He wrote:

Most such knowledge is practical in character: it is inherent in the capability to "go on" within the routines of social life. The line between the discursive and practical consciousness is fluctuating and permeable, both in the experience of the individual agent and as regards comparisons between actors in different contexts of social activity. There is no bar between these, however, as there is between the unconscious and discursive consciousness. The unconscious includes those forms of cognition and impulsion which are either wholly repressed from consciousness or appear in consciousness only in distorted form. Unconscious motivational components of action, as psychoanalytic theory suggests, have an internal hierarchy of their own, a hierarchy which expresses the "depth" of the life history of the individual actor. (pp. 4-5)

Narrative theories suggest that storytelling serves the cultural function of encouraging audience enactment (Lucaites & Condit, 1985). "Notwithstanding the debates about its factual grounding, informative value, or linkage to personal identity," stated Lieblich, Tuval-Mashiach, and Zilber (1998), "the life story constructs and transmits individual and cultural meanings. People are meaning-generating organisms; they construct their identities and self-narratives from building blocks available in the common culture, above and beyond their individual experience" (pp. 8-9).

Griffin (1990) suggested that autobiographical narratives create myths of self that provide accounts for behavior, an assertion that can be readily applied to drinking stories where the reenactment of a performance (or the acceptance of another's reenactment) serves as a construction of the identity of self. Narrative also serves to perpetuate a specific reality, presenting a preferred frame for performances that best meet the needs of the culture. Thus, stories become an essential tool to develop interpretations of social actions and situate the actions into a specific construction of reality. As a deeply entrenched form of cultural reproduction, the drinking story serves as both a *mirror* and a *cue* for social behavior, instructing the rules of social interaction and the context of consumption (Workman, 2001a). Narratives told in commercial and personal settings become the molecules of popular culture, expressing the essence of the beliefs, values, rules, and tensions of the culture.

## LESSONS OF DRINKING IN POPULAR CULTURE

The dog collar story referenced at the beginning of this chapter could easily be labeled an archetype for adolescent behavior, as it appears often in popular culture, particularly in the commodification of alcohol. Even a cursory examination of advertising images and texts produces a clear understanding that alcohol consumption has been associated with aspects of recreation and pleasure. Alcohol advertisements most commonly associate drinking with friendship, sexual pleasure, masculine play, physical strength, success, and relaxation (Berger, 1996; Grube & Wallack, 1994; Jhally, 1990; Kilbourne, 1999; Postman, Nystrom, Strate, & Weingartner, 1988). Luik (1999) described the "paradox of pleasure" in Western culture, where pleasure "has always required permission" (p. 25). Advertising, as a socializing force (Leiss et al., 1997), may serve as the American culture's source for permission, normalizing the pursuit of pleasure through the consumption of goods and providing a social authority that permits indulgence. A study of college drinking stories found that many of the personal stories circulating among students were also common themes in television and magazine advertisements for alcohol (Workman, 2001b). In those collected stories, behaviors like the dog collar experiment were common. Students readily told stories about their own embarrassing actions or the embarrassing actions of others. In fact, the more dramatic the action, the more likely the individual was given "hero" status. In the drinking stories told by college students, however, behaviors like the dog collar experiment all occurred when the students were intoxicated. It is difficult, then, to determine if the storytelling is a celebration of the learning through foolish error or a celebration of drunkenness. In focus groups, fraternity men commented that the two were indistinguishable; drinking and drunkenness were the same thing, and the behaviors shared in stories would rarely be attempted without some level of intoxication (Workman, 2001a).

Intoxicated behaviors—the stuff that drinking stories are made of—are mirrored often in other popular cultural texts. Student most often cite *Animal House*, a film made before many of the students were even born, as the classic narrative about college drinking and drunken behavior. Other films, such as *Road Trip* and *Old School*, maintain the same signification for drinking as a conduit to "story-worthy" behavior. Like the dog collar advertisement, the behaviors are retold as ultimately nonconsequential, more funny than serious, and framed within the natural lessons of life. The behaviors are framed as heroic and worthy of imitation.

Likewise, television commercials for beer continue to associate consumption with a set of behaviors that would not occur without consumption. In one television advertising campaign for Bud Lite, the men dressed up as women in order to get the drinking specials on "Ladies Night"; in another for Coors, the commercial equates partying with a man, shirt off and chest painted, who makes a spectacle of himself in front of his friends. A magazine ad series entitled "Real Friends. Real Bourbon." for Jim Beam, featured a variety of situations where the men engaged in behaviors that, as one tag line suggested, could only be shown on cable TV.

For college students, the search for pleasure is also socially sanctioned, often labelled as "sowing one's wild oats" and encouraged as a privilege of youth. "Sowing one's oats" revolves around social interaction. It is a quest for identity and esteem through successful interaction in social settings and the discovery of the sexual self. It also involves the use of "adult" products such as tobacco and alcohol. One need only turn to the many post-adolescent films of the past decade (*Pretty in Pink, Porky's, St. Elmo's Fire, The Breakfast Club, Say Anything, American Pie*, and *Road Trip* to name a few) to see a young lifestyle surrounded by an angst-ridden quest for adult identity that is found only through social and sexual interaction, much of which includes alcohol consumption. These films also represent a lifestyle focused around multiple opportunities for pleasure and social/sexual interaction rather than work, family, community, or other responsibilites.

The popular film *American Pie* is a perfect example. Within the first 10 minutes of the film, the audience watches a high school party where the men (all graduating seniors) drink to excess, attempt some form of sexual conquest over the young women at the party (unsuccessfully), and make a pact to "get laid" before the end of the semester. The scene's message mirrors cable's MTV and VH-1, where spring break shows dwarf the reality of jobs, classes, career development, and other burdens of student life, favoring the "party" as the central locus of activity. The February 2000 issue of *Rolling Stone* features its annual "Spring Break" story and, like the MTV program, focuses its attention entirely on a single representation of spring break— week off from classes for college students, a beach party somewhere on the southeast coast of the United States, complete with images and stories of excessive alcohol consumption and anonymous sex. As if to confirm the true meaning of "break," attached to the list of recommended activities and lodgings are maps to Florida from various locations, complete with a state-by-state listing of age-of-consent and sodomy laws. Semiotically, *Rolling Stone* and MTV's "Spring Break" serve as a referent to hedonistic consumption.

Both of these texts are mirrored in actual drinking stories exchanged among college students. Drinking stories collected at fraternites found themes of sexual exploration and exploitation, along with a host of other behaviors that serve as "once in a lifetime" adventures connected to youth and to the college experience (Workman, 2001a). Rather than a rite of passage, drinking is socially situated as a route to learning about ones limits, abilities, and identity. Excessive drinking is also a sign of class, an enactment of recreation over work, of conspicuous consumption via discretionary income.

The consumption of pleasure as a form of consumerist entitlement is signified within alcohol commercials targeted at young adults. These referents are often framed humorously. The essential need for pleasure ("fun") over other goods or actions is presented as comic irony. Unlike the class distinctions often found in alcohol advertising in *Cosmopolitan* or *Men's*

*Journal* where class is signified through clothing, setting, or activities (golfing, dinner parties, formal events), advertising for college students utilizes referents that legitimize pleasure within the economic and social context of young adulthood. "Fun" is still the ultimate goal, yet it is presented as an expectation of American life. Most importantly, the signification of "fun" references the consumption of alcohol. Alcohol provides the door to instant social, sexual, and physical gratification.

Read in this light, the "dog collar experiment" is an experience of the wealthy who have the time and the resources to experiment with technological gizmos (like electronic fences for dogs) and sit chatting about their results with friends. Other mediated drinking narratives follow this same class distinction; those who party have the time, the money, and the opportunity to engage in social recreation and consumption rather than work. It is no wonder, then, that the highest rates of alcohol abuse in the United States occur among White, middle- to upperclass students who are members of fraternities and sororities (Wechsler, Isaac, Grodstein, & Sellers, 1994; Wechsler, Lee, Kuo, & Lee, 2000; Wechsler, Molnar, Davenport, & Baer, 1999).

Williamson (1978) suggested that audiences of advertisements "mediate" the missing elements of commercial messages, allowing audiences to personalize the message by connecting the commercial images with examples from their own memory. This may best explain why socially situated learning, when surrounded by the reinforced messages of popular culture texts, continues to occur within cultural groups rather than across racial or socioeconomic boundaries. Messages from popular culture reinforce the idea that only members of certain social classes are entitled to these behaviors.

Messages from popular culture also reinforce that the behaviors are ultimately nonconsequential, as the stories never depict real harm coming from the consumption or the associated behavior. Students, likewise, never circulate drinking stories with negative consequences, because, as one student stated, "It would bring everybody down" (Workman, 2001a). It is not surprising, then, that persuasive health campaigns attempting to warn students of the impending doom of excessive consumption have had little effect on drinking rates; they contradict the frame of the culture and the lessons learned within social settings.

## CULTURAL INTERVENTION:
## SOCIAL NORMS AS REMEDY

Taken together, this body of research suggests that popular culture plays a critical role in the development and uncritical reproduction of meaning and ultimately, social practices like excessive alcohol consumption. The larger perceptual frames provided by popular culture have a direct impact on the ways in which SSEL occurs. This analysis supports the notion that interventions must be based in social ecology in order to be effective.

"Social ecology" concentrates on pro-health messages or normative/misperception campaigns that reduce expectancies and misperceptions, offering what Berkowitz described as "proactive prevention." This model has been rapidly adopted on a number of college campuses (Berkowitz, 1997; Haines, 1996; Johannessen et al., 1999; Lederman et al., 2001; Perkins, 2003c; University of Michigan, 1993) because of growing evidence that "an exclusive emphasis on abuse and problem behavior may unintentionally serve to perpetuate problem alcohol and other drug use" (Berkowitz, 1998, p. 119). Normative campaigns work to employ messages that "not everyone" is engaged in binge drinking. Evidence from studies suggests that, when student misperceptions of the frequency and intensity of peer drinking are corrected, drinking rates across the population decrease (Berkowitz, 1998; Haines, 1996; Johannessen et al., 1999).

More importantly, the field has evolved rapidly, moving from simplistic mass messages to sophisticated campaigns that work within specific groups and through specific experiences. Normative campaigns like the RU SURE Campaign (see Chapter 4) and the Small Group Norms Challenging Intervention (Far & Miller, 2001) provide new and innovative approaches to the basic theory. These programs offer several critical elements that serve as interventions to the interpretive frames of popular culture.

The first is the need for programs to move individuals into a conscious state of critical reflection, what Prochaska (Prochaska, DiClemente, & Norcross, 1992; Migneault, Velicer, Prochaska, & Stevenson, 1999) called moving from pre-cognition to cognition. Norms programs must acknowledge the messages and images of popular culture and then create opportunities for students to become aware of those meanings at a conscious level. Media literacy may be a critical first step in socially situated experiential learning, as students reflect on where the assignment of meanings originate. Though difficult, students can recognize the similarities of their lessons learned to those learned by mediated personas.

Second, normative programs can provide a sense of dissonance with the dominant narratives of popular culture, offering an opportunity for students to determine the representation of the narratives they consume from the media and their social groups. In fact, it is the messages of popular culture that offer counterargument for behavior-based norms messages ("Most students drink four or fewer drinks when they party"); stories about moderation are never told either in mediated or personal settings. Especially in group-based feedback data, popular cultural narratives can be seen as myths rather than as reflections of reality; behaviors like the dog collar experiment become isolated incidents that live outside of the norm rather than archetypes.

Finally, there is a key role in environmental management to address the types of stories that enter popular culture. A number of groups, including the Center for Alcohol Marketing to Youth and the Action Coalition for Media Education, have begun addressing the "media environment" as part of the landscape that impacts health behaviors in ways similar to how laws, policies, and enforcement impact the physical environment of drinking on campuses and in communities. Limiting the messages that young adults consume surrounding nonconsequential consumption and intoxicated behavior would certainly impact socially situated experiential learning, and needs to be further explored.

This research, however, also raises an important caution in the evolution of social norms programming. As suggested by cultural theory, social identity is a key aspect of the stories we tell. Norms programs and media environmentalism work to bring a critical question to the college drinking story yet offer no viable, functional alternative to help college students form their identity. We have yet to ask the difficult questions: What happens to a culture when their stories die? Can new stories (of social, academic, even civic success) serve as adequate replacements? It is essential that norms programs begin to grapple with these difficult questions, determining what types of behaviors (and the stories that follow) can serve as valid experiential learning opportunities.

# REFERENCES

Agostinelli, G., Brown, J. M., & Miller, W.R. (1995). Effects of normative feedback on consumption among heavy drinking college students. *Journal of Drug Education, 25,* 31-40.

Agostinelli, G., & Miller, W. R. (1994). Drinking and thinking: How does personal drinking affect judgements of prevalence and risk? *Journal of Studies on Alcohol, 55,* 327-337.

American Council on Education (ACE). (1988, August). *Self-regulation initiatives: Resource documents for colleges and universities. Alcohol and other substance abuse: Resources for institutional action.* Washington, DC: American Council on Education.

American College Health Association (ACHA). (2001). *Standards of practice for health promotion in higher education.* Bloomington: Indiana University Press.

Anderson, D. S., & Milgram, G. G. (1997). *Promising practices: Campus alcohol strategies.* Fairfax, VA: George Mason University.

Asch, S. E. (1951). Effects of group pressure on the modification and distortion of judgements. In H. Guetzkow (Ed.), *Groups, leadership and men: Research in human relations* (pp. 177-190). Pittburgh, PA: Carnegie Press.

Asch, S. E. (1952). *Social psychology.* Englewood Cliffs, NJ: Prentice-Hall.

Baer, J. S. (1994). Effects of college residence on perceived norms for alcohol consumption: An examination of the first year of college. *Psychology of Addictive Behaviors, 8,* 43-50.

Baer, J. S. (2002). Student factors: Understanding individual variation in college drinking. *Journal of Studies on Alcohol, Supplement No. 14,* 40-53.

Baer, J. S., & Carney, M. M. (1993). Biases in the perceptions of the consequences of alcohol use among college students. *Journal of Studies on Alcohol, 54,* 54-60.

Baer, J. S., Kivlahan, D.R., & Marlatt, G. A. (1995). High-risk drinking across the transition from high school to college. *Alcoholism: Clinical and Experimental Research, 19,* 54-61.

Baer, J., Stacy, A., & Larimer, M. (1991). Biases in the perception of drinking norms among college students. *Journal of Studies on Alcohol, 52,* 580-586.

Bandura, A. (1986). *The social foundation of thought and action: A social cognitive theory.* Englewood Cliffs, NJ: Prentice-Hall.

Barnett, L. A., Far, J. M., Maus, A. L., & Miller, J. A. (1996). Changing perceptions of peer norms as a drinking reduction program for college students. *Journal of Alcohol and Drug Education, 41*(2), 39-61.

Baudrillard, J. (1988). Consumer society. In M. Poster (Ed.), *Selected writings* (pp. 29-56). Stanford, CA: Stanford University Press.

Bauerle, J. (2003). The University of Virginia's social norms marketing campaign. *The Report on Social Norms: Working Paper No. 11.* Little Falls, NJ: PaperClip Communications.

Bauerle, J., Burwell, C., & Turner, J. C. (2002, May). *Social norms marketing at the University of Virginia.* Paper presented at the annual meeting of the American College Health Association, Washington, DC.

Beck, K. H., & Treiman, K. A. (1996). The relationship of social context of drinking, perceived social norms, and parental influence to various drinking patterns of adolescents. *Addictive Behaviors, 21,* 633-644.

Bennett, M. E., McCrady, B. S., Frankenstein, W., Laitman, L. A., Van Horn, D. H. A., & Keller, D. S. (1993). Identifying young adult substance abusers: The Rutgers collegiate substance abuse screening test. *Journal of Studies on Alcohol, 54,* 522-527.

Berger, A. A. (1996). *Manufacturing desire: Media, popular culture, and everyday life.* New Brunswick, NJ: Transaction Books.

Berkowitz, A. D. (1997). From reactive to proactive prevention: Promoting an ecology of health on campus. In P. C. Rivers & E. Shore (Eds.), *A handbook on substance abuse for college and university personnel* (pp. 140-199). Westport, CT: Greenwood Press.

Berkowitz, A. D. (1998, September/October). The proactive prevention model: Helping students translate healthy beliefs into healthy actions. *About Campus,* pp. 26-27.

Berkowitz, A. D. (2002a). Fostering men's responsibility for preventing sexual assault. In P. A. Schewe (Ed.), *Preventing intimate partner violence: Developmentally appropriate interventions across the life span* (pp. 163-196). Washington, DC: American Psychological Press.

Berkowitz, A. D. (2002b). Responding to the critics: Answers to common questions and concerns about the social norms approach. *The Report on Social Norms: Working paper no. 7.* Little Falls, NJ: PaperClip Communications.

Berkowitz, A. D. (2003b). *The social norms approach: Theory, research and annotated bibliography.* Posted on the Web site of the Higher Education Center, Newton, MA. (Available from http://www.edc.org/hec)

Berkowitz, A. D. (2003a). Applications of social norms theory to other health and social justice issues. In H. W. Perkins (Ed.), *The social norms approach to preventing school and college age substance abuse: A handbook for educators, counselors, and clinicians* (pp. 259-279). San Francisco, CA: Jossey-Bass.

Berkowitz, A. D., & Perkins, H. W. (1986a). Problem drinking among college students: A review of recent research. *Journal of American College Health, 35,* 21-28.

Berkowitz, A. D., & Perkins, H. W. (1986b). Resident advisors as role models: A comparison of drinking patterns of resident advisors and their peers. *Journal of College Student Personnel, 27*, 146-153.

Berkowitz, A.D., & Perkins, H. W. (1987). Current issues in effective alcohol education programming. In J. S. Sherwood (Ed.), *Alcohol policies and practices on college and university campuses* (pp. 69-85). Washington, DC: National Association of Student Personnel Administrators.

Bigsby, M. J. (2002). Seeing eye to eye? Comparing students' and parents' perceptions of bullying behavior. *School Social Work, 27*(1), 37-57.

Botvin, G. J., Griffin, K. W., Diaz, T., & Ifill-Williams, M. (2001). Preventing binge drinking during early adolescence: One- and two-year follow-up of a school-based preventive intervention. *Psychology of Addictive Behaviors, 15*, 360-365.

Bourdieu, P. (1984). *Distinction: A social critique of the judgment of taste* (R. Nice, Trans.). Cambridge, MA: Harvard University Press.

Bourgeois, M. J., & Bowen, A. (2001). Self-organization of alcohol-related attitudes and beliefs in a campus housing complex: An initial investigation. *Health Psychology, 20*(6), 1-4.

Bowen, A. M., & Bourgeois, M. J. (2001). Attitudes towards lesbian, gay, and bisexual college students: The contribution of pluralistic ignorance, dynamic social impact, and contact theories. *Journal of American College Health, 50*, 91-96.

Bredemeier, M. E., & Greenblat, C. S. (1981). The educational effectiveness of simulation games: A synthesis of findings. *Simulation and Games, 12*, 307-332.

Brooker, P. (1999). *A concise glossary of cultural theory.* London: Arnold.

Brower, A. (2002). Are college students alcoholics? *Journal of American College Health, 50*, 253-255.

Brown, R. (1973). *A first language: The early stages.* Cambridge, MA: Harvard University Press.

Bruce, S. (2002). The "A Man" campaign: Marketing social norms to men to prevent sexual assault. *The Report on Social Norms: Working Paper No. 5.* Little Falls, NJ: PaperClip Communications.

Burns, W. D., Ballou, J., & Lederman, L. (1991). *Perceptions of alcohol use and policy on the college campus: Preventing alcohol/drug abuse at Rutgers University.* Unpublished manuscript, U.S. Department of Education Fund for the Improvement of Post Secondary Education (FIPSE) conference paper.

Burns, W. D., & Goodstadt, M. (1989). *Alcohol use on the Rutgers University campus: A study of various communities.* Unpublished manuscript, U.S. Department of Education Fund for the Improvement of Post Secondary Education (FIPSE) conference paper.

Burns, W. D., & Klawunn, M. (1997). The web of caring: An approach to accountability in alcohol policy. In *Designing alcohol and other drug prevention programs in higher education: Bringing theory into practice* (pp. 49-124). Washington, DC: U.S. Department of Education. (Available at http://www.edc.org/hec/pubs/theorybook/burns.html)

Butcher, A. H., Manning, D. T., & O'Neal, E. C. (1991). HIV-related sexual behaviors of college students. *Journal of American College Health, 40*, 115-118.

Butler, E. R. (1993). Alcohol use by college students: A rite of passage ritual. *NASPA Journal, 31*(1), 48-55.

Calder, B. (1977). Focus groups and the nature of qualitative marketing research. *Journal of Marketing Research, 14*, 353-364.

Cappella, J. (2003). Editor's introduction: Theoretical approaches to communication campaigns. *Communication Theory, 13*, 160-163.

Carbaugh, D. (1990). *Situating selves: The communication of social identities in American scenes.* Albany: State University of New York Press.

Carbaugh, D., & Hastings, S. O. (1992). A role for communication theory in ethnography and cultural analysis. *Communication Theory, 2*, 156-165.

Carey, K. B. (1995a). Alcohol-related expectancies predict quantity and frequency of heavy drinking among college students. *Psychology of Addictive Behaviors, 9*, 236-241.

Carey, K. B. (1995b). Heavy drinking contexts and indices of problem drinking among college students. *Journal of Studies on Alcohol, 56*, 287-292.

Carter, C. A., & Kahnweiler, W. M. (2000). The efficacy of the social norms approach to substance abuse prevention applied to fraternity men. *Journal of American College Health, 49*, 66-71.

Cimini, M. D., Page, J. C., & Trujillo, D. (2002). Using peer theater to deliver social norms information: The Middle Earth Players program. *The Report on Social Norms: Working Paper No. 8.* Little Falls, NJ: PaperClip Communications.

Clapp, J. D., & McDonnell, A. L. (2000). The relationship of perceptions of alcohol promotion and peer drinking norms to alcohol problems reported by college students. *Journal of College Student Development, 41*(1), 20-26.

Cohen, D. J, & Lederman, L. C. (1998). Navigating the freedom of college life: Students talk about alcohol, gender, and sex. In N. Roth & L. Fuller (Eds.), *Women and AIDS: Negotiating safer practices, care, and representation* (pp. 101-126). New York: Haworth Press.

The Core Institute (1996). *Campus survey of alcohol and other drug norms.* Carbondale: The Core Institute, Southern Illinois University.

The Core Institute (2003). About the Core Institute. Retrieved July 13, 2003, from http://www.siu/edu/departments/coreinst/public.html.

Cunningham, J. A., Wild, T. C., Bondy, S. J., & Lin, E. (2001). Impact of normative feedback on problem drinkers: A small-area population study. *Journal of Studies on Alcohol, 62*, 228-233.

D'Amico, E. J., Metrik, J., McCarthy, D. M., Frissell, K. C., Appelbaum, M., & Brown, S. A. (2001). Progression into and out of binge drinking among high school students. *Psychology of Addictive Behaviors, 15*, 341-349.

Danish, S. J., Petitpas, A. J., & Hale, B. D. (1993). Life development intervention for athletes: Life skills through sports. *Counseling Psychologist, 21*, 352-385.

DeJong, W. (2003). An interview with William DeJong, Ph.D. *The Report on Social Norms, 3*(1), 1, 5-8.

DeJong, W., Vince-Whitman, C., Colthurst, T., Cretella, M., Rosati, M., & Zweig, K. (1998). *Environmental management: A comprehensive strategy for reducing alcohol and other drug use on college campuses.* Newton, MA: The Higher Education Center for Alcohol and Other Drug Prevention.

Delia, J. G. (1987). Interpersonal cognition, message goals, and organization of communication: Recent constructivist research. In D. L. Kincaid (Ed.),

*Communication theory: Eastern and western perspectives* (pp. 255-274). San Diego, CA: Academic.

Dewey, J. (1929). *Experience and education.* New York: Harper.

Dimeff, L., Baer, J., Kvilahan, D., & Marlatt, G. A. (1999). *Brief alcohol screening and intervention for college students (BASICS): A harm reduction approach.* New York: Guilford.

Dubuque, E., Ciano-Boyce, C., & Shelley-Sireci, L. (2002). Measuring misperceptions of homophobia on campus. *The Report on Social Norms: Working Paper No. 4.* Little Falls, NJ: PaperClip Communications.

Eagly, A. H., & Chaiken, S. (1993). *The psychology of attitudes.* New York: Harcourt, Brace, & Jovanovich.

Engs, R. C. (1977). Drinking patterns and drinking problems of college students. *Journal of Studies on Alcohol, 38,* 2144-2156.

Erikson, E. H. (1968). *Identity: Youth and crisis.* New York: Norton.

Fabiano, P. M. (2003). Applying the social norms model to universal and indicated alcohol interventions at Western Washington University. In H. W. Perkins (Ed.), *The social norms approach to preventing school and college age substance abuse: A handbook for educators, counselors, and clinicians* (pp. 83-99). San Francisco, CA: Jossey-Bass.

Fabiano, P. M., & Lederman, L. C. (2002). *Top ten misperceptions of focus group research.* The Report on Social Norms: Working paper no. 3. Little Falls, NJ: PaperClip Communications.

Fabiano, P. M., McKinney, G., Hyun, Y. R., Mertz, H., & Rhoads, K. (1999). *WWU Lifestyles Project III: Patterns of alcohol and drug consumption and consequences among Western Washington University students.* Bellingham, WA: WWU Office of Institutional Assessment and Testing Report no. 1999-01, Western Washington University.

Fabiano, P. M., Perkins, H.W., Berkowitz, A.D., Linkenbach, J., & Stark, C. (2003). Engaging men as social justice allies in ending violence against women: Evidence for a social norms approach. *Journal of American College Health, 52,* 105-112.

Far, J. (2001). The small groups norms-challenging model. *The Report on Social Norms, 1*(1), 4-5. Little Falls, NJ: PaperClip Communications.

Far, J., & Miller, J. (2003). The small group norms challenging model: Social norms interventions with targeted high risk groups. In H. W. Perkins (Ed.), *The social norms approach to preventing school and college age substance abuse: A handbook for educators, counselors, and clinicians* (pp. 111-132). San Francisco, CA: Jossey-Bass.

Festinger, L. (1957). *A theory of cognitive dissonance.* Stanford, CA: Stanford University Press.

Fishbein, M., & Ajzen, I. (1975). *Belief, attitude, intention and behavior: An introduction to theory and research.* Reading, MA: Addison-Wesley.

Fisher, W. R. (1987). *Human communication as narration: Toward a philosophy of reason, value, and action.* Columbia: University of South Carolina Press.

Fiske, J. (1989a). *Reading the popular.* London, UK: Routledge.

Fiske, J. (1989b). *Understanding popular culture.* London, UK: Routledge.

Giddens, A. (1984). *The constitution of society: Outline of the theory of structuration.* Cambridge, UK: Polity Press.

Gladwell, M. (2000). *The tipping point.* Boston, MA: Little, Brown.

Glaser, B. G., & Strauss, A. L. (1967). *The discovery of grounded theory: Strategies for qualitative research.* Chicago, IL: Aldine.

Glider, P., Midyett, S., Mills-Novoa, B., Johannessen, K., & Collins, C. (2001). Challenging the collegiate rite of passage: A campus-wide social marketing media campaign to reduce binge drinking. *Journal of Drug Education, 31,* 207-220.

Goldman, M. S. (2002). Introduction. *Journal of Studies on Alcohol, Supplement No. 14,* 5.

Goree, C. T., & Szalay, L. B. (1996). *Rethinking the campus environment: A guide for substance abuse prevention.* Newton, MA: Higher Education Center.

Gouran, D. (1982). *Making decision in groups.* Glenview, IL: Scott, Foresman.

Granfield, R. (2002). Can you believe it? Assessing the credibility of a social norms campaign. *The Report on Social Norms: Working Paper No. 2.* Little Falls, NJ: PaperClip Communications.

Greenbaum, T. L. (1994). *The handbook for focus group research* (2nd ed.). Thousand Oaks, CA: Sage.

Griffin, C. J. G. (1990). The rhetoric of form in conversion narratives. *Quarterly Journal of Speech, 76,* 152-163.

Grube, J. W., & Wallack, L. (1994). Television beer advertisements and drinking knowledge, beliefs, and intentions among schoolchildren. *American Journal of Public Health, 84,* 254-259.

Haines, M. P. (1993). Using media to change student norms and prevent alcohol abuse: A tested model. *Oregon Higher Education Alcohol & Drug Newsletter, 1,* 1-3.

Haines, M. P. (1996). *A social norms approach to preventing binge drinking at colleges and universities.* Newton, MA: The Higher Education Center for Alcohol and Other Drug Prevention (U.S. Department of Education, Publication No. ED/OPE/96-18).

Haines, M. P., & Barker, G. P. (2003). The Northern Illinois University experiment: A longitudinal case study of the social norms approach. In H.W. Perkins (Ed.), *The social norms approach to preventing school and college age substance abuse: A handbook for educators, counselors, and clinicians* (pp. 21-34). San Francisco, CA: Jossey-Bass.

Haines, M. P., Barker, G. P., & Rice, R. (2003). Using social norms to reduce alcohol and tobacco use in two midwestern high schools. In H. W. Perkins (Ed.), *The social norms approach to preventing school and college age substance abuse: A handbook for educators, counselors, and clinicians* (pp. 235-244). San Francisco, CA: Jossey-Bass.

Haines, M. P., & Spear, S. F. (1996). Changing the perception of the norm: A strategy to decrease binge drinking among college students. *Journal of American College Health, 45,* 134-140.

Hall, S. (1996). Cultural studies: Two paradigms. In J. Storey (Ed.), *What is cultural studies? A reader* (pp. 31-48). London: Arnold.

Hancock, L. (2002). Social norms and prayer. *The Report on Social Norms, 2(3),* 4-6.

Hancock, L., Abhold, J., Gascoigne, J., & Altekruse, M. (2002). Applying social norms marketing to tobacco cessation and prevention: Lessons learned from three campaigns. *The Report on Social Norms: Working Paper No. 6*. Little Falls, NJ: PaperClip Communications.

Hancock, L., & Henry, N. (2003). Perceptions, norms and tobacco use in college residence hall freshmen: Evaluation of a social norms marketing intervention. In H. W. Perkins (Ed.), *The social norms approach to preventing school and college age substance abuse: A handbook for educators, counselors, and clinicians* (pp. 135-153). San Francisco, CA: Jossey-Bass.

Hansen, W. B., & Graham, J. W. (1991). Preventing alcohol, marijuana, and cigarette use among adolescents: Peer pressure resistance training versus establishing conservative norms. *Preventive Medicine, 20*, 414-430.

Hanson, D. J. (1984). College students' drinking attitudes: 1970-1982. *Psychological Reports, 54*, 300-302.

Harper, N. L., Lederman, L. C., Stewart, L. P., Yee, M., Kennedy, L., Galen, L., Winebarger, A., Barr, S., Powell, R., Laitman, L., & Goodhart, F. (1999). *A study of drinking among Grand Valley State University and Rutgers University students: Preliminary results of the personal report of student perceptions (PRSP)*. CHI Research Series: Report no. 7. New Brunswick, NJ: Center for Communication and Health Issues, Rutgers University.

Herndon, S. L. (2001). Using focus group interviews for preliminary investigation. In S. L. Herndon & G. L. Kreps (Eds.), *Qualitative research: Applications in organizational life* (pp. 63-72). Cresskill, NJ: Hampton Press.

Higher Education Center for Alcohol and Other Drug Prevention. (2002, July). *Prevention updates: Environmental management—An approach to alcohol and other drug prevention*. Newton, MA: Author.

Hingson, R., Heeren, T., Zakocs, R., Kopstein, A., & Wechsler, H. (2002). Magnitude of alcohol-related mortality and morbidity among U.S. college students ages 18-24. *Journal of Studies on Alcohol, 63*, 136-144.

Hyun, Y. R., Snyder, E., Harwick, E., & Fabiano, P. M. (1998). *Assessing the role of alcohol among students at Western Washington University: A qualitative study*. Bellingham, WA: Prevention and Wellness Services/Project WE CAN 2000, Western Washington University.

Institute of Medicine (1990). *Broadening the base of treatment for alcohol problems*. Washington, DC: National Academy Press.

Jacob, T., & Leonard, K. (1991). Experimental drinking procedures in the study of alcoholics and their families: A consideration of ethical issues. *Journal of Consulting and Clinical Psychology, 59*, 249-255.

Jaksa, J. A., & Pritchard, M. S. (1988). *Communication ethics: Methods of analysis*. Belmont, CA: Wadsworth.

Jameson, F. (1998). *The cultural turn: Selected writings on the postmodern 1983-1998*. London: Verso.

Jeffrey, L. R., & Negro, P. (1996). *Contemporary trends in alcohol and other drug use by college students in New Jersey*. Trenton, NJ: New Jersey Higher Education Consortium on Alcohol and Other Drug Prevention and Education.

Jeffrey, L. R., Negro, P., Demond, M., & Frisone, J. D. (2003). The Rowan University social norms project. In H. W. Perkins (Ed.), *The social norms approach to preventing school and college age substance abuse: A handbook for educators, counselors, and clinicians* (pp. 100-110). San Francisco, CA: Jossey-Bass.

Jhally, S. (1990). *The codes of advertising: Fetishism and the political economy of meaning in the consumer society.* London, UK: Routledge.

Johannessen, K. J., Collins, C., Mills-Novoa, B. M., & Glider, P. (1999). *A practical guide to alcohol abuse prevention: A campus case study in implementing social norms and environmental management approaches.* Tempe, AZ: Campus Health Service, the University of Arizona. (Available from The Higher Education Center for Alcohol and Other Drug Prevention, http://www.edu.org/hec orhttp://www.socialnorms.CampusHealth.net)

Johannessen, K.J., & Dude, K. (2003). Is your campus ready for a social norms marketing campaign? *The Report on Social Norms, 2*(5), 1,6-8.

Johannessen, K.J., & Glider, P. (2003). The University of Arizona's campus health social norms media campaign. In H.W. Perkins (Ed.), *The social norms approach to preventing school and college age substance abuse: A handbook for educators, counselors, and clinicians* (pp. 65-82). San Francisco, CA: Jossey-Bass.

Johannesen, R. L. (1990). *Ethics in human communication* (3rd ed.). Prospect Heights, IL: Waveland.

Johnson, R. (1996). What is cultural studies anyway? In J. Story (Ed.), *What is cultural studies: A reader* (pp. 75-114). London, UK: Arnold.

Kandel, D. B., & Andrews, K. (1987). Processes of adolescent socialization by parents and peers. *International Journal of the Addictions, 22,* 319-342.

Keeling, R. P. (2003, January 31). *Drug prevention programs: Methods and context.* Paper presented at the Drugs on Campus Seminar, Rutgers University, New Brunswick, NJ.

Kilbourne, J. (1999). *Deadly persuasion: Why women and girls must fight the addictive power of advertising.* New York: The Free Press.

Kilmartin, C. (2003). A visit to the archive: Applications of classic social psychology to social norms interventions. *The Report on Social Norms, 2*(9), 1, 7-8.

Kilmer, J. R., & Cronce, J. M. (2003). Do your data do you justice? *The Report on Social Norms, 2*(7), 1, 8.

Klein, H. (1992). Self-reported reasons for why college students drink. *Journal of Alcohol and Drug Education, 37*(2), 14-28.

Kolb, D. (1984). *Experiential learning: Experience as a source of learning.* Englewood Cliffs, NJ: Prentice Hall.

Korcuska, J. S., & Thombs, D. L. (2003). Gender role conflicts and sex-specific drinking norms: Relationships to alcohol use in undergraduate women and men. *Journal of College Student Development, 44,* 204-215.

Kreps, G. L., Bonaguro, E. W., & Query, J. L. (1998). The history and development of the field of health communication. In L. D. Jackson & B. K. Duffy (Eds.), *Health communication research: A guide to developments and directions* (pp. 1-15). Westport, CT: Greenwood.

Kusch, J. (2002). *Test of a social norms approach to understanding disordered eating practices in college women.* Unpublished doctoral dissertation, Washington State University, Pullman, WA.

Laitman, L. (1987). An overview of a university student assistance program. *Journal of American College Health, 36,* 103-108.

Larimer, M. E., & Cronce, J. M. (2002). Identification, prevention and treatment: A review of individual-focused strategies to reduce problematic alcohol consumption by college students. *Journal of Studies on Alcohol, Supplement No. 14*, 148-163.

Larimer, M. E., Irvine, D. L., Kilmer, J. R., & Marlah, G. A. (1997). College drinking and the Greek system: Examining the role of perceived norms for high-risk behavior. *Journal of College Student Development, 38*, 587-598.

Larimer, M. E., & Neighbors, C. (2003). Normative misperception and the impact of descriptive and injunctive norms on college student gambling. *Psychology of Addictive Behaviors, 17*, 235-243.

Lederman, L. C. (1983a). Differential learning outcomes in an instructional simulation: Exploring the relationship between designated role and perceived-learning outcome. *Communication Quarterly, 32*, 198-204.

Lederman, L. C. (1983b). High apprehensives talk about communication apprehension. *Communication Quarterly, 32*, 233-238.

Lederman, L. C. (1990). Assessing educational effectiveness: The focus group interview as a technique for data collection. *Communication Education, 39*, 117-127.

Lederman, L. C. (1991). *IMAGINE THAT! A simulation of drinking and dating decisions.* New Brunswick, NJ: Rutgers University Health Services.

Lederman, L. C. (1992). Debriefing: Towards a theory of the post-experience analytic process and learning. *Simulation & Gaming, 23*, 145-160.

Lederman, L. C. (1993). Friends don't let friends beer goggle: A case study in the use and abuse of alcohol and communication among college students. In E. B. Ray (Ed.), *Case studies in health communication* (pp. 161-174). Hillsdale, NJ: Erlbaum.

Lederman, L. C. (1995). *Asking questions, listening to answers and talking to people.* Dubuque, IA: Kendall Hunt.

Lederman, L. C. (1996). Internal muzak: An exploration of intrapersonal communication. In H. B. Mokros (Ed.), *Interaction & identity: Information & behavior* (Vol. 5, pp. 197-214). New Brunswick, NJ: Transaction Books.

Lederman, L. C. (1999). *Focus group interviews for alcohol prevention campaigns on the college campus: A manual for use in preparing, conducting, and analyzing data from focus group research.* New Brunswick, NJ: Center for Communication and Health Issues, Rutgers University.

Lederman, L. C. (2002a). Alcohol abuse and college students. In J. R. Schement (Ed.), *Encyclopedia of communication and information* (pp. 16-18). New York: Macmillan.

Lederman, L. C. (2002b). Intrapersonal communication. In J. R. Schement (Ed.), *Encyclopedia of communication and information* (pp. 490-492). New York: Macmillan.

Lederman, L. C., Powell, R., Stewart, L. P., Goodhart, F., & Laitman, L. (2001). *RU SURE? A game of decisions and consequences.* New Brunswick, NJ: Center for Communication and Health Issues, Rutgers University.

Lederman, L. C., & Ruben, B. D. (1978). Construct validity in communication simulations, *Simulation and Games, 9*, 259-274.

Lederman, L. C., & Ruben, B. D. (1982). Instructional simulation gaming: Validity, reliability, and utility. *Simulation and Games, 13*, 233-243.

Lederman, L. C., & Ruben, B. D. (1984). Systematic assessment of communication simulations and games. *Communication Education, 33,* 151-159.

Lederman, L. C., & Stewart, L. P. (1983). *The SIMCORP simulation participant's manual.* Princeton, NJ: Total Research Corporation.

Lederman, L. C., & Stewart, L. P. (1985). Pass it on: Simulating organizational communication. In J. W. Pfeiffer (Ed.), *A handbook of structured experiences for human relations training* (Vol. 10, pp. 68-75). San Diego, CA: University Associates.

Lederman, L. C., & Stewart, L. P. (1987). THE MARBLE COMPANY: A case study in the design of a simulation board game. *Simulation and Games, 18,* 57-81.

Lederman, L. C., & Stewart, L. P. (1991). The rules of the game. *Simulation & Gaming, 22,* 502-507.

Lederman, L. C., & Stewart, L. P. (1998). *Addressing the culture of college drinking through correcting misperceptions: The socially situated experiential learning (SSEL) model.* Paper presented at the annual meeting of the National Communication Association, New York. (CHI Research Series: Report no. 4. New Brunswick, NJ: Center for Communication and Health Issues, Rutgers University.)

Lederman, L. C., & Stewart, L. P., with students in Advanced Health Communication. (2001). RU SURE BINGO. In D. S. Anderson & G. G. Milgram (Eds.), *Promising practices: Campus alcohol strategies* (p. 83). Fairfax, VA: George Mason University.

Lederman, L. C., Stewart, L. P., Barr, S., & Perry, D. (2001). RU SURE?: Using the AHC simulation in a dangerous drinking prevention campaign. *Simulation & Gaming, 101,* 228-239.

Lederman, L. C., Stewart, L. P., Barr, S. L., Powell, R., Laitman, L., & Goodhart, F. W. (2000). RU SURE?: The role of communication theory and experiential learning in addressing dangerous drinking on the college campus. In L. C. Lederman & D. W. Gibson (Eds.), *Communication theory: A casebook approach* (pp. 325-335). Dubuque, IA: Kendall Hunt.

Lederman, L. C., Stewart, L. P., Barr, S. L., Powell, R., Laitman, L., & Goodhart, F. W. (2001). RU SURE? Using communication theory to reduce dangerous drinking on a college campus. In R. E. Rice & C. K. Atkin (Eds.), *Public communication campaigns* (3rd ed., pp. 295-299). Thousand Oaks, CA: Sage.

Lederman, L. C., Stewart, L. P., & Golubow, M. (2002). Using debriefing interviews to collect qualitative data on dangerous drinking: A case study. *Qualitative Research Reports, 2,* 1-8.

Lederman, L. C., Stewart, L. P., Goodhart, F. W., & Laitman, L. (2003). A case against "binge" as the term of choice: Convincing college students to personalize messages about dangerous drinking. *Journal of Health Communication, 8,* 79-91.

Lederman, L. C., Stewart, L. P., Kennedy, L., Donovan, B. W., Powell, R., Laitman, L., Goodhart, F., Barr, S., & McLaughlin, P. (2001). Using qualitative and quantitative methods to triangulate the research process: The role of communication in perpetuating the myth of dangerous drinking as the norm on college campuses. In S. L. Herndon & G. L. Kreps (Eds.), *Qualitative research: Applications in organizational life* (2nd ed., pp. 251-268). Cresskill, NJ: Hampton Press.

Lederman, L. C., Stewart, L. P., Kennedy, L., Powell, R., Goodhart, F. W., & Laitman, L. (1998). *Personal report of student perceptions (PRSP): An alcohol awareness measure* (CHI Research Series: Report no. 2). New Brunswick, NJ: Center for Communication and Health Issues, Rutgers University.

Lederman, L. C., Stewart, L. P., Laitman, L., Goodhart, F., & Powell, R. (2000). *A case against "binge" as the term of choice: How to get college students to personalize messages about dangerous drinking* (CHI Research Series: Report no. 15). New Brunswick, NJ: Center for Communication and Health Issues, Rutgers University.

Leiss, W., Kline, S., & Jhally, S. (1997). *Social communication in advertising: Persons, products and images of well-being* (2nd ed.). London, UK: Routledge.

Lewis, M. A., & Neighbors, C. (in press). Gender-specific misperceptions of college student drinking norms. *Psychology of Addictive Behaviors.*

Lieblich, A., Tuval-Mashiach, R., & Zilber, T. (1998). *Narrative research: Reading, analysis, and interpretation.* Thousand Oaks, CA: Sage.

Lindlof, T. R. (1995). *Qualitative communication research methods.* Thousand Oaks, CA: Sage.

Linkenbach, J. (2003). The Montana model: Development and overview of a seven-step process for implementing macro-level social norms campaigns. In H. W. Perkins (Ed.), *The social norms approach to preventing school and college age substance abuse: A handbook for educators, counselors, and clinicians* (pp. 182-206). San Francisco, CA: Jossey-Bass.

Linkenbach, J., & Perkins, H. W. (2003a). Most of us are tobacco free: An eight-month social norms campaign reducing youth initiation of smoking in Montana. In H. W. Perkins (Ed.), *The social norms approach to preventing school and college age substance abuse: A handbook for educators, counselors, and clinicians* (pp. 224-234). San Francisco, CA: Jossey-Bass.

Linkenbach, J., & Perkins, H. W. (2003b). Misperceptions of peer alcohol norms in a statewide survey of young adults. In H. W. Perkins (Ed.), *The social norms approach to preventing school and college age substance abuse: A handbook for educators, counselors, clinicians* (pp. 173-181). San Francisco, CA: Jossey-Bass.

Linkenbach, J., Perkins, H. W., & DeJong, W. (2003). Parent's perceptions of parenting norms: Using the social norms approach to reinforce effective parenting. In H. W. Perkins (Ed.), *The social norms approach to preventing school and college age substance abuse: A handbook for educators, counselors, and clinicians* (pp. 247-258). San Francisco, CA: Jossey-Bass.

Littlejohn, S. W. (1996). *Theories of human communication* (5th ed.). Belmont, CA: Wadsworth.

Lo, C. C., & Globetti, G. (1993). A partial analysis of the campus influence on drinking behavior: Students who enter college as non-drinkers. *Journal of Drug Issues, 23,* 715-725.

Lucaites, J. L., & Condit, C. M. (1985). Re-constructing narrative theory: A functional perspective. *Journal of Communication, 35,* 90-108.

Luik, J. (1999). Wardens, abbots, and modest hedonists: The problem of permission for pleasure in a democratic society. In S. Peele & M. Grant (Eds.), *Alcohol and pleasure: A health perspective* (pp. 25-36). Philadelphia, PA: Taylor & Francis.

Maggs, J. L. (1997). Alcohol use and binge drinking as goal-directed action during the transition to postsecondary education. In J. Schulenberg, J. L. Maggs, & K. Horrelmann (Eds.), *Health risks and development transitions during adolescence* (pp. 345-371). New York: Cambridge University Press.

Manis, J. G., & Meltzer, B. N. (1978). *Symbolic interaction.* Boston: Allyn & Bacon.

Marks, G., Graham, J. W., & Hansen, W. B. (1992). Social projection and social conformity in adolescent alcohol use: A longitudinal analysis. *Personality and Social Psychology Bulletin, 18,* 96-101.

Marlatt, G. A., & Baer, J. S. (1997). Harm reduction and alcohol abuse: A brief intervention for college student binge drinking: Results from a two-year follow-up assessment. In P. G. Erickson, D. M. Riley, Y. W. Cheung, & P. A. O'Hare (Eds.), *Harm reduction: A new direction for drug policies and programs* (pp. 245-262). Toronto: University of Toronto Press.

Marlatt, G. A., Baer, J. S., Kivlahan, D. R., Dimeff, L. A., Larimer, M. E., Quigley, L. A., Somers, J. A., & Williams, E. (1998). Screening and brief intervention for high-risk college student drinkers: Results from a 2-year follow-up assessment. *Journal of Consulting and Clinical Psychology, 66,* 604-615.

Marshall, A., Scherer, C. W., & Real, K. (1998). The relationship between students' social networks and engaging in risky behaviors: The college tradition of "drink 'til you drop." *Journal of Health Communication, 11*(2), 34-41.

McLeroy, K., Bibeau, D., Steckler, A., & Glanz, K. (1988). An ecological perspective on health promotion programs. *Health Education Quarterly, 15,* 351-377.

Meilman, P. W., Cashin, J. R., McKillip, J., & Presley, C. A. (1998). Understanding the three national databases on collegiate alcohol use. *Journal of American College Health, 46,* 159-162.

Meilman, P. W., Leichliter, J. S., & Presley, C. A. (1999). Greeks and athletes: Who drinks more? *Journal of American College Health, 47,* 187-190.

Merton, R., Fiske, M., & Kendall, P. (1952). *The focused interview.* New York: Bureau of Applied Social Research, Columbia University.

Migneault, J. P., Velicer, W. F., Prochaska, J. O., & Stevenson, J. F. (1999). Decisional balance for immoderate drinking in college students. *Substance Use and Misuse, 34,* 1325-1346.

Milgram, G. G. (1993). Adolescents, alcohol and aggression. *Journal of Studies on Alcohol, 54,* 53-61.

Milgram, G. G., & Anderson, D. S. (2000). *Action planner: Steps for developing a comprehensive campus alcohol abuse prevention program.* Fairfax, VA: George Mason University.

Miller, D. T., & McFarland, C. (1987). Pluralistic ignorance: When similarity is interpreted as dissimilarity. *Journal of Personality and Social Psychology, 53*(2), 298-305.

Miller, D. T., & McFarland, C. (1991). When social comparison goes awry: The case of pluralistic ignorance. In J. Suls & T.A. Wills (Eds.), *Social comparison: Contemporary theory and research* (pp. 287-313). Hillsdale, NJ: Erlbaum.

Miller, W. R. (2000). Rediscovering fire: Small interventions, large effects. *Psychology of Addictive Behaviors, 14,* 6-18.

Miller, W. R., & Rollnick, S. (2002). *Motivational interviewing: Preparing people for change* (2nd ed.). New York: Guilford Press.

Modeste, N. N. (1996). *Dictionary of public health promotion and education: Terms and concepts.* Thousand Oaks, CA: Sage.

Morgan, D. L. (1988). *Focus groups as qualitative research.* Newbury Park, CA: Sage.

Murphy, J. G., Duchnick, J. J., Vuchinich, R. E., Davison, J. W., Karg, R. S., Olson, A. M., Smith, A. F., & Cottey, T. (2001). Relative efficacy of a brief motivational intervention for college student drinkers. *Psychology of Addictive Behaviors, 15,* 373-379.

National Institute on Alcohol Abuse and Alcoholism (NIAAA). (2002). *A call to action: Changing the culture of drinking at U.S. colleges.* Washington, DC: National Institute on Alcohol Abuse and Alcoholism/National Institutes of Health.

Neighbors, C., Larimer, M. E., & Lewis, M. A. (in press). Targeting misperceptions of descriptive drinking norms: Efficacy of a computer delivered personalized normative feedback intervention. *Journal of Consulting and Clinical Psychology.*

Neighbors, C., & Lewis M. A. (2003). The impact of computer delivered, personalized normative feedback. *The Report on Social Norms,* no. 2, pp. 4-5. Little Falls, NJ: PaperClip Communications.

Nezlek, J. B., Pilkington, C. J., & Bilbro, K. G. (1994). Moderation in excess: Binge drinking and social interaction among college students. *Journal of Studies on Alcohol, 55,* 342-351.

O'Malley, P. M., & Johnston, L. D. (2002). Epidemiology of alcohol and other drug use among American college students. *Journal of Studies on Alcohol, Supplement No. 14,* 23-39.

Page, R. M., Scanlan, A., & Gilbert, L. (1999). Relationship of the estimation of binge-drinking among college students and personal participation in binge drinking: Implications for health education and promotion. *Health Education, 30,* 98-103.

Pasavac, E. J. (1993). College students' views and excessive drinking and the university role. *Journal of Drug Education, 23,* 237-245.

Paschall, M., & Flewelling, R. (2002). Postsecondary education and heavy drinking by young adults: The moderating effect of race. *Journal of Studies on Alcohol, 63,* 447-455.

Pearson, M., & Smith, D. (1986). Debriefing in experience-based learning. *Simulation/Games for Learning, 16,* 155-172.

Peeler, C. M., Far, J., Miller, J., & Brigham, T. (2000). An analysis of the effects of a program to reduce heavy drinking among college students. *Journal of Alcohol and Drug Education, 45,* 39-54.

Perkins, H. W. (1985). Religious traditions, parents, and peers as determinants of alcohol and drug use among college students. *Review of Religious Research, 27,* 15-31.

Perkins, H. W. (1987). Parental religion and alcohol use problems as intergenerational predictors of problem drinking among college youth. *Journal for the Scientific Study of Religion, 26,* 340-357.

Perkins, H. W. (1992). Gender patterns in consequences of collegiate alcohol abuse: A 10-year study of trends in an undergraduate population. *Journal of Studies on Alcohol, 53,* 458-462.

Perkins, H. W. (1994). Confronting misperceptions of peer drug use norms among college students: An alternative approach for alcohol and other drug education programs. In L. Grow (Ed.), *FIPSE drug prevention programs in higher education training institute manual* (4th ed., pp. 453-473). Washington, DC: U.S. Department of Education.

Perkins, H. W. (1997). College student misperceptions of alcohol and other drug norms among peers: Exploring causes, consequences, and implications for prevention programs. In *Designing alcohol and other drug prevention programs in higher education: Bringing theory into practice* (pp. 177-206). Washington, DC: U.S. Department of Education

Perkins, H. W. (2002a). Social norms and the prevention of alcohol misuse in collegiate contexts. *Journal of Studies on Alcohol, Supplement No. 14*, 164-172.

Perkins, H. W. (2002b). Surveying the damage: A review of research on consequences of alcohol misuse in college populations. *Journal of Studies on Alcohol, Supplement No. 14*, 91-100.

Perkins, H. W. (2003a). The emergence and evolution of the social norms approach to substance abuse prevention. In H. W. Perkins (Ed.), *The social norms approach to preventing school and college age substance abuse: A handbook for educators, counselors, and clinicians* (pp. 3-18). San Francisco, CA: Jossey-Bass.

Perkins, H. W. (2003b). The promise and challenge of future work on the social norms model. In H. W. Perkins (Ed.), *The social norms approach to preventing school and college age substance abuse: A handbook for educators, counselors, and clinicians* (pp. 280-295). San Francisco, CA: Jossey-Bass.

Perkins, H. W. (Ed.). (2003c). *The social norms approach to preventing school and college age substance abuse: A handbook for educators, counselors, and clinicians.* San Francisco, CA: Jossey-Bass.

Perkins, H. W., & Berkowitz, A. D. (1986). Perceiving the community norms of alcohol use among students: Some research implications for campus alcohol education programming. *International Journal of Addictions, 21*, 961-976.

Perkins, H. W., & Craig, D. A. (2002). *A multi-faceted social norms approach to reduce high-risk drinking: Lessons from Hobart and William Smith Colleges.* Newton, MA: The Higher Education Center for Alcohol and Other Drug Prevention and the U.S. Department of Education.

Perkins, H. W., & Craig, D. A. (2003a). The Hobart and William Smith Colleges experiment: A synergistic social norms approach using print, electronic media and curriculum infusion to reduce collegiate problem drinking. In H. W. Perkins (Ed.), *The social norms approach to preventing school and college age substance abuse: A handbook for educators, counselors, and clinicians* (pp. 35-64). San Francisco, CA: Jossey-Bass.

Perkins, H. W., & Craig, D. A. (2003b). The imaginary lives of peers: Patterns of substance use and misperceptions of norms among secondary school students. In H. W. Perkins (Ed.), *The social norms approach to preventing school and college age substance abuse: A handbook for educators, counselors, and clinicians* (pp. 209-223). San Francisco, CA: Jossey-Bass.

Perkins, H. W., Meilman, P. W., Leichliter, J. S., Cashin, J. R., & Presley, C. A. (1999). Misperceptions of the norms for the frequency of alcohol and other drug use on college campuses. *Journal of American College Health, 47*, 253-258.

Perkins, H. W., & Wechsler, H. (1996). Variation in perceived college drinking norms and its impact on alcohol abuse: A nationwide study. *Journal of Drug Issues, 26,* 961-974.

Petty, R. E., & Cacioppo, J. T. (1986). *Communication and persuasion: Central and peripheral routes to attitude change.* New York: Springer-Verlag.

Philipsen, G. (1997). A theory of speech codes. In G. Philipsen & T. L. Albrecht (Eds.), *Developing human communication theory* (pp. 119-156). Albany: State University of New York Press.

Pierfy, D. A. (1977). Comparative simulation game research. *Simulation & Games, 8,* 255-268.

Pintrich, P. R., & Schrauben, B. (1992). Students' motivational beliefs and their cognitive engagement in classroom tasks. In D. Schunk & J. Meece (Eds.), *Student perceptions in the classroom: Causes and consequences* (pp. 149-183). Hillsdale, NJ: Erlbaum.

Pollard, J. W., Freeman, J. E., Ziegler, D. A., Hersman, M. N., & Goss, C. W. (2000). Predictions of normative drug use by college students: False consensus, false uniqueness, or just plain accuracy? *Journal of College Student Psychotherapy, 14*(3), 5-12.

Postman, N., Nystrom, C., Strate, L., & Weingartner, C. (1988). *Myths, men and beer: An analysis of beer commercials on broadcast television.* Falls Church, VA: AAA Foundation for Traffic Safety.

Prentice, D. A., & Miller, D. T. (1993). Pluralistic ignorance and alcohol use on campus: Some consequences of misperceiving the social norm. *Journal of Personality and Social Psychology, 64,* 243-256.

Presley, C. A., Meilman, P. W., & Cashin, J. R. (1996). *Alcohol and other drugs on American campuses: Use, consequences, and perceptions of the campus environment, Volume 4, 1992-1994.* Cardondale: Core Institute, Southern Illinois University.

Presley, C. A., Meilman, P. W., & Cashin, J. R. (1997). Weapon carrying and substance abuse among college students. *Journal of American College Health, 46,* 3-8.

Prochaska, C. A., & DiClemente, C. C. (1984). *The transtheoretical approach: Crossing traditional boundaries of therapy.* Homewood IL: Dow Jones/Irwin.

Prochaska, J. O., DiClemente, C. C., & Norcross, J. C. (1992). In search of how people change: Applications to addictive behaviors. *American Psychologist, 47,* 1102-1114.

Rabow, J., & Duncan-Schill, M. (1995). Drinking among college students. *Journal of Alcohol and Drug Education, 40*(3), 52-64.

Rapaport, R. J., Minelli, M. J., Angera, J. J., & Thayer, J. E. (1999). Using focus groups to quickly assess students' opinions about alcohol issues and programs. *Journal of College Student Development, 40,* 311-314.

Raths, J. (1987, October). Enhancing understanding through debriefing. *Educational Leadership,* pp. 25-27.

Rice, R. (2002). Some notes on methodological and other issues. In A. Berkowitz, Responding to the critics: Answers to some common questions and concerns about the social norms approach. *The Report on Social Norms: Working Paper No. 7,* 3. Little Falls, NJ: PaperClip Communications.

Rice, R. E., & Atkin, C. K. (Eds.). (2001). *Public communication campaigns* (3rd ed.). Thousand Oaks, CA: Sage.

Ruben, B. D., & Lederman, L. C. (1982). Instructional simulations: Validity, reliability and utility. *Simulation and Games, 13,* 233-243.

Rutgers University Health Services (RUHS). *Commitment to student health and education.* New Brunswick, NJ: Author.

Sacks, P. (1996). *Generation X goes to college: A journey into teaching in postmodern America.* Chicago: Open Court.

Salmon, C. T., & Murray-Johnson, L. (2001). Communication campaign effectiveness. In R. E. Rice & C. K. Atkin (Eds.), *Public communication campaigns* (3rd ed., pp. 168-180). Thousand Oaks, CA: Sage.

Schall, M., Kemeny, A., & Maltzman, I. (1992). Factors associated with alcohol use in university students. *Journal of Studies on Alcohol, 53,* 122-136.

Schroeder, C. M., & Prentice, D. A. (1998). Exposing pluralistic ignorance to reduce alcohol use among college students. *Journal of Applied Social Psychology, 28,* 2150-2180.

Senchak, M., Leonard, K. E., & Greene, B. W. (1998). Alcohol use among college students as a function of their typical social drinking context. *Psychology of Addictive Behaviors, 12,* 62-70.

Sher, K., Bartholow, B. D., & Nanda, S. (2001). Short- and long-term effects of fraternity and sorority membership on heavy drinking: A social norms perspective. *Psychology of Addictive Behaviors, 15,* 42-51.

Sherif, M. (1972). Experiments on norm formation. In E. P. Hollander & R. G. Hunt (Eds.), *Classic contributions to social psychology* (pp. 320-329). New York: Oxford University Press.

Simons-Morton, B. G., Donohew, L., & Crump, A. D. (1997). Health communication in the prevention of alcohol, tobacco, and drug use. *Health Education & Behavior, 24,* 544-554.

Snyder, L. B. (2001). How effective are mediated health campaigns? In R. E. Rice & C. K. Atkin (Eds.), *Public communication campaigns* (3rd ed., pp. 180-190). Thousand Oaks, CA: Sage.

Steffian, G. (1999). Correction of normative misperceptions: An alcohol abuse prevention program. *Journal of Drug Education, 29,* 115-138.

Stewart, L. P. (1987). Testing a model of organizational simulations: The influence of participant sex and sex role on participativeness. In L. B. Nadler, M. K. Nadler, & W. R. Todd-Mancillas (Eds.), *Advances in gender and communication research* (pp. 363-376). Lanham, MD: University Press of America.

Stewart, L. P. (1992). Ethical issues in postexperimental and postexperiential debriefing. *Simulation & Gaming, 23,* 197-212.

Stewart, L. P., & Lederman, L. C. (1988). THE MARBLE COMPANY: A simulation game for organizational communication and information management. *Organizational Behavior Teaching Review, 13,* 96-105.

Stewart, L. P., & Lederman, L. C. (2003). *Intercept interviews for evaluation data* (CHI Research Series: Report no. 18). New Brunswick, NJ: Center for Communication and Health Issues, Rutgers University.

Stewart, L. P., & Lederman, L. C., with Golubow, M., Cattafesta, J. L., Goodhart, F. W., Powell, R., & Laitman, L. (2002). Applying communication theories to prevent dangerous drinking among college students: The RU SURE campaign. *Communication Studies, 53,* 381-399.

Stewart, L. P., & Shafer, M. (2002). *Voicing the concerns of the community: An example of communication in action in a service learning program.* Paper presented at the National Communication Association Conference, New Orleans, LA.

Storey, J. (1993). *An introductory guide to cultural theory and popular culture.* Athens: University of Georgia Press.

Strauss, A. L., & Corbin, J. M. (1998). *Basics of qualitative research: Techniques and procedures for developing grounded theory.* Thousand Oaks, CA: Sage.

Substance Abuse and Mental Health Services Administration (SAMSHA). (2001). *Results from the 2001 National Household Survey on Drug Abuse: Volume I. Summary of National Findings.* (Available at http://www.csattce.samhsa. gov/OAS/NHSDA.htm).

Sullivan, M. C., Myers, R. A., Bradfield, C. D., & Street, D. L. (1999). *Service-learning: Educating students for life.* Harrisonburg, VA: Institute for Research in Higher Education, James Madison University.

Sussman, S., Dent, C. W., Mestel-Rauch, J., Johnson, C. A., Hansen, W. B., & Flay, B. R. (1988). Adolescent nonsmokers, triers and regular smokers' estimates of cigarette smoking and prevalence: When do overestimations occur and by whom? *Journal of Applied Social Psychology, 18,* 537-551.

Tansey, P. J. (1971). *Educational aspects of simulation.* Maidenhead, England: McGraw Hill.

Tesch, F. E. (1977). Debriefing research participants: Though this may be method there is madness to it. *Journal of Personality and Social Psychology, 35,* 217-224.

Thombs, D. L. (1999). Alcohol and motor vehicle use: Profiles of drivers and passengers. *American Journal of Health and Behavior, 23,* 13-24.

Thombs, D. L. (2000). A test of the perceived norms model to explain drinking patterns among university student athletes. *Journal of American College Health, 49,* 75-83.

Thombs, D. L., Mahoney, C. A., & Olds, R. S. (1998). Application of a bogus testing procedure to determine college students' utilization of genetic screening for alcoholism. *Journal of American College Health, 47,* 103-112.

Thombs, D. L., Wolcott, B. J., & Farkash, L. G. E. (1997). Social context, perceived norms and drinking behavior in young people. *Journal of Substance Abuse, 9,* 257-267.

Thornton, G. C., & Cleveland, J. N. (1990). Developing managerial talent through simulation. *American Psychologist, 45,* 190-199.

Thurman, R. (1993). Instructional simulation from a cognitive psychology viewpoint. *Educational Technology Research & Development, 41*(4), 75-89.

Toch, H., & Klofas, J. (1984). Pluralistic ignorance, revisited. In G. M. Stephenson & J. H. Davis (Eds.), *Progress in applied social psychology* (Vol. 2, pp. 129-159). New York: Wiley.

Trockel, M., Williams, S., & Reis, J. (2003). Considerations for more effective social norms based alcohol education on campus: An analysis of different theoretical conceptualizations in predicting drinking among fraternity men. *Journal of Studies on Alcohol, 64,* 50-59.

University of Michigan. (1993). *University of Michigan survey regarding alcohol and other drugs.* Ann Arbor, MI: UM Initiative on Alcohol and Other Drugs.

Walters, S. T. (2000). In praise of feedback: An effective intervention for college students who are heavy drinkers. *Journal of American College Health, 48,* 235-238.

Watzlawick, P., Beavin Bavelas, J., & Jackson, D. D. (1967). *Pragmatics of human communication: A study of interactional patterns, pathologies, and paradoxes.* New York: Norton.

Wechsler, H. (1996). Alcohol and the American college campus: A report from the Harvard School of Public Health. *Change, 28*(4), 20-25, 60.

Wechsler, H., Davenport, A., Dowdall, G., Moeykens, B., & Castillo, S. (1994). Health and behavior consequences of binge drinking in college. *Journal of the American Medical Association, 272,* 1672-1677.

Wechsler, H., Fulop, M., Padilla, A., Lee, H., & Patrick, K. (1997). Binge drinking among college students: A comparison of California and other states. *Journal of American College Health, 45,* 273-278.

Wechsler, H., Isaac, N., Grodstein, F., & Sellers, D.E. (1994). Continuation and initiation of alcohol use from the first to the second year of college. *Journal of Studies on Alcohol, 55,* 41-46.

Wechsler, H., & Kuo, M. (2000). College students define binge drinking and estimate its prevalence: Results of a national survey. *Journal of American College Health, 49,* 57-64.

Wechsler, H., Kuh, G., & Davenport, A. (1996). Fraternities, sororities, and binge drinking: Results from a national study of American colleges. *NASPA Journal, 33,* 260-279.

Wechsler, H., Lee, J. E., Kuo, M., & Lee, H. (2000). College binge drinking in the 1990s: A continuing problem. *Journal of American College Health, 48,* 199-210.

Wechsler, H., Lee, J. E., Kuo, M., Seibring, M., Nelson, T. F., & Lee, H. (2002). Trends in college binge drinking during a period of increased prevention efforts. *Journal of American College Health, 50,* 203-217.

Wechsler, H., Lee, J. E., Meichun, K. & Lee, H. (2000). College binge drinking in the 1990's — A continuing problem; Results of the Harvard School of Public Health 1999 college alcohol study. *Journal of American College Health, 48,* 211-215.

Wechsler, H., Molnar, B., Davenport, A., & Baer, J. (1999). College alcohol use: A full or empty glass? *Journal of American College Health, 47,* 247-252.

Weitzman, E. R., Nelson, T. F., & Wechsler, H. (2003). Taking up binge drinking in college: The influences of person, social group, and environment. *Journal of Adolescent Health, 32,* 26-35.

Wenzel, M. (2001). *Misperceptions of social norms about tax compliance* (Working paper no. 7 [a prestudy] and working paper no. 8 [a field experiment]). Centre for Tax System Integrity, Australian National University.

Werch, C. C. E., Pappas, D. M., Carlson, J. M. , DiClemente, C. C., Chally, P. S., & Sinder, J. A. (2000). Results of a social norm intervention to prevent binge drinking among first-year residential college students. *Journal of American College Health, 49,* 85-92.

White, J., Williams, L. V., & Cho, D. (2003). A social norms intervention to reduce coercive behaviors among deaf and hard-of-hearing college students. *The*

*Report on Social Norms: Working Paper No. 9.* Little Falls, NJ: PaperClip Communications.

Whorf, B. L. (1956). *Language, thought, and reality.* Cambridge, MA: MIT Press.

Williams, R. (1965). *The long revolution.* Harmondsworth, England: Penguin Books.

Williamson, J. (1978). *Decoding advertisements.* London: Marion Boyars.

Witte, K., Meyer, G., & Martell, D. (2001). *Effective health risk messages.* Thousand Oaks, CA: Sage.

Wolfson, S. (2000). Student's estimates of the prevalence of drug use: Evidence for a false consensus effect. *Psychology of Addictive Behaviors, 14,* 295-298.

Workman, T.A. (1999). *Constructions from within the collegiate drinking culture: An analysis of fraternity drinking stories.* A paper presented at the annual meeting of the National Communication Association, New York.

Workman, T. A. (2001a). Finding the meanings of college drinking: An analysis of fraternity drinking stories. *Health Communication, 13,* 427-447.

Workman, T. A. (2001b). An intertextual analysis of the collegiate drinking culture. Unpublished doctoral dissertation, University of Nebraska-Lincoln.

Yanovitzky, I., Lederman, L. C., & Stewart, L. P. (2002). *College experience survey.* Unpublished.

Yanovitzky, I., Stewart, L. P., & Lederman, L. C. (in press). Social distance, perceived drinking by peers, and alcohol use by college students. *Health Communication.*

# ABOUT THE AUTHORS

**Linda Costigan Lederman, PhD,** professor of communication and co-founder and director of the Center for Communication Health Issues (CHI) at Rutgers University, specializes in experiential learning and qualitative research in communication and health issues. Lederman holds a joint appointment with the Rutgers Center of Alcohol Studies as well as an Associate Faculty Appointment in the Rutgers Graduate School of Education. She is also an associate (emeritus) of the Center of Higher Education. Professor Lederman has written or co-authored nine books. In 2003, she received the Rutgers College Class of 1962 Presidential Public Service Award in recognition of distinguished service. Lederman is currently a co-principal investigator on a $6 million grant awarded to Rutgers by the National Institute on Drug Abuse for the establishment of the Rutgers Transdisciplinary Prevention Research Center that will be located at the Rutgers Center of Alcohol Studies.

**Lea P. Stewart, PhD,** professor of communication and co-founder and director of the Center for Communication Health Issues (CHI) at Rutgers University, specializes in gender and ethical issues in communication and health as well as higher education curriculum development. She holds a joint appointment with the Rutgers Center of Alcohol Studies and is a Rutgers University Citizenship and Service Education (CASE) advisor. Stewart has written or co-authored 11 books. In 2003, she received the Rutgers University Warren I. Susman Award for Excellence in Teaching, the university's highest honor in achieving excellence in the classroom. Professor Stewart is currently a co-principal investigator on a $6 million grant awarded to Rutgers by the National Institute on Drug Abuse for the establishment of the Rutgers Transdisciplinary Prevention Research Center that will be located at the Rutgers Center of Alcohol Studies. In 2002, she was listed in the *International Who's Who of Professional and Business Women.*

## ABOUT THE CONTRIBUTING AUTHORS

**Alan David Berkowitz, PhD,** is co-founder of the social norms approach and the editor of the *Report on Social Norms.* He works as an independent consultant who helps colleges, universities, and communities design programs that address health and social justice issues. He is the recipient of five national awards, is well known for his scholarship and innovative programming, and frequently serves as an expert advisor to organizations and federal agencies.

**Patricia Fabiano, PhD,** has been at Western Washington University for 13 years as the program director of Prevention and Wellness Services, where she has developed a model college health promotion program. She has been in college student services for nearly 20 years (first at Southern Illinois University at Carbondale and then at Stanford University) and has made research and program development contributions to her profession throughout that time. Fabiano has authored an innovative social norms marketing grant, funded by the U.S. Department of Education, which demonstrated significant outcomes in reducing high-risk alcohol consumption on her campus. She is also the author of a recent violence prevention grant funded by the U.S. Department of Justice. Fabiano has taken a lead in thinking about the application of social norms marketing to social justice issues.

**Fern Walter Goodhart, MS, CHES,** director of health education for the Rutgers University Health Services, has been a public health educator since 1977, in both state government and at large public universities, and has taught as an adjunct professor for the Rutgers University School of Public Health and the University of Massachusetts. Goodhart has presented more than 70 papers, reviewed manuscripts for health education and college health journals, served as associate editor of *JACH,* authored or co-authored 20 articles, book chapters or book reviews, and received numerous awards including the Society for Public Health Education Program Excellence Award, the NJ Society for Public Health Education Louise Chut Program Excellence Award, and the SOPHE "Profiles in Courage" Award, 2000. In 1999, she served as a Northeast Regional Public Health Leadership Institute Fellow, and was inducted as an ACHA Fellow in 1994.

**Linda Jeffrey, PhD,** is a professor of psychology at Rowan University, Glassboro, New Jersey where she directs the Center for Addiction Studies, and a licensed clinical psychologist. She teaches alcohol and other drug treatment and prevention courses at the undergraduate and graduate levels, and serves as project director for the NJ Higher Education Consortium on Alcohol and Other Drug Prevention and Education.

**Lisa Laitman, MSEd, CADC,** has been director of the Alcohol and Other Drug Assistance Program for Students (ADAPS) at Rutgers University since 1983. In that capacity she developed a program for college students that specifically addresses the needs of this population. The goals of ADAPS are to intervene with high-risk alcohol and drug use, provide counseling services for children of alcoholics/drug addicts, and provide recovery support services for students who are alcohol or drug dependent or in recovery. ADAPS has operated Recovery Housing, an on-campus living environment for recovering students for 16 years. Laitman has been a member of CHI since its inception. Additionally, she has been on the University Alcohol Policy Committee and participated in other campus activities that assist with the issues related to alcohol and drug use at Rutgers.

**Pamela Negro, MSW, CADC,** is the associate director of the Center for Addiction Studies, Rowan University, Glassboro, New Jersey. She co-directs the state-wide initiative on alcohol abuse for the New Jersey Higher Education Consortium on Alcohol and Other Drug Use.

**Thomas Workman, PhD,** is the assistant director of student involvement, which is the home of NU Directions, the campus-community coalition to reduce high-risk drinking at the University of Nebraska-Lincoln. He oversees the department's Information Strategies area. He has maintained an active research agenda in health communication and cultural studies since 1997 and has served as the communications coordinator for NU Directions since 1999. In 2002, Workman received a special award of appreciation from the University of Nebraska Board of Regents for his work with students surrounding alcohol issues.

# AUTHOR INDEX

**A**

Abhold, J., 198, *260-261*
Agostinelli, G., 200(*t*), 210, *255*
Ajzen, I., 34, *259*
Altekruse, M., 198, 201(*t*), 206, 208(*t*), *260-261*
American College Health Association (ACHA), 186, *255*
American Council on Education (ACE), 180, 182, 183, *255*
Anderson, D. S., 51, 146, 219, *255, 266*
Andrews, K., 239, *262*
Angera, J. J., 53, *269*
Appelbaum, M., 201(*t*), 204, 204(*t*), *258*
Asch, S. E., 32, 220, *255*
Atkin, C. K., 3, 27, *270*

**B**

Baer, J. S., 14, 21, 36, 190, 191, 198, 200(*t*), 202(*t*), 210, 236, 237, 239, 241, 251, *255, 259*
Ballou, J., 7, 13, 15, 33, 39, 51, 52, 53, 54, 55, 167, *257*
Bandura, A., 33, 34, *256*

Barker, G. P., 197, 198, 200(*t*), 201(*t*), 205, 207(*t*), 208(*t*), 234, 235, *260*
Barnett, L. A., 200(*t*), 209, *256*
Barr, S. L., 51, 52, 54, 73(*n*1), 77, 81, 101, 166, 252, *261, 264*
Bartholow, B. D., 200(*t*), 202(*t*), 203, 204(*t*), *270*
Baudrillard, J., 246, *256*
Bauerle, J., 209, 210, *256*
Beavin Bavelas, J., 31, *272*
Beck, K. H., 201v 203, 204(*t*), *256*
Bennett, M. E., 18, *256*
Berger, A. A., 249, *256*
Berkowitz, A.D., 14, 20, 35, 39, 55, 62, 194, 195, 196(*t*), 197, 199, 200(*t*), 202(*t*), 203, 205, 212, 213, 220, 223, 235, 241, 252, *256, 257, 268*
Bibeau, D., 183, *266*
Bigsby, M. J., 201(*t*), *257*
Bilbro, K. G., 51, 52, *267*
Bonaguro, E. W., 3, 4, *262*
Bondy, S. J., 210, *258*
Botvin, G. J., 201(*t*), 204, 204(*t*), *257*
Bourdieu, P., 247, *257*

Bourgeois, M. J., 35, 39, 41, 195, 200(*t*), 201(*t*), 203, *257*

Bowen, A. M., 35, 39, 41, 195, 200(*t*), 201(*t*), 203, *257*

Bradfield, C. D., 87, *271*

Bredemeier, M. E., 77, 147, *257*

Brigham, T., 200(*t*), 209, *267*

Brooker, P., 245, *257*

Brower, A., 190, *257*

Brown, J. M., 200(*t*), 210, *255*

Brown, R., 8, *257*

Brown, S. A., 201(*t*), 204, 204(*t*), *258*

Bruce, S., 198, 201(*t*), *257*

Burns, W. D., 7, 13, 14, 15, 33, 39, 50, 51, 52, 53, 54, 55, 75, 167, 179, *257*

Burwell, C., 209, 210, *256*

Butcher, A. H., 52, *257*

Butler, E. R., 35, 51, 52, *257*

**C**

Cacioppo, J. T., 34, 35, *269*

Calder, B., 138, *258*

Cappella, J., 27, *258*

Carbaugh, D., 32, *258*

Carey, K. B., 50, 51, *258*

Carlson, J. M., 200(*t*), *272*

Carney, M. M., 200(*t*), *255*

Carter, C. A., 200(*t*), 202(*t*), *258*

Cashin, J. R., 7, 50, 200(*t*), 201(*t*), 223, 234. *266, 268, 269*

Castillo, S., 8, 41, *272*

Cattafesta, J. L., 19, 32, 145, *270-271*

Chaiken, S., 34, *259*

Chally, P. S., 200(*t*), *272*

Cho, D., 198, 202(*t*), 209, *272-273*

Ciano-Boyce, C., 195, 201(*t*), *259*

Cimini, M. D., 209, *258*

Clapp, J. D., 200(*t*), 204(*t*), 203, *258*

Cleveland, J. N., 147, *271*

Cohen, D. J., 7, 15, 17, 33, 39, 40, 41, 52, 54-55, 75, *258*

Collins, C., 74, 197, 200(*t*), 205, 207(*t*), 223, 234, 235, 252, *260, 262*

Colthurst, T., 180, *258*

Condit, C. M., 248, *265*

Corbin, J. M., 140, *271*

Core Institute, The, 19, 122, 130, 169, *258*

Cottey, T., 210, *267*

Craig, D. A., 197, 200(*t*), 201(*t*), 205, 206, 207(*t*), 210, 233, *268*

Cretella, M., 180, *258*

Cronce, J. M., 210, 212, *262, 263*

Crump, A. D., 4, *270*

Cunningham, J. A., 210, *258*

**D**

D'Amico, E. J., 201(*t*), 204, 204(*t*), *258*

Danish, S. J., 6, *258*

Davenport, A., 8, 41, 235, 251, *272*

Davison, J. W., 210, *267*

DeJong, W., 180, 202(*t*), 212, *258, 265*

Delia, J. G., 51, *258-259*

Demond, M., 6, 198, 200(*t*), 205, 207(*t*), *261*

Dent, C. W., 201(*t*), *271*

Dewey, J., 32, 145, *259*

Diaz, T., 201(*t*), 204, 204(*t*), *257*

DiClemente, C. C., 200(*t*), 238, 239, 252, *269, 272*

Dimeff, L. A., 190, 191, 198, 210, 236, 237, 239, 241, *259, 266*

Donohew, L., 5, *270*

Donovan, B. W., 52, 54, 81, 252, *264*

Dowdall, G., 8, 41, *272*

Dubuque, E., 195, 201(*t*), *259*

Duchnick, J. J., 210, *267*

Dude, K., 211, *262*

Duncan-Schill, M., 51, *269*

**E**

Eagly, A. H., 34, *259*

Engs, R. C., 51, *259*

Erikson, E. H., 7, *259*

**F**

Fabiano, P. M., 170, 195, 197, 200(*t*) 205, 207(*t*), 223, 234, 35, 239, *259, 261*

Far, J. M., 39, 198, 200(*t*), 202(*t*), 209, 210, 252, *256, 259, 267*

Farkash, L. G. E., 51, 200(*t*), 201(*t*), 202(*t*), 203, 204(*t*), *271*

Festinger, L., 34, 36, *259*

Fishbein, M., 34, *259*

Fisher, W. R., 32, *259*

Fiske, J., 245, *259*

Fiske, M., 138, *266*

Flay, B. R., 201(*t*), *271*

Flewelling, R., 6, *267*

Frankenstein, W., 18, *256*

Freeman, J. E., 200(*t*), 201(*t*), *269*

Frisone, J. D., 6, 198, 200(*t*), 205, 207(*t*), *261*

Frissell, K. C., 201(*t*), 204, 204(*t*), *258*

Fulop, M., 50, *272*

**G**

Galen, L., 51, 54, 166, *261*

Gascoigne, J., 198, 201(*t*), 206, 208(*t*), *260-261*

Giddens, A., 247, 248, *257*

Gilbert, L., 200(*t*), 203, 204(*t*), *267*

Gladwell, M., 230, *260*

Glanz, K., 183, *266*

Glaser, B. G., 27, *260*

Glider, P., 74, 197, 200(*t*), 205, 207(*t*), 223, 234, 235, 252, *260, 262*

Globetti, G., 14, *265*

Goldman, M. S., 6, *260*

Golubow, M., 19, 32, 133, 145, 163, 170, *264, 270-271*

Goodhart, F. W., 5, 7, 19, 32, 35, 36, 39, 49(*n*1), 50, 51, 52, 53, 54, 55, 62, 75, 81, 122, 131, 136, 145, 146, 149, 166, 169, 180, 252, *261, 265, 270-271*

Goodstadt, M., 7, 13, 14, 15, 39, 50, 52, 75, *257*

Goree, C. T., 179, *260*

Goss, C. W., 200(*t*), 201(*t*), *269*

Gouran, D., 159, *260*

Graham, J. W., 201(*t*), 204, 204(*t*), *261, 266*

Granfield, R., 212, *260*

Greenbaum, T. L., 138, *260*

Greenblat, C. S., 77, 147, *257*

Greene, B. W., 52, *270*

Griffin, C. J. G., 248, *260*

Griffin, K. W., 201(*t*), 204, 204(*t*), *257*

Grodstein, F., 251, *272*

Grube, J. W., 249, *260*

**H**

Haines, M. P., 6, 14, 20, 22, 35, 39, 52, 62, 74, 197, 198, 200(*t*), 201(*t*), 205, 207(*t*), 208(*t*), 223, 234, 235, 252, *260*

Hale, B. D., 6, *258*

Hall, S., 245, *260*

Hancock, L., 198, 201(*t*), 206, 208(*t*), *260-261*

Hansen, W. B., 201(*t*), 204, 204(*t*), *261, 266, 271*

Hanson, D. J., 51, *261*

Harper, N. L., 51, 54, 166, *261*

Harwick, E., 235, 239, *261*

Hastings, S. O., 32, *258*

Heeren, T., 7, *261*

Henry, N., 198, 201(*t*), 206, 208(*t*), *261*

Herndon, S. L., 138, 139, *261*

Hersman, M. N., 200(*t*), 201(*t*), *269*

Higher Education Center for Alcohol and Other Drug Prevention, 183, *261*

Hingson, R., 7, *261*

Hyun, Y. R., 223, 235, 239, *259, 261*

**I**

Ifill-Williams, M., 201(*t*), 204, 204(*t*), *257*

Institute of Medicine, 236, 238, *261*
Irvine, D. L., 200(*t*), 202(*t*), *263*
Isaac, N., 251, *272*

**J**

Jackson, D. D., 31, *272*
Jacob, T., 239, *261*
Jaksa, J. A., 157, 158, *261*
Jameson, F., 245, *261*
Jeffrey, L. R., 6, 20, 22, 35, 62, 198,
    200(*t*), 205, 207(*t*), *261*
Jhally, S., 244, 246, 249, *262*
Johannesen, R. L., 157, *262*
Johannessen, K. J., 74, 197, 200(*t*),
    205, 207(*t*), 211, 223, 234, 235,
    252, *260, 262*
Johnson, C. A., 201(*t*), *271*
Johnson, R., 246, *262*
Johnston, L. D., 6, *267*

**K**

Kahnweiler, W. M., 200(*t*), 202(*t*),
    *258*
Kandel, D. B., 239, *262*
Karg, R. S., 210, *267*
Keeling, R. P., 183, *262*
Keller, D. S., 18, *256*
Kemeny, A., 52, *270*
Kendall, P., 138, *266*
Kennedy, L., 5, 7, 19, 35, 36, 39, 50,
    51, 52, 53, 54, 55, 62, 75, 81, 122,
    131, 136, 166, 169, 252, *261, 265*
Kilbourne, J., 249, *262*
Kilmartin, C., 197, *262*
Kilmer, J. R., 200(*t*), 202(*t*), 212, *262,*
    *263*
Kivlahan, D. R., 239, 241, *255, 266*
Klawunn, M., 179, *257*
Klein, H., 51, 53, *262*
Kline, S., 246, 249, *265*
Klofas, J., 194, 196(*t*), 199, *271*
Kolb, D., 32, 145, *262*
Kopstein, A., 7, *261*

Korcuska, J. S., 202(*t*), 203, 204(*t*),
    *262*
Kreps, G. L., 3, 4, *262*
Kuh, G., 235, *272*
Kuo, M., 5, 6, 7, 20, 51, 52, 62, 63,
    189, 251, *272*
Kusch, J., 202(*t*), *262*
Kvilahan, D., 190-, 191, 198, 236,
    237, 239, *259*

**L**

Laitman, L. A., 5, 7, 18, 19, 32 35, 36,
    39, 49(*n*1), 50, 51, 52, 53, 54, 55,
    62, 75, 81, 122, 131 136, 145, 146,
    149, 166, 169, 180, 188, 200(*t*),
    *256, 261, 262, 263, 265, 270-271*
Larimer, M. E., 14, 21, 199, 200(*t*),
    202(*t*), 210, 239, 241, *255*, 263,
    *266, 267*
Lederman, L. C., 1, 2, 4, 5, 7, 8, 9, 13,
    14, 15, 17, 19, 27, 28, 30, 32, 34, 35,
    36, 39, 40, 41, 45, 49(*n*1), 50, 51,
    52, 53, 54-55, 57, 59, 62, 70,
    73(*n*1), 75, 77, 78, 79, 80, 81, 87,
    101, 108, 122, 124, 145, 146, 147,
    148, 149, 153, 154, 162, 163, 166,
    167, 169, 170, 175, 180, 244, 245,
    252, *257, 258, 261, 263, 264, 265,*
    *270-271*
Lee, H., 5, 6, 7, 20, 36, 50, 51, 189,
    251, *272*
Lee, J. E., 5, 6, 7, 20, 36, 50, 51, 189,
    251, *272*
Leichliter, J. S., 7, 200(*t*), 201(*t*), 223,
    235, *266, 268*
Leiss, W., 246, 249, *265*
Leonard, K. E., 52, *270*
Leonard, K., 239, *261*
Lewis, M. A., 199, 202(*t*), 241, *265*
Lieblich, A., 248, *265*
Lin, E., 210, *258*
Lindlof, T. R., 162, *265*
Linkenbach, J., 195, 198, 201(*t*),
    202(*t*), 205, 206, 208(*t*), *259, 265*

Littlejohn, S. W., 51, *265*
Lo, C. C., 14, *265*
Lucaites, J. L., 246, *265*
Luik, J., 249, *265*

**M**

Maggs, J. L., 6, *266*
Mahoney, C. A., 50, *271*
Maltzman, I., 52, *270*
Manis, J. G., 32, *266*
Manning, D. T., 52, *257*
Marks, G., 204, 204(*t*), *266*
Marlah, G. A., 200(*t*), 202(*t*), *263*
Marlatt, G. A., 190, 191, 198, 209,
    236, 237, 239, *271*, *255*, *259*, *266*
Marshall, A., 8, 51, *266*
Martell, D., 31, 120, 122, 175, *273*
Maus, A. L., 200(*t*), 209, *256*
McCarthy, D. M., 201(*t*), 204, 204(*t*),
    *258*
McCrady, B. S., 18, *256*
McDonnell, A. L., 200(*t*), 203,
    204(*t*), *258*
McFarland, C., 36, 40, 194, 196(*t*),
    199, *266*
McKillip, J., 50, *266*
McKinney, G., 223, 235, *259*
McLaughlin, P., 52, 54, 81, 252, *264*
McLeroy, K., 183, *266*
Meichun, K., 36, *272*
Meilman, P. W., 7, 50, 200(*t*), 201(*t*),
    223, 234, 235, *266*, *268*, *269*
Meltzer, B. N., 32, *266*
Merton, R., 138, *266*
Mertz, H., 223, 235, *259*
Mestel-Rauch, J., 201(*t*), *271*
Metrik, J., 201(*t*), 204, 204(*t*), *258*
Meyer, G., 31, 120, 122, 175, *273*
Midyett, S., 197, 200(*t*), 205, 207(*t*),
    260
Migneault, J. P., 252, *266*
Milgram, G. G., 51, 146, 219, *255*,
    *266*

Miller, D. T., 36, 40, 194, 196(*t*), 199,
    200(*t*), 203, 204(t), *266*, *269*
Miller, J. A., 39, 198, 200(*t*), 202(*t*),
    209, 210, 252, *256*, *259*, *267*
Miller, W. R., 200(*t*), 210, 238, *255*,
    *266*
Mills-Novoa, B. M., 74, 197, 200(*t*),
    205, 207(*t*), 223, 234, 235, 252,
    *260*, *262*
Minelli, M. J., 53, *269*
Modeste, N. N., 236, *267*
Moeykens, B., 8, 41, *272*
Molnar, B., 251, *272*
Morgan, D. L., 138, 139, *267*
Murphy, J. G., 210, *267*
Murray-Johnson, L., 3, 4, *270*
Myers, R. A., 87, *271*

**N**

Nanda, S., 200(*t*), 202(*t*), 203, 204(*t*),
    *270*
National Institute on Alcohol Abuse
    and Alcoholism, 4, 6, 146, 242,
    *267*
Negro, P., 6, 20, 22, 35, 62, 198,
    200(*t*), 205, 207(*t*), *261*
Neighbors, C., 199, 202(*t*), 241, 263,
    *265*, *267*
Nelson, T. F., 5, 6, 20, 189, *272*
Nezlek, J. B., 51, 52, *267*
Norcross, J. C., 252, *269*
Nystrom, C., 249, *269*

**O**

O'Malley, P. M., 6, *267*
O'Neal, E. C., 52, *257*
Olds, R. S., 50, *271*
Olson, A. M., 210, *267*

**P**

Padilla, A., 50, *272*
Page, J. C., 209, *258*
Page, R. M., 200(*t*), 203, 204(*t*), *267*
Pappas, D. M., 200(*t*), *272*
Pasavac, E. J., 50, *267*

Paschall, M., 6, *267*
Patrick, K., 50, *272*
Pearson, M., 139, 162, 163, *267*
Peeler, C. M., 200(*t*), 209, *267*
Perkins, H. W., 6, 7, 14, 20, 22, 35, 36, 39, 40, 41, 50, 52, 55, 62, 74, 134, 194, 195, 197, 198, 199, 200(*t*), 201(*t*), 202(*t*), 203, 204(*t*), 205, 206, 207(*t*), 208(*t*), 210 212, 220, 223, 233, 235, 236, 241, 242, 252, *256, 257, 265, 267, 268, 269*
Perry, D., 73(*n*1), 77, 101, *264*
Petipas, A. J., 6, *258*
Petty, R. E., 34, 35, *269*
Philipsen, G., 32, *269*
Pierfy, D. A., 77, 148, *269*
Pilkington, C. J., 51, 52, *267*
Pintrich, P. R., 147, *269*
Pollard, J. W., 200(*t*), 201(*t*), *269*
Postman, N., 249, *269*
Powell, R. 5, 7, 19, 32, 35, 36, 39, 50, 51, 52, 53, 54, 55, 62, 75, 81, 122, 131, 136, 145, 146, 149, 166, 169, 252, *261, 265, 270-271*
Prentice, D. A., 40, 200(*t*), 203, 204(t), 209, *269, 270*
Presley, C. A., 7, 50, 200(*t*), 201(*t*), 223, 234, 235, *266, 268, 269*
Pritchard, M. S., 157, 158, *261*
Prochaska, C. A., 238, 239, *269*
Prochaska, J. O., 252, *266 269*

**Q**

Query, J. L., 3, 4, *262*
Quigley, L. A., 241, *266*

**R**

Rabow, J., 51, *269*
Rapaport, R. J., 53, *269*
Raths, J., 157, *269*
Real, K., 8, 51, *266*
Reis, J., 202(*t*), 203, 204(*t*), *271*
Rhoads, K., 223, 235, *259*

Rice, R. E., 3, 27, 198, 201(*t*), 205, 207(*t*), 208(*t*), 212, *260, 269, 270*
Rollnick, S., 238, *266*
Rosati, M., 180, *258*
Ruben, B. D., 77, 78, 80, 147, 148, *263, 264, 270*
Rutgers University Health Services (RUHS), 183, *270*

**S**

Sacks, P., 246, *270*
Salmon, C. T., 3, 4, *270*
Scanlan, A., 200(*t*), 203, 204(*t*), *267*
Schall, M., 52, *270*
Scherer, C. W., 8, 51, *266*
Schrauben, B., 147, *269*
Schroeder, C., M., 200(*t*), 209, *270*
Seibring, M., 6, 20, 189, *272*
Sellers, D. E., 251, *272*
Senchak, M., 52, *270*
Shafer, M., 168, *271*
Shelley-Sireci, L., 195, 201(*t*), *259*
Sher, K., 200(*t*), 202(*t*), 203, 204(*t*), *270*
Sheriff, M., 220, *270*
Simons-Morton, B. G., 4, *270*
Sinder, J. A., 200(*t*), *272*
Smith, A. F., 210, *267*
Smith, D., 139, 162, 163, *267*
Snyder, E., 235, 239, *261*
Snyder, L. B., 3, *270*
Somers, J. A., 241, *266*
Spear, S. F., 14, 20, 22, 35, 62, 197, 200(*t*), 205, (*t*), 223, *260*
Stacy, A., 14, 21, 200(*t*), 202(*t*), 239, 241, *255*
Stark, C., 195, *259*
Steckler, A., 183, *266*
Steffian, G., 200(*t*), 203, 204(*t*), 209, *270*
Stevenson, J. F., 252, *266*
Stewart, L. P., 2, 5, 7, 9, 19, 28, 32, 35, 36, 39, 40, 41, 45, 49(*n*1), 50, 51, 52, 53, 54, 55, 57, 59, 62, 70,

73($n$1), 75, 77, 79, 81, 87,101, 108, 122, 124, 131, 133, 136, 137, 139, 144, 145, 146, 148, 149, 157, 163, 166, 167, 168, 169, 170, 175, 180, 244, 252, *261, 264, 265, 270-271*
Storey, J., 245, 246, *271*
Strate, L., 249, *269*
Strauss, A. L., 27, 140, *260, 271*
Street, D. L., 87, *271*
Substance Abuse and Mental Health Services Administration (SAMSHA), 189, *271*
Sullivan, M. C., 87, *271*
Sussman, S., 201($t$), *271*
Szalay, L. B., 179, *260*

**T**

Tansey, P. J., 147, *271*
Tesch, F. E., 139, *271*
Thayer, J. E., 53, *269*
Thombs, D. L., 50, 51, 200($t$), 201($t$), 202($t$), 203, 204, 204($t$), *262, 271*
Thornton, G. C., 147, *271*
Thurman, R., 147, *271*
Toch, H., 194, 196($t$), 199, *271*
Treiman, K. A., 201($t$), 203, 204($t$), *256*
Trockel, M., 202($t$), 203, 204($t$), *271*
Trujillo, D., 209, *258*
Turner, J. C., 209, 210, *256*
Tuval-Mashiach, R., 248, *265*

**U**

University of Michigan, 252, *272*

**V**

Van Horn, D. H. A., 18, *256*
Velicer, W. F., 252, *266*
Vince-Whitman, C., 180, *258*
Vuchinich, R. E., 210, *267*

**W**

Wallack, L., 249, *260*
Walters, S. T., 190, *272*
Watzlawick, P., 31, *272*
Wechsler, H., 5, 6, 7, 8, 20, 36, 40, 41, 50, 51, 52, 56, 62, 63, 189, 201($t$), 203, 204($t$), 223, 235, 251, *261, 272*
Weingartner, C., 249, *269*
Weitzman, E. R., 5, *272*
Wenzel, M., 202, *272*
Werch, C. C. E., 200($t$), *272*
White, J., 198, 202($t$), 209, *272-273*
Whorf, B. L., 7, *273*
Wild, T. C., 210, *258*
Williams, E., 241, *266*
Williams, L. V., 198, 202($t$), 209, *272-273*
Williams, R., 245, *273*
Williams, S., 202($t$), 203, 204($t$), *271*
Williamson, J., 244, 251, *273*
Winebarger, A., 51, 54, 166, *261*
Witte, K., 31, 120, 122, 175, *273*
Wolcott, B. J., 51, 200($t$), 201($t$), 202($t$), 203, 204($t$), *271*
Wolfson, S., 201($t$), *273*
Workman, T. A., 17, 32, 51, 248, 249, 250, 251, *273*

**Y**

Yanovitzky, I., 167, 169, *273*
Yee, M., 51, 54, 166, *261*

**Z**

Zakocs, R., 7, *261*
Ziegler, D. A., 200($t$), 201($t$), *269*
Zilber, T., 246, *265*
Zweig, K., 180, *258*

# SUBJECT INDEX

**A**

Action Coalition for Media
Education, 253
ADAPS. *See* Alcohol and Other
Drug Assistance Program for
Students
ADAwGS. *See* Alcohol and Other
Drug Awareness Generated by
Students
ADEPT. *See* Alcohol and Other
Drug Education Program for
Training
Adoption, beginning with needs
assessment
assessing and testing key mes-
sages, 170-171
discovering drinking-related atti-
tudes, behaviors, and percep-
tions, 170
gathering baseline data, 169-171
Advanced Health Communication
(AHC), 99
changes in reported drinking by
students in, 138
as a subdivision of CHI, 79

Advanced Health Communication
(AHC) course assignments,
89-91
briefing document and formal
presentation, 90
environmental scan work plan, 90
final paper, 91
formal presentations/report on
Environmental Scan and collection data, 91
formal presentations to CHI, 91
individual papers, 90-91
intercept interview questionnaire,
90
preliminary presentation/report
on implementation/materials
development strategies, 91
work ethic, 92
Advanced Health Communication
(AHC) Simulation, 77-83
interactions, 80-82
outcome criteria, 83
roles, 79-80
rules, 80
simulation characteristics of
AHC, 78

Agostinelli, Gina, 198
AHC. *See* Advanced Health
 Communication
Alcohol, 16-17
 documentation of misperceptions
  regarding, 200-201
 experimentation with, 13
 rules for using, 17-18
Alcohol and Other Drug Assistance
 Program for Students (ADAPS),
 182, 188-191
Alcohol and Other Drug Awareness
 Generated by Students
 (ADAwGS), 184-185
Alcohol and Other Drug Education
 Program for Training (ADEPT),
 181, 183-184, 189
Alcohol Fact Sheet, 153, 156
Alcohol Skills Training Program
 (ASTP), 198-199, 210, 237-238
*Alcoholism and Drug Abuse*
 *Weekly*, 72
American College Health
 Association, 186
American Council on Education,
 182
*American Pie* (film), 250
Analytical skills, developing, 158
Anecdotal findings
 perceptions of others, 135-136
 qualitative study exploring, 139-143
 students' self-comments, 136-137
 suggesting impact of campaign on
  campaign workers, 135-137
*Animal House* (film), 4, 249
Artifacts, distributed in process eval-
 uation, 121
Assessment
 of key messages, 170-171
 of messages and media, 172
Assumptions, of social norms theory, 196

ASTP. *See* Alcohol Skills Training
 Program
Attitude problems, 54
Attitudes
 discovery of drinking-related, 170
 toward drinking, 23
Audience, selecting the target, 171-
 172

B

Background of the RU SURE
 Campaign, 1-45
 the conceptual model, 27-45
 conducting a needs assessment
  before designing a health communication campaign, 11-25
 culture of college drinking—a
  health communication issue, 3-10
Baseline data collection, 62, 169-171
 conducting a needs assessment
  before designing a health communication campaign, 1, 11-25
 earliest comprehensive study at
  Rutgers, 12-18
 focus group interviews, 14-18
 implications for a new era of prevention on campus, 24-25
 prevention efforts based on findings, 18-24
 Rutgers Student Alcohol and
  Drug Survey, 12-14
 survey of parents, 14
Behavioral data, using the simulation
 game to collect, 160-163
Behaviors
 discovery of drinking-related, 170
 drinking-related, 20-22
Believability issue, 211-212
Berkowitz, Alan D., 10, 178, 193-214
Binge drinking, 50, 52-53, 56, 62-63
Bingo. *See* RU SURE Bingo
Bloustein, Edward J., 181
Brief Intervention Model, 191

Briefing document, 84
    and formal presentation, assignment in AHC course, 90
    sample, 93-95
Burns, W. David, 12, 181

**C**

Campaign activities, 84-85
Campaign language, 48-58
    advantages of the term "dangerous drinking," 56-57
    background, 50-51
    getting students to personalize campaign messages, 49-58
    how college students think about drinking, 51-53
    implications of what we learned from students, 55-56
    what students think problem drinking is, 53-55
Campaign materials, 84
Campaign media, selecting, 68, 173-174
Campaign messages
    dissemination of, 68-69, 174-175
    personalization by students, 49-58
    phrasing and pilot-testing of key, 64-65
Campaign workers, impact of campaign on, 135-137
*The Campus Survey of Alcohol and Other Drug Norms*, 19, 224, 228
Carriers, of misperceptions, 134
Case study, in using a social norms approach for high-risk students, 178, 233-242
    discussion of the infusion of social norms data into brief motivational interventions, 241
    high-risk drinkers, 236-237
    implications, 241-242
    infusion of social norms into brief interventions, 237-238
    motivational interviews, 238

    results, 240-241
    WWU environment and perceptions of the frequency of peer alcohol use, 234-236
    WWU's brief motivational intervention, 239-240
Center for Alcohol Marketing to Youth, 253
Center for Communication and Health Issues (CHI), 77, 85, 180
Center of Alcohol Studies, 187
Centers for Disease Control, 193
Challenges and issues, 210-213
    combining social norms with other approaches to drug prevention, 213
    creating credible messages in terms of message, source, and explanation of data (believability issue), 211-212
    deciding which messages are appropriate and relevant for which audience (salience issue), 211
    developing the necessary infrastructure to support a social norms campaign ("readiness" issue), 211
    issues of replicability, 213
    making sure program evaluations are thorough and reveal any successes (evaluation issue), 212
    responding to critics, 212-213
CHI. *See* Center for Communication and Health Issues
Chip Score Sheets, 151, 153
Coalition building, 71
Coffee Breaks. *See* RU SURE Coffee Breaks
Collection
    of baseline data, 224
    of data to evaluate, 175
College Alcohol Study, 199

College drinking
  reality of, 4-7
  as socially situated experiential
    learning, 2, 28-29
College Experience Survey, 169
College students, their thinking
  about drinking, 51-53
Communication, ethnography of, 32
Communication theory, research-
  driven, 11
Complacency, 220
Components, of process evaluation,
  121
Components of the campaign, 61
  environmental scan, 101
  RU SURE Bingo, 108-110
  RU SURE Coffee Breaks, 116
  RU SURE Video, 114
  RU SURE Word Scramble, 111-
    112
  Table Talks, 105
  the Walk About, 102-103
The conceptual model of college
  drinking as socially situated expe-
  riential learning, 27-45
  application to the culture of col-
    lege drinking, 30-37
  evaluation of the RU SURE
    Campaign's impact, 43-45, 49,
    59, 119, 133, 146, 165
  a five-step model, 29-45
  formulation of the RU SURE
    Campaign, 42
  implementation of the RU SURE
    Campaign, 42-43, 73, 97, 100
  research, observation, and formu-
    lation of, 37-41
Consensus, false, 195, 239
Consortia, and change, 220-221
Continuous evaluation of the campaign, 98, 122-132
  Core surveys, 129-131
  intercept interviews, 124-129

personal report of student percep-
    tions, 131-132
  quantitative data collection, 122-
    123
Control, drinking to loss of, 53
Coordination of program elements,
  230
Core Alcohol and Drug Survey, 129
Core Institute, 129
The Core Survey, 129-131, 169, 199
*Cosmopolitan*, 250
Course assignments, 89-91
  briefing document and formal
    presentation, 90
  environmental scan work plan, 90
  final paper, 91
  formal presentations/report on
    Environmental Scan and collec-
    tion data, 91
  formal presentations to CHI, 91
  individual papers, 90-91
  intercept interview questionnaire,
    90
  and objectives, 76
  preliminary presentation/report
    on implementation/materials
    development strategies, 91
  and requirements, 76-77
  work ethic, 92
Course products, 84-85
  campaign activities, 84-85
  campaign materials, 84
  instruments for data collection, 85
  presentation materials, 85
  training document (briefing docu-
    ment), 84
Creation
  of a campaign logo for RU SURE,
    66-68, 173-174
  of credible messages in terms of
    message, source, and explana-
    tion of data (believability), 211-
    212

of a formula for the *Top Ten Misperceptions at Rutgers*, 65-66
Cue cards, 153
Cultural intervention, social norms as remedy, 251-253
Cultural theory, and socially situated experiential learning, 244-248
Culture of college drinking, 4, 27, 30-37
  a health communication issue, 3-10
  images and reality of, 4-7
  learning the norms about, 7-9
Curriculum infusion, 70-71
  AHC as a subdivision of CHI, 79
  AHC Simulation, 77-83
  in college classrooms, 74-75
  course products (campaign materials, activities, reports), 84-85
  design of, 76-83
  goals, 82-83
  institutional setting for, 75-76
  and participation in the simulation and the RU SURE Campaign, 83-86
  pre- and postexperience self-report of drinking attitudes, perceptions, and behaviors, 86
  process outcomes, 85-86

**D**

"Dangerous drinking," 5, 8, 23
  advantages of the term, 56-57
Data
  baseline, 169-171
  instruments for collecting, 85
  observational, 161-162
  quantitative, 122-123
Debriefing interviews, 86, 138-139, 153-157, 162
  guide to, 153
  positioning, 155
  scheduling, 155
  suggested questions, 155-157

  as a three-phase stepwise process, 163
Decisions
  about which messages are appropriate and relevant for which audience (salience), 211
  charting, 153
Demographics, of students as drinkers, 20
Design of the RU SURE Campaign, 27, 48, 59-72
  components of the campaign, 61
  creation of a campaign logo, 66-68
  creation of a formula for, 65-66
  design of the media component, 64
  development of the campaign theme, 64
  dissemination of the campaign messages, 68-69
  goal of the campaign, 60-62
  identification of target population, 62-63
  interpersonal components of the RU SURE Campaign, 69-72
  phrasing and pilot-testing key campaign messages, 64-65
  review of baseline data, 62
  RU SURE logo, 68
  selection of campaign media, 68
  the *Top Ten Misperceptions at Rutgers*, 64, 67
Development
  of the campaign theme, 64, 171
  of the necessary infrastructure to support a social norms campaign ("readiness"), 211
*Diagnostic and Statistical Manual of Mental Disorders—IV*, 189
Disagreement, tolerating, 158
Discovery, of drinking-related attitudes, behaviors, and perceptions, 170

Dissemination, of the campaign messages, 68-69, 174-175
Documentation of misperceptions, 199-202
  regarding alcohol, 200-201
  regarding illegal drug use, 201
  regarding other behaviors, 201-202
  regarding tobacco, 201
  in specific populations, 202
"Dog collar experiment," 243-244, 248-249, 251
Dosage issues, in media campaigns, 229
Drinkers
  demographics of students as, 20
  heavy, 20, 23
  high risk, 50, 52, 56, 236-237
Drinking
  attitudes toward, 23
  binge, 50, 52-53, 56, 62-63
  "dangerous," 5, 8, 23, 56-58
  excessive, 56
  frequency of, 53
  learning the norms about, 7-9
  to loss of control, 53
  negative consequences of, 6-7
  in popular culture, lessons of, 248-251
  problematic, 56
  respondents' comparison of their drinking to others' drinking, 22
Drinking-related behaviors, 20-22
  perceptions of alcohol use as compared to others, 21
  respondents' comparison of their drinking to others' drinking, 22
Drinking stories as learning tools, 178, 243-253
  cultural intervention, 251-253
  cultural theory and socially situated experiential learning, 244-248
  lessons of drinking in popular culture, 248-251
  social norms as remedy, 251-253

E
Eagleton Institute for Public Opinion Polling, 12
Educational plans, 183-185
Enforcement issues, 192
Environmental management approach, 180
Environmental scan, 101-102
  for campaign message dissemination, 101-102
  description of, 101
  implementation of, 101-102
  potential problems and their solutions, 102
  preparation needed for, 102
  work plan assignment in AHC course, 90
Ethical issues, 87-88, 157-159
  recognition of, 158
Ethnography of communication, 32
Evaluation
  of AHC Simulation, 83
  of the campaign, continuous, 98, 122-132
  formative, 120, 175
  outcome, 175
  process, 120-122, 175
  of the RU SURE Campaign's impact and socially situated experiential learning, 43-45, 49, 59, 119, 133, 146, 165, 212
  summative, 122-132
Events, held in process evaluation, 121
Excessive drinking, 56
Experiential learning theory, 33
Experimentation with alcohol, 13
Extension of the campaign and its socially situated experiential learning approach to other campuses, 98, 165-175
  background, 166-168

replicating the *Top Ten Misperceptions at Rutgers* media component of the campaign, 166-168

**F**

Fabiano, Patricia, 10, 178, 233-242
Fact Sheet, 153
False consensus, 195, 239
Far, Jeanne, 198
"Fast Food Approach to Alcohol Prevention," 168
Final paper, assignment in AHC course, 91
FIPSE. *See* Fund for the Improvement of Post-Secondary Education
Five-step model, 29-45
*The Focus*, 72
Focus group interviews, 14-18, 170
    role alcohol plays in students' lives, 15-17
    rules for alcohol use, 17-18
Formal presentations to CHI, assignment in AHC course, 83, 91
Formative evaluation, of the campaign, 120, 175
Formulation
    of college drinking as SSEL, 37-41
    of the RU SURE Campaign, 42
Frech, Alfred, 216
Frequency, of drinking, 53
Fund for the Improvement of Post-Secondary Education (FIPSE), 12, 216-218

**E**

Game materials, 152-153
    Alcohol Fact Sheet, 153
    chip score sheets, 153
    cue cards, 153
    debriefing guide, 153
    decision charts, 153
    plastic chips, 152-153
    scenario guide, 152

Game of Choices and Consequences. *See* RU SURE Game of Choices and Consequences
Generation X, 246
Gladwell, Malcolm, 230-231
Goals, of the campaign, 60-62
Goals of AHC Simulation, 82-83
    evaluation phase, 83
    planning and implementation phase, 82-83
    training phase, 82
Goodhart, Fern Walter, 10, 177, 179-192
Goodstadt, Michael, 12
Guided discussions (debriefing sessions), 86

**H**

Haines, Michael, 197
Hastings Center, 157
Health Belief Model (HBM), 31
Health communication, the issue of college drinking, 3-10
Heavy drinkers, 20, 23
High-risk drinkers, 50, 52, 56, 236-237
Higher Education Center for Alcohol and Other Drug Prevention, 182-183, 198, 219
History
    of alcohol awareness at Rutgers University, 181-182
    of debriefing interviews, 163
    of the social norms approach, 197-199

**I**

Identification
    of students for intervention, 189-190
    of target population, 62-63
    of young adult substance abusers, 18

Ignorance, pluralistic, 36, 194-195

Illegal drug use, documentation of misperceptions regarding, 201

Images of college drinking, 4-7

*Imagine That!* game, 149

Impact of campaign on campaign workers, anecdotal evidence suggesting, 135-137

Implementation of the RU SURE Campaign, 42-43, 48, 73-98, 100

   AHC course assignments, 89-91

   of AHC Simulation, 80-83

   curriculum infusion and participation, 83-86

   the curriculum infusion design, 76-83

   curriculum infusion in college classrooms, 74-75

   of environmental scan, 101-102

   ethical issues, 87-88

   institutional setting for curriculum infusion, 75-76

   objectives of, 76

   requirements of, 76-77

   of RU SURE Bingo, 108

   of RU SURE Coffee Breaks, 116-117

   of RU SURE Video, 114

   of RU SURE Word Scramble, 111-112

   sample briefing document, 93-95

   of the Walk About, 103

Indicated prevention (individualized social norms interventions), 205, 209-210

Individualized social norms interventions, 209-210

Infusion of social norms into brief interventions, 237-238, 241

Institute of Medicine, 238

Institutional setting for curriculum infusion, 75-76

Instruments for data collection, 85

Integrated environmental framework (education, prevention, intervention, treatment, and enforcement), 177-192

   history of alcohol awareness at Rutgers University, 181-182

   Rutgers' five-pronged approach—education, prevention, intervention, treatment, and enforcement, 183-191

   setting policy, 181-182

Intercept Interview Survey, 137, 169

Intercept interviews, 124-129

   questionnaire as an assignment in AHC course, 90

   results, 126-129

   sampling protocol, 125

   students learning about RU SURE Campaign message through various media, 128

   training of interviewers, 125-126

Interpersonal components of the RU SURE Campaign, 69-72

   coalition building, 71

   curriculum infusion, 70-71

   interpersonally based strategies for experiential learning, 69-70

   public relations campaign, 71-72

   Web site, 71

Interpersonally based strategies for campaign message dissemination, 48, 99-118

   environmental scan, 101-102

   RU SURE Bingo, 108-111

   RU SURE Coffee Breaks, 116-118

   RU SURE Video, 114-116

   RU SURE Word Scramble, 111-113

   Table Talks, 105-107

   the Walk About, 102-105

Interpersonally based strategies for experiential learning, 69-70

"Intertextual" meaning-making, 244-245
Interventions, 188-191
  identification of students for, 189-190
  policy and staff training for, 188-189
  and treatment, 188-191
Interventions successfully utilizing the social norms approach, 205-210
  indicated prevention (individualized social norms interventions), 209-210
  selective prevention—targeted social norms interventions, 208-209
  universal prevention—social norms marketing campaigns, 205-208
Interviews
  focus group, 14-18
  intercept, 124-129
  motivational, 238
  postexperience, 162-163
Issues. See also Challenges and issues of replicability, 213

J

Jeffrey, Linda R., 10, 178, 215-232

K

Keeling, Richard P., 183
Key campaign messages, phrasing and pilot-testing of, 64-65

L

Laitman, Lisa, 10, 177, 179-192
Language, of the campaign, 48-58
Learning theory, experiential, 33
Learning tools, drinking stories as, 178, 243-253
Lederman, Linda, 180
Lifestyles Survey administration, 235

Logo creation, for RU SURE, 66-68, 173-174
Loss of control, drinking to, 53

M

Management. See Environmental management approach
Management of multicampus campaigns using a social norms approach, 178, 215-232
  finding the "tipping" point— transforming campus climate, 230-232
  launching a multicampus social norms project, 223-230
  the social norms approach, 219-223
Marketing campaigns, and social norms, 205-208
Marlatt, Alan, 198
Materials
  in assignments in AHC course, development strategies for, 91
  presentation, 85
Media campaigns, 228-229
  dosage, 229
  media messages, 229
  message testing, 229
"Media environment," 253
Media messages, 229
Men's Journal, 250-251
Message testing, 229
Milgram, Gail, 219
Miller, John, 198
Miller, William, 198
Minority groups, 5
Misperceptions, 199-202
  carriers of, 134
  predicting behavior, 203-204
  regarding alcohol, 200-201
  regarding illegal drug use, 201
  regarding other behaviors, 201-202
  regarding tobacco, 201

and social change, 223
in specific populations, 202
Moral imagination, stimulating, 157
Motivation problem, 54
Motivational interviews, 238
Multicampus social norms projects
collection of baseline data, 224
coordination of program elements, 230
launching, 223-230
media campaigns, 228-229
New Jersey collegiate drinking
patterns, 225-228
outcome measurement, 230
Myers, Peter, 216

**N**

National Committee on Alcohol and
Drug Dependence, 71
National Institute on Alcohol Abuse
and Alcoholism (NIAAA), 146,
193
Task Force on College Drinking,
5-6
National Research Council,
Committee on Techniques for the
Enhancement of Human
Performance, 147
National Social Norms Resource
Center, 198, 205
Negro, Pamela, 10, 178, 215-232
New Brunswick Responsible
Hospitality Resource Panel, 71
New Jersey collegiate drinking pat-
terns, 225-228
perceived norms vs. actual norms,
225-227
student misperceptions of college
drinking norms, 227-228
New Jersey Department of Health
and Senior Services, Division of
Addiction Services, 223
New Jersey Division of Acohol
Beverage Control, 71

New Jersey Higher Education
Consortium on Alcohol and
Other Drug Prevention and
Education, 166, 180, 215-222, 224
*The New York Times*, 72
*New Yorker*, 230
NIAAA. *See* National Institute on
Alcohol Abuse and Alcoholism
NIU. *See* Northern Illinois
University
Norms
about drinking, learning, 7-9
saliency of, 202-203
"Norms Correction Efforts," 219
Northern Illinois University (NIU),
197

**O**

Observational data
for collecting behavioral data,
161-162
of college drinking as SSEL, 37-41
*Old School* (film), 249
Outcomes
of AHC Simulation, 83
evaluating, 175
of marketing campaigns, 207-208
measurement of, 230
process, 85-86
of social norms marketing campaigns, 207-208
Outcomes of the campaign, 97-175
continuous evaluation, 119-132
extending to other campuses, 165-
175
interpersonal strategies for message dissemination, 99-118
RU SURE Game of Choices and
Consequences, 145-164
unanticipated, 133-144

**P**

Pandina, Robert J., 187
Papers, assigned in AHC course, 90-
91

Perceived norms *vs.* actual norms, in
New Jersey collegiate drinking
patterns, 225-227
Perception
of alcohol use and abuse, 23-24
compared to others', 21, 135-136
discovery of drinking-related, 170
*vs.* reality, 221-223
Perkins, H. Wesley, 197, 213, 220
The Personal Report of Student
Perceptions (PRSP), 19, 24, 62,
131-132
Personalization of campaign mes-
sages, by students, 49-58
Personalized Feedback Profile, 237-
241
Phrasing, of key campaign messages,
64-65
Pilot-testing
of key campaign messages, 64-65
of messages and media, 172
Planning phase, of AHC Simulation,
82-83
Plastic chips, 152-153
Pluralistic ignorance, 36, 194-195
Policy, and staff training, 188-189
The popular culture, lessons of
drinking in, 248-251
Populations, documentation of misperceptions about specific, 202
Positioning, 155
Postexperience interviews, 162-163
for collecting behavioral data,
162-163
debriefing interview as a three-
phase stepwise process, 163
history of debriefing interviews,
163
Potential problems and their solutions
for environmental scan, 102
for RU SURE Bingo, 110-111
for RU SURE Coffee Breaks,
117-118

for RU SURE Video, 115-116
for RU SURE Word Scramble, 113
for Table Talks, 107
for the Walk About, 104-105
Preexperience self-report of drinking
attitudes, perceptions, and behaviors, 86
Preparation needed
for environmental scan, 102
for RU SURE Bingo, 108-110
for Table Talks, 106-107
to use RU SURE Coffee Breaks,
117
to use RU SURE Video, 114-115
to use RU SURE Word Scramble,
113
for the Walk About, 103-104
Presentation materials, 85
Prevention
indicated, 205
selective, 205
Prevention efforts, 18-24, 186-187
attitudes toward drinking, 23
demographics of students as
drinkers, 20
drinking-related behaviors, 20-22
identifying young adult substance
abusers, 18
indicated, 209-210
perceptions of alcohol use and
abuse, 23-24
the Personal Report of Student
Perceptions, 19
results, 20-24
the Rutgers Collegiate Substance
Abuse Screening Test, 18
selective, 208-209
universal, in social norms marketing campaigns, 205-208
Prevention in the larger context,
177-253
case study in using a social norms
approach within a brief inter-

vention for identified high-risk
students, 178, 233-242
drinking stories as learning
tools—socially situated experiential learning and popular culture, 178, 243-253
integrated environmental frame
work—education, prevention,
intervention, treatment, and
enforcement, 179-192
managing multicampus cam-
paigns using a social norms
approach, 178, 215-232
overview of the social norms
approach, 178, 193-214
"Preventive ethics," 158
Problem drinking, 56
students thoughts about, 53-55
Process evaluation, 120-122, 175
artifacts distributed in, 121
of the campaign, 120-122
components, 121
events held in, 121
number of events held and artifacts distributed, 121
Process learning, 85
Process outcomes, 85-86
guided discussions (debriefing
sessions), 86
reflection papers, 85-86
Program elements, coordination of,
230
Program evaluations, thoroughness
of, 212
Promising Practices: Campus Alcohol
Strategies, 219
Protocol, for sampling, 125
PRSP. See The Personal Report of
Student Perceptions
Public health campaigns, 3
Public relations campaigns, 71-72

Q
Qualitative study exploring the
anecdotal findings, 11, 139-143
findings, 140-143
impact on others, 140-141
impact on self, 141-143
procedures, 139-140
Quantitative data collection, 11, 122-
123
Questionnaire
for intercept interview, in AHC
course, 90
suggested questions for, 155-157

R
"Readiness" issue, 211
The Real World, 4
Recognition, of ethical issues, 158
Recovery Housing, 191
Reflection papers, 85-86
Replicating the Top Ten
Misperceptions at Rutgers media
component of the campaign,
166-168, 213
assessing and pilot-testing messages and media, 172
collecting data to evaluate, 175
determining the campaign
approach and selecting the target
audience, 171-172
developing the campaign theme,
171
disseminating messages, 174-175
selecting media and creating logo,
173-174
using the formula created for,
172-173
Report on Environmental Scan, and
collection data, assignment in
AHC course, 91
Research on social norms, 199-204
of college drinking as SSEL, 37-41
documentation of misperceptions, 199-202

misperceptions predicting behavior, 203-204
saliency of norms, 202-203
Responsible Hospitality Resource Panel, 187
Road Trip (film), 249-250
Rochester Institute of Technology, 209
Rolling Stone, 250
Rowan University, 10, 197
RSCAT. See The Rutgers Collegiate Substance Abuse Screening Test
RU AWARE campaign, 18
RU SURE Bingo, 69-70, 83, 108-111
    for campaign message dissemination, 108-111
    description of, 108-110
    implementation of, 108
    potential problems and their solutions, 110-111
    preparation needed for, 108-110
The RU SURE Campaign, 9-10, 28-29, 82, 252
    AHC course assignments, 89-91
    AHC Simulation, 80-82
    background of, 1-45
    components of, 61
    course description and objectives, 76
    course description and requirements, 76-77
    creation of a logo for, 66-68
    curriculum infusion and participation in the simulation and, 83-86
    the curriculum infusion design, 76-83
    curriculum infusion in college classrooms, 74-75
    design of, 59-72
    development of the theme for, 64
    dissemination of the messages, 68-69

ethical issues, 87-88
goal of, 60-62
identification of target population, 62-63
implementation of, 73-98
institutional setting for curriculum infusion, 75-76
interpersonal components of, 69-72
phrasing and pilot-testing key messages of, 64-65
review of baseline data, 62
sample briefing document, 93-95
selection of media for, 68
and the Top Ten Misperceptions at Rutgers, 64-67
RU SURE Coffee Breaks, 116-118
    for campaign message dissemination, 116-118
    description of, 116
    implementation of, 116-117
    potential problems and their solutions, 117-118
    preparation needed to use, 117
RU SURE Game of Choices and Consequences, 9, 44, 98, 145-164
    background, 146-147
    brief history of simulation games, 147-148
    using the simulation game as a 1-hour prevention tool, 150-160
    using the simulation game to collect behavioral data, 160-163
RU SURE Video, 114-116
    for campaign message dissemination, 114-116
    description of, 114
    implementation of, 114
    potential problems and their solutions, 115-116
    preparation needed to use, 114-115

RU SURE Word Scramble, 83, 111-
113
    for campaign message dissemina-
    tion, 111-113
    description of, 111-112
    implementation of, 111-112
    potential problems and their solu-
    tions, 113
    preparation needed to use, 113
RUHS. *See* Rutgers University
    Health Services
Rules
    of AHC Simulation, 80
    for alcohol use, 17-18
Rutgers Board of Governors, 182
The Rutgers Collegiate Substance
    Abuse Screening Test (RSCAT),
    18
Rutgers' five-pronged approach—
    education, prevention, interven-
    tion, treatment, and enforcement,
    183-191
    education, 183-185
    enforcement, 192
    intervention and treatment, 188-
    191
    prevention, 186-187
Rutgers University, 11, 179-180. *See
    also* Student Alcohol and Drug
    Survey (1987)
    Center for Communication and
    Health Issues (CHI), 77
    Center of Alcohol Studies, 187,
    191
    Department of Communication,
    75-76, 180
    Eagleton Institute for Public
    Opinion Polling, 12
    earliest comprehensive study at,
    12-18
    School of Communication,
    Information and Library Studies
    Research Subgrant Program, 12n

Teaching Excellence Center, 12n
University Personnel Counseling
    Service, 188
Rutgers University Health Services
    (RUHS), 10, 12n, 71, 183, 191

S
Sacks, Peter, 246
Safe and Drug-Free Schools and
    Communities Act of 1994, 186
Safe and Drug-Free Schools
    Program, 180
Salience, 211
    of norms, 202-203
Sample briefing document, 93-95
Sampling protocol, 125
Saturation, 172
Scenario guide, 152
School of Communication,
    Information and Library Studies
    Research Subgrant Program, 12n
Secondary target audience, systemat-
    ic evaluation impact on, 137-139
Selective prevention, 205
    targeted social norms interven-
    tions, 208-209
"Self-fulfilling prophecies," 39
Self-report of drinking attitudes,
    perceptions, and behaviors, pre-
    and postexperience, 86
SGNM. *See* Small Group Norms
    Model
Shalala, Donna, 216
SIMCORP, 79
Simulation characteristics of AHC,
    78
The simulation game, 150
    behavioral records in, 160-163
    debriefing, 153-157
    ethical considerations of, 157-159
    game materials, 152-153
    how the simulation game is
    played, 151-153
    objectives, 150-151

observational data in, 161-162
postexperience interviews in, 162-163
using as a 1-hour prevention tool, 150-160
using to collect behavioral data, 160-163
Simulation games
  brief history of, 147-148
  playing, 151-153
Small Group Norms Challenging Intervention, 252
Small Group Norms Model (SGNM), 198, 209
SNM. *See* Social norms marketing
Social cognitive theory, 34
"Social ecology," 252
Social interaction perspectives, 31
The social norms approach, 178, 193-214, 219-223
  combining with other approaches to drug prevention, 213
  consortia and change, 220-221
  emerging challenges and issues, 210-213
  history of, 197-199
  individualized interventions, 209-210
  infusion of data, 241
  marketing campaigns, 205-208
  misperceptions and social change, 223
  perception *vs.* reality, 221-223
  as remedy for cultural intervention, 251-253
  research on social norms, 199-204
  successful interventions utilizing the social norms approach, 205-210
Social norms marketing (SNM), 197
Social norms theory, 35, 193-197
  assumptions of, 196

Socially Situated Experiential Learning (SSEL) model, 148, 167, 245
  college drinking in, 2, 28-29
  cultural theory and SSEL, 244-248
  five steps in, 28-45
  lessons of drinking in popular culture, 248-251
  and popular culture, 177, 243-253
  social norms as a remedy, 251-253
SSEL. *See* Socially Situated Experiential Learning (SSEL) model
Staff training, policy and, 188-189
Stewart, Lea, 180
"Stickiness factor," 231
Stolberg, Victor, 216
Student Alcohol and Drug Survey (1987), 12-14, 19
Students
  as drinkers, demographics of, 20
  learning about RU SURE Campaign message through various media, 128
  misperceptions of college drinking norms by, 227-228
  role alcohol plays in their lives, 15-17
  self-comments by, 136-137
Summative evaluation of the campaign, 122-132
  Core surveys, 129-131
  intercept interviews, 124-129
  Personal report of Student Perceptions, 131-132
  quantitative data collection, 122-123
Surveys
  Core, 129-131
  measures of, 137-138
  of parents, 14

Systematic evaluation impact on the secondary target audience, 137-139
  changes in reported drinking by students in Advanced Health Communication, 138
  debriefing interviews, 138-139
  survey measures, 137-138

**T**

Table Talks, 83, 105-107
  for campaign message dissemination, 105-107
  description of, 105
  implementation of, 105-106
  potential problems and their solutions, 107
  preparation needed for, 106-107
Target audience, selecting, 171-172
Task Force on College Drinking, 5-6
Testing, of key messages, 170-171
Theory of social norms, 193-197
  assumptions of, 196
"Tipping" point, transforming campus climate, finding, 230-232
*The Tipping Point*, 230
Tobacco
  agenda of manufacturers of, 231
  documentation of misperceptions regarding, 201
The *Top Ten Misperceptions at Rutgers* (media component of the campaign), 9-10, 67
  adapting to other campuses, 175
  replicating, 166-168
  using the formula created for, 172-173
Training
  of AHC Simulation, 82
  documents for (briefing document), 84
  of interviewers, 125-126
  of staff, and policy issues, 188-189

Treatment, 188-191
  policy and staff training for, 188-189
  treatment of alcohol/drug problems, 190-191

**U**

Unanticipated impact of campaign messages on the messengers, 98, 133-144
  anecdotal evidence suggesting, 135-137
  lessons learned, 143-144
  qualitative study exploring, 139-143
  systematic evaluation impact on the secondary target audience, 137-139
Universal prevention, in social norms marketing campaigns, 205-208
University of Nebraska—Lincoln, 10
University Personnel Counseling Service (UPCS), 188
UPCS. *See* University Personnel Counseling Service
U.S. Department of Education, 72, 166, 193, 215
  Fund for the Improvement of Post-Secondary Education, 12
  Higher Education Center for Alcohol and Other Drug Prevention, 182
  Safe and Drug-Free Schools Program, 180
U.S. Department of Justice, 193
U.S. Surgeon General, 5

**V**

Video. *See* RU SURE Video

**W**

The Walk About, 83, 102-105
  for campaign message dissemination, 102-105

description of, 102-103
implementation of, 103
potential problems and their solutions, 104-105
preparation needed for, 103-104
"We Check for 21" program, 71
Web sites, 71, 198
Western Washington University (WWU), 10, 197, 205, 233-242
brief motivational intervention, 239-240
environment and perceptions of the frequency of peer alcohol use, 234-236

Word Scramble. *See* RU SURE Word Scramble
Work ethic, for assignments in AHC course, 92
Workman, Thomas A., 10, 178, 243-253
WWU. *See* Western Washington University

**Y**

You're Not What You Think When You Drink campaign, 18

Printed in the United States
24494LVS00004B/115-234

9 781572 735934